APR 16 1999

Psychopharmacology of Animal Behavior Disorders

Psychopharmacology of Animal Behavior Disorders

edited by

Nicholas H. Dodman, BVMS, MRCVS
Professor and Head
Section of Animal Behavior
Tufts University School of Veterinary Medicine
Department of Clinical Studies
North Grafton, Massachusetts

Louis Shuster, PhD
Professor of Pharmacology, Biochemistry, and Neuroscience
Tufts University School of Medicine
Boston, Massachusetts
Tufts University School of Veterinary Medicine
Department of Pharmacology and Experimental Therapeutics
North Grafton, Massachusetts

Blackwell Science

© 1998 by Blackwell Science, Inc.
Editorial Offices:
350 Main Street, Malden, MA 02148-5018, USA
Osney Mead, Oxford OX2 0EL, England
25 John Street, London WC1N 2BL, England
23 Ainslie Place, Edinburgh EH3 6AJ, Scotland
54 University Street, Carlton, Victoria 3053, Australia

Other Editorial Offices:
Blackwell Wissenschafts-Verlag GmbH
Kurfürstendamm 57
10707 Berlin, Germany

Blackwell Science KK
MG Kodenmacho Building
7–10 Kodenmacho Nihombashi
Chuo-ku, Tokyo 104, Japan

First published 1998

Acquisitions: Nancy Hill Wilton
Production: Ellen Samia
Manufacturing: Lisa Flanagan
Typeset by Best-set Typesetter Ltd., Hong Kong
Printed in the United States of America
98 99 00 01 5 4 3 2

The Blackwell Science logo is a trade mark of Blackwell Science Ltd, registered at the United Kingdom Trade Marks Registry

Distributors

Marston Book Services Ltd
PO Box 269
Abingdon, Oxon OX14 4YN
England
(*Orders*: Tel: 44-01235-465500
         Fax: 44-01235-465555)

USA
Blackwell Science, Inc.
Commerce Place
350 Main Street
Malden, MA 02148-5018
(*Orders*: Tel: 800-759-6102
              617-388-8250
         Fax: 617-388-8255)

Canada
Copp Clark Professional
200 Adelaide Street, West, 3rd Floor
Toronto, Ontario M5H 1W7
(*Orders*: Tel: 800-815-9417
              416-597-1616
         Fax: 416-597-1617)

Australia
Blackwell Science Pty Ltd
54 University Street
Carlton, Victoria 3053
(*Orders*: Tel: 3-9347-0300
         Fax: 3-9349-3016)

Library of Congress Cataloging-in-Publication Data

Psychopharmacology of animal behavior disorders/edited by Nicholas H. Dodman and Louis Shuster
     p. cm.
  Includes bibliographical references and index.
  ISBN 0-632-04358-X
   1. Veterinary psychopharmacology. I. Dodman, Nicholas H. II. Shuster, Louis
SF756.84.P79 1997
636.089'578–dc21

97-27824

CIP

Contents

Preface

Behavior problems, the leading cause of death in the pet population, are responsible for the euthanasia of between 3 and 6 million dogs and cats annually. It is now known that many of these problems are potentially treatable by behavior modification, with or without various forms of supportive therapy. Supportive therapy takes the form of attention to exercise requirements, appropriate nutrition, clearer communication between the owner and the pet, environmental enrichment, and when indicated, pharmacotherapy.

The first steps in evaluating a behavior case involve obtaining a detailed history and conducting a clinical examination of the patient. Medical causes of behavior problems must be sought early in the process and treated accordingly; pure behavior diagnoses warrant a somewhat different approach. Once a behavior diagnosis is reached, treatment can begin. It is important to realize that without a diagnosis, treatment can be only symptomatic, a sad state of affairs in any branch of medicine. In addition, a behavior diagnosis should not simply be a description of what is happening, it should address the underlying cause. For example, barking excessively is not an acceptable diagnosis, but separation anxiety or hyperactivity might be, depending on the circumstances.

Although most simple, recently acquired behavior problems can often be treated successfully by non-pharmacologic behavior modification therapy, many of the more complex and ingrained behaviors can be extremely difficult to treat by this means alone. Dominance aggression in dogs, for example, can be improved by behavior modification alone, but only to a degree, and the degree of improvement may not be acceptable to the owner (1). Likewise, fear-based conditions, like fear aggression and thunderstorm phobia, can be refractory to treatment, and some compulsive disorders can be virtually indelible (Uchida Y, Dodman NH, unpublished data, 1977). It is such cases that adjunctive pharmacologic therapy can help greatly by facilitating and expediting otherwise lengthy or ineffective treatment programs.

In the past, pharmacologic therapy for behavior problems was rather crude, relying on sedation rather than specific drug effects to achieve results. Unfortunately, this legacy is still with us, and serves to discourage many veterinarians and owners from venturing into the realms of more targeted, modern therapy. It is interesting to note that older drugs aroused just as much interest—though not as much controversy—as safer and more specific contemporary drugs. We can, at least, credit earlier drugs for paving the way for today's more precise pharmacologic approach.

Barbiturates were first on the scene, and were investigated extensively in the first half of this century. As important as barbiturates were in anesthesia and epilepsy management, it was the phenothiazines, notably chlorpromazine, launched in the 1950s that caused the most significant changes in behavior modification. Veterinarians at last had a way to render their patients more tractable without anesthetizing them. Terms like ataractic and tranquilizer were coined to describe the state of mind produced by such agents. A few years later, in the 1960s, the progestins entered in veterinary behavioral medicine, joining acepromazine and phenobarbital as the mainstays of veterinary behavioral pharmacology. The breakthrough discovery of the benzodiazepines in the late 1950s did not make much impact in the veterinary arena until much later, but these drugs, particularly diazepam, gradually found a niche for the treatment of anxiety-based conditions. Veterinarians tended to confine themselves to these classes of drugs for management of behavior problems throughout the 1970s and 1980s, but then some alternatives started to become available.

In the early 1980s we were researching the effect of opioid antagonists on stereotypic behavior in horses, and discovered that cribbing was temporarily abolished by treatment with the opioid antagonists naloxone, naltrexone, and nalmefene (2). This observation implicated endogenous opioids in the propagation of cribbing, and possibly other stall vices, and paved the way for pharmacologic treatment of these behaviors. Unfortunately, a utilizable form of the compounds was never produced for logistical reasons, but our scientific interest in this type of treatment had been piqued. A year later we extended our observations to include successful opioid antagonist treatment of dogs with acral lick dermatitis (ALD) and other self-directed behaviors (3). One popular press journal illustrated our findings with the analogy that if endogenous opioids were the lock, then opioid antagonists were the key to controlling these behaviors. The great advantage of opioid antagonists is that they are safe, efficacious, and relatively free from unwanted side effects. In effect, we had discovered the veterinary equivalent of what in human medicine are called "smart drugs"—drugs that target specific receptors without producing appreciable "collateral damage."

Our next venture involved investigating a human anxiolytic drug, buspirone. We set about evaluating its role in treating anxiety-related problems, like fear aggression, thunderstorm phobia, and separation anxiety. From the pharmacologic description, buspirone seemed ideal: no organ toxicity, no addiction potential or withdrawal, few side effects, and a pure anxiety relieving (anxiolytic) pharmacologic profile. Buspirone proved to be effective in a number of these conditions in dogs, cats, and horses. Dr. Benjamin Hart joined us in exploring the veterinary applications of buspirone and published an extensive clinical study documenting buspirone's efficacy in anxiety-related inappropriate urine-marking behavior in cats (4).

As we were investigating buspirone, other researchers substantiated the role of antidepressants and antiobsessional agents in veterinary psychopharmacology. In 1989, the treatment of canine ALD with fluoxetine, a selective serotonin reuptake inhibitor was described (5). Two years later, another (primarily) serotonin reuptake blocking agent, clomipramine, was found effective in ALD (6). The rationale was that ALD might represent a canine form of obsessive-compulsive disorder. The following year the definitive work was published on the subject confirming unequivocally, in a double-blind placebo-controlled study, the successful use of a variety of human antiobsessional medications in the treatment of ALD (7). This work redefined ALD and heralded a new era in the treatment of compulsive behaviors in animals.

As the 1990s progressed, we and others began to explore other clinical applications of antiobsessional and other human psychotrophic medication in a variety of veterinary behavioral conditions, and pharmaceutical companies began to take an interest in what was happening. Recently, there have been corporately funded clinical investigations into the use of buspirone, novel benzodiazepenes, opioid antagonists, clomipramine, and L-deprenyl in various veterinary behavioral conditions, ranging from separation anxiety and compulsive behaviors to the so-called cognitive dysfunction syndrome of older dogs. More studies are on the way, despite the reduced incentive for pharmaceutical companies to develop veterinary drugs because of a recent (October 1996) interpretation of the Animal Medicinal Drug Use Clarification Act of 1994. As we approach the end of the second millennium, veterinary behavioral pharmacology is alive and well despite such obstacles and most likely will continue to grow.

Now is the perfect time to crystallize current knowledge in the form of a textbook to inform and educate veterinary students, practitioners, and animal scientists about the rapid expansion of knowledge in this field. Perhaps more important than the specifics of the drugs themselves is the philosophy of how and when to intervene, what to anticipate, and the neurophysiology and neuropharmacology relevant to the conditions. We asked our authors to adopt this approach so that the principles of treatment, not simply recipes for the use of drugs in behavior modification, would become the focus of the contributions.

In the introduction, research psychiatrist Dr. Dan Stein discusses the classification of veterinary behavior problems. He refers to the human psychiatric classification to illustrate that approach and then provides what could be a more appropriate way of objectively classifying veterinary behavior problems. He also reviews the main classes of drugs employed in psychopharmacology, including fundamentals of their modes of action, providing good groundwork for the pharmacologic discussions featured in later chapters.

Five main sections follow: aggression, fear and anxiety, compulsive behavior, sexual behavior, and geriatric behavior. Between them, these five sections encompass most of the major behavior problems seen in veterinary practice.

Part One, Aggression, begins with a chapter describing the basic mechanisms of aggression. Immediately following is a clinical discussion of aggression-modifying drugs. Because behavior modification alone is not always completely successful in treating these conditions, this chapter should be of great value to practitioners trying to deal with refractory problems of this nature. The third chapter in this section deals with the systemic causes of aggression, which might be confused with pure behavioral diagnoses, and details their medical management.

Part Two, Fear and Anxiety, contains chapters on basic mechanisms of fear and anxiety-related conditions, pharmacologic treatment of fear and anxiety, and the pharmacologic treatment of phobias. Although anxiety, fears, and phobias are related conditions, we believed discussions of these conditions would be useful because of the unique phenotypic expressions of the resulting behaviors, their classification, and to some extent their pharmacologic responsiveness.

Part Three, Compulsive Behavior, starts out with a chapter detailing basic mechanisms of underlying compulsive disorders. This chapter is designed to provide a framework for the chapters that follow. The first discusses pharmacologic treatment of compulsive disorders and the second deals with self-injurious behavior. Although the clinical syndromes usually appear reasonably distinct (and medically are classified separately), some overlap is apparent in these two chapters because self-injurious behavior is regarded primarily as a compulsive behavior manifestation in this rendition.

In the appendix, Dr. Ben Hart discusses the design and conduct of experimental trials for behavioral drugs. Even for those with a more clinical bent, this discussion will assist in interpreting published clinical studies meaningfully. For those who wish to conduct trials themselves, it also provides a valuable starting point.

Psychopharmacology of Animal Behavior Disorders should enable readers to familiarize themselves with the latest pharmacologic treatments for commonly encountered behavior problems and provides an academic framework from which to build. We wish to emphasize that although behavior modification therapy and pharmacologic therapy each can be effective in their own right, a combination of these approaches is frequently more successful than either therapy alone for treatment of refractory behavior problems. This does not mean that drug treatment should always accompany behavior modification therapy; rather, conditions that respond poorly to nonpharmacologic treatment can usually be resolved more satisfactorily if a pharmacologic adjunctive treatment is simultaneously employed. Effective pharmacologic treatment often allows an owner to observe an earlier response to therapy, which in itself encourages continued owner compliance with a concurrent behavior modification program. Owner compliance (or lack of it) is a major factor determining success of behavior modification programs. Whatever the rationale behind its success in any particular case, pharmacologic treatment does assist in behavior problem management and does save animal lives. It is a subject with which every veterinarian should be familiar.

Nicholas H. Dodman and Louis Shuster

References

1. Dodman NH, Moon R, Zelin M. Influence of owner personality type on expression and treatment outcome of dominance aggression in dogs. JAVMA 1996;209:1107–1103.
2. Dodman NH, Shuster L, Court MH, Dixon R. Investigation into the use of narcotic antagonists in the treatment of stereotypic behavior pattern (crib-biting) in the horse. Am J Vet Res 1987;48:311–319.
3. Dodman NH, Shuster L, White SD, et al. Use of narcotic antagonists to modify stereotypic self-licking, self-chewing, and scratching behavior in dogs. JAVMA 1988;193:815–819.
4. Hart BL, Eckstein RA, Powell KL, Dodman NH. Effectiveness of buspirone on urine spraying and inappropriate urination in cats. J Am Vet Med Assoc 1993;203(2):254–258.
5. Shoulberg N. The efficacy of fluoxetine (Prozac) in the treatment of acral lick and inhalant dermatitis in canines. Proceedings of the American College of Veterinary Dermatologists. San Francisco, CA. 1990;31–32.
6. Goldberger E, Rapoport J. Canine acral lick dermatitis: response to the anti-obsessional drug clomipramine. J Am Hosp Assoc 1991;22:179–182.
7. Rapoport J, Ryland DH, Kriete M. Drug treatment for canine acral lick: an animal model of obsessive-compulsive disorder. Arch Gen Psychiatry 1992;49:517–521.

Contributors

Linda P. Aronson, DVM
Tufts University School of Veterinary Medicine
Department of Surgery
North Grafton, Massachusetts

Kelly D. Cliff, DVM
Staff Research Associate
Veterinary Medical Teaching Hospital
University of California
Davis, California

Nicholas H. Dodman, BVMS, MRCVS
Professor and Head
Section of Animal Behavior
Tufts University School of Veterinary Medicine
Department of Clinical Studies
North Grafton, Massachusetts

Robert A. Eckstein, DVM
Professor of Biology
Warren Wilson College
Asheville, North Carolina

Benjamin L. Hart, DVM, PhD
Professor of Physiology and Behavior
Chief, Behavior Service
Veterinary Medical Teaching Hospital
University of California
Davis, California

U.A. Luescher, DVM, PhD
Department of Population Medicine
University of Guelph
Guelph, Ontario
Canada

Petra A. Mertens, TA, Dr. Med Vet, FTAV
Institute for Animal Hygiene, Ethology, and Animal Welfare
Ludwig-Maximilians University
Munchen
Germany

Klaus A. Miczek, PhD
Moses Hunt Professor of Psychology, Psychiatry, and Pharmacology
Tufts University
Medford, Massachusetts

Berend Oliver, PhD
Professor of Psychopharmacology
University of Utrecht
Utrecht
The Netherlands

Karen L. Overall, MA, VMD, PhD
Diplomate, ACVB
ABS Certified Applied Animal Behaviorist
University of Pennsylvania School of Veterinary Medicine
Philadelphia, Pennsylvania

William W. Ruehl, VMD, PhD
Diplomate, ACVP
Vice President of Scientific Affairs
Deprenyl Animal Health Inc.
Overland Park, Kansas
Clinical Assistant Professor
Department of Pathology
Stanford University School of Medicine
Stanford, California

Louis Shuster, PhD
Professor of Pharmacology, Biochemistry, and Neuroscience
Tufts University School of Medicine
Boston, Massachusetts
Tufts University School of Veterinary Medicine
Department of Pharmacology and Experimental Therapeutics
North Grafton, Massachusetts

Dan J. Stein, MB
Director of Research
Department of Psychiatry
University of Stellenbosch
Tygerberg
South Africa

Steven B. Thompson, DVM
Clinical Assistant Professor
Director, Outpatients, Department of Veterinary Clinical Sciences
The Ohio State University College of Veterinary Medicine
Columbus, Ohio

Introduction: Steps Toward a Comparative Clinical Psychopharmacology

Dan J. Stein

Although psychopharmacology is a relatively young field, it has matured rapidly. Basic laboratory research conducted in the last few decades has led to important advances in our understanding of the pharmacodynamics and pharmacokinetics of a broad range of psychotropic agents. During the same period, clinical research in humans with various psychiatric disorders has produced an enormous database of open and controlled trials of many of these agents. The scientific and medical rewards of this increased knowledge of psychopharmacology have been enormous (1).

Nevertheless, despite psychopharmacologic investigation of laboratory animals and human patients, an area that might be termed *comparative clinical psychopharmacology* remains underresearched. While many areas of comparative science and medicine have shown steady advances, our understanding of converging and diverging psychopharmacologic mechanisms in different species is relatively undeveloped.

In this introduction, some of the theoretical and practical considerations that must be addressed to consolidate a comparative clinical psychopharmacology are described. Discussed in turn are the classification of behavior disorders, the classification of psychotropic agents, some basic questions for a comparative clinical psychopharmacology, and the mind-body question.

Classification of Behavior Disorders

Medical disorders can be classified in a variety of ways. First, categories of illness may rely on clinically observable features of the disorder; for example, diarrheal conditions may be clustered together. There are also categories that emphasize the underlying pathogenic mechanisms of the disorder; for example, conditions resulting from tuberculosis infection might be grouped together. In developing a comparative clinical psychopharmacology, we must first determine how best to delineate the various kinds of behavior disorders.

In work on animal behavior disorders, evolutionary and ethologic theory has explicitly or implicitly played a significant role in nosology. Thus, disorders are typically related to dysfunctional aberrations of important species-specific behaviors. For example, a well-known textbook divides animal behavior disorders into those relating to sexual dysfunction, eating dysfunction, and so forth (2). Similarly, a category of grooming disorders has been proposed that includes acral lick dermatitis (ALD) in dogs, psychogenic alopecia in cats, feather-picking in birds, and compulsive grooming (trichotillomania) in humans (3).

In contrast, the most influential diagnostic system in contemporary psychiatry, the *Diagnostic and Statistical Manual of Mental Disorders* (DSM), has explicitly focused on signs and symptoms that can be readily observed or reported. Each disorder is defined in terms of particular diagnostic criteria, which typically attempt to provide operational definitions of the symptoms of the disorder. The architects of this classification system argued that such diagnostic criteria were theory-free and would allow clinicians to diagnose disorders with a high degree of reliability, no matter what their theoretical view of the pathogenesis of these conditions. Indeed, DSM-III (the third edition of DSM) was particularly important, precisely because it allowed psychiatry to claim a diagnostic rigor equal to that of other branches of medicine, and because it provided clinicians from various theoretical schools with a common language.

Although it may be argued that data from biologic psychiatry have in fact impacted on the DSM (4), from the perspective of a comparative clinical psychopharmacology, this nosologic system is likely to be viewed with reservation. First, given the fact that veterinary diagnosis relies primarily on objective rather than subjective data, diagnostic reliability has perhaps been an assumption rather than a goal of work on animal behavior disorders. Second, given the importance of evolutionary and ethologic theory in comparative biology, a comparative clinical psychopharmacology might immediately move toward classification systems that rely on these theories.

Nevertheless, it might be argued that comparative clinical psychopharmacology has much to learn from the conservative approach taken by the DSM system, which emphasizes operational definition while gradually moving toward a classification system that includes biologic theory. In particular, it is of paramount importance to develop rigorous diagnostic criteria for the various behavior disorders seen in veterinary practice. For example, the development of rigorous diagnostic criteria for separation anxiety is an important first step in planning studies of the psychopharmacology of this disorder (5).

Similarly, given the underdeveloped state of current comparative clinical psychopharmacology, basing classification solely on theoretical considerations may provide only a rough guide for clinicians. For example, a category of grooming disorders might suggest that they have an overlapping neurobiology in different species. And, given the importance of serotonin in grooming, it might be expected that the selective serotonin reuptake inhibitors would be useful for ALD, psychogenic alopecia, feather-picking, and obsessive-compulsive disorder (3,6,7). On the other hand, these conditions might also have significant differences in their phenomenology and neurobiology, with varying involvement of the dopaminergic (8), opioid (9), or other systems. Other disorders, such as disorders of aggression, may differ even more significantly in phenomenology and psychopharmacology across species.

At the same time, it might be argued that a comparative clinical psychopharmacology that turns to evolutionary and ethologic theory for its classification system will ultimately contribute to the revision and improvement of the DSM system. Too often, in its reliance on overt phenomena, the DSM seems to ignore obvious underlying neurobiologic commonalities between disorders (for example, several disorders with stereotypic features are classified under entirely separate divisions). Indeed, several authors have suggested that the DSM should base its concepts explicitly on those of evolutionary dysfunction (10). A challenge for the field of comparative clinical psychopharmacology will be to provide sufficient empirical evidence for diagnostic categories based on evolutionary and ethologic theory (11).

As a preliminary step toward a nosology for a comparative clinical psychopharmacology, a number of evolutionarily important behaviors likely to have specific neurobiologic underpinnings may be listed. Each of these behaviors can show abnormalities, for which it will be necessary to formulate diagnostic criteria. Such a list of abnormal behaviors might include:

1. *Disorders of Grooming.* Grooming is an important activity in a variety of domestic animals and, as an evolutionarily preserved behavior, is likely to have similar neurobiologic underpinnings. More specifically, grooming seems to involve dopamine, opioid, and serotonin systems. Excessive grooming may present in a) dogs (ALD), b) cats (psychogenic alopecia), c) birds (excessive feather-picking), and other animals (3). Lack of self-grooming has also been noted in animals (12).

2. *Disorders of Sexual Behavior.* Sexual activity is another clearly important category of behavior that is likely to be mediated by overlapping neurobiologic mechanisms. Hormonal factors play a particularly important role in this system. Disorders of sexual activity can broadly be classified into a) hypersexual disorders, b) hyposexual disorders, and c) inappropriately directed sexual behavior. In many cases of hypersexuality, these are not so much disorders as normal behaviors that are problematic for companion-animal owners. Conversely, hyposexuality is likely to be a problem for breeders and owners of farm animals (2).

3. *Disorders of Eating.* The neurobiology of appetite and appetite disorders has received a good deal of investigation. Serotonin and the opioids appear to play particularly important roles in the control of appetite. Eating disorders comprise a) hyperphagic disorders, b) hypophagic disorders, and c) stereotypic

disorders of eating or *pica* (excessive eating of nonfood objects). In animals, it is of paramount importance to rule out general medical conditions that sometimes underlie such behaviors (2).

4. *Disorders of Locomotion.* A number of behavior disorders of locomotion exist, particularly in animals that normally show a great deal of locomotor behavior. The dopaminergic system is particularly important here. Hyperactivity may be a problem in some animal species, such as dogs. In addition, stereotypic locomotor behaviors are common in horses (13) and caged exotic animals (14,15).

5. *Disorders of Elimination.* These are reportedly the most common behavior problems in dogs and cats. Problems of house training, including litter-box aversion in cats, are well known. Although treating such behavior often falls within the domain of traditional behavior modification therapy, psychopharmacotherapy may also have a role in certain cases (16). Urine-marking in dogs and urine-spraying/marking in cats are sexually dimorphic, predominantly male behaviors that often present for treatment. These behaviors sometimes continue even after castration and may require medication (16).

6. *Phobic/Anxiety Disorders.* Evolution has created a number of brain-alarm systems. The noradrenergic, serotonergic, and GABA (gamma-aminobutyric acid)-ergic neurotransmitter systems appear to play a particularly important role in mediating the anxiety induced by such alarms. Dysfunction of these alarm systems may manifest in behavior disorders such as noise/thunder phobias (17).

7. *Disorders of Attachment/Separation.* Separation anxiety is seen when animals manifest various abnormal behaviors when left alone. This is included as a separate category based on a range of primate studies on separation (18) as well as on studies of infants from different species (19). Monoamine and opioid systems are likely to mediate such behavior.

8. *Disorders of Aggression.* Aggression has commonly been divided into specific forms, each of which may have underlying neurobiologic characteristics. For example, Moyer (20) described seven classes of aggression (predatory, intermale, fear-induced, irritable, territorial, maternal, and instrumental), while Reis (21) divided aggression into affective (offensive or defensive) and predatory forms. The serotonin system has often been implicated in aggression. As in other categories of behavioral disorders, aggression secondary to a general medical disorder (e.g., seizure disorder, thyroid dysfunction, dementia) must be ruled out (22).

9. *Disorders of Trainability.* Dogs raised without human contact may later be difficult to train (23,24). Although prophylactic measures to avoid such conditions are the obvious intervention, it is possible that isolation may be associated with specific neurobiologic changes (25) that are modifiable by pharmacotherapy. A number of general medical disorders may also result in

untrainability. A residual set of animals may have idiopathic learning difficulties (2).

10. *Disorders of Sleep*. Sleep disorders can be divided into a) hypersomniac disorders, b) hyposomniac disorders, and c) other disorders such as narcolepsy. Narcolepsy is characterized by sleep attacks and may be seen in both dogs and cats (26,27).

Additional categories of behavior that have not been well studied by psychopharmacologists include deviations in care-giving behavior, deviations in denning and nesting instincts, and others (11). Learned helplessness and spontaneous "depressive" symptoms (28) have received more attention from psychopharmacologists, and perhaps this will lead to the delineation of a category of animal mood disorders.

The classification previously given does not include a separate section for "organic" behavior disorders. Indeed, in DSM-IV (the fourth edition of DSM) a decision was made to omit any reference to the term "organic"—a word which implies, falsely, that nonorganic behavior disorders are not mediated by brain systems. Instead, for example, a depression that is secondary to a brain tumor is classified on one axis (Axis I) as Major Depression, and the general medical disorder is noted on another axis (Axis III). Similar principles would seem to apply to a classification of animal behavior disorders.

Still another axis (Axis II) in DSM is used to classify personality disorders, which differ from many discrete psychiatric disorders in that they comprise enduring patterns of behavior. In the case of domestic animals, where breeding for specific temperaments has taken place, problems may arise with exaggerated behavioral patterns (e.g., nervousness, aggressiveness). As in humans, there are neurobiologic mechanisms mediating these characteristics, and psychopharmacotherapy may be able to play a role in their modification (29,30).

Classification of Psychotropic Agents

As in the case of medical disorders, psychotropic agents can be classified in a number of different ways. Categories of these medications may emphasize clinical use (e.g., antidepressants, antipsychotics, anxiolytics), chemical structure (e.g., tricyclics, tetracyclics), or neurochemical effects (e.g., serotonin reuptake blockers, dopamine blockers). Once again, comparative clinical psychopharmacology must formulate how best to approach the agents that are central to the field.

The bulk of clinical psychopharmacology has been undertaken in humans. Thus, despite increased understanding of the neurochemical effects of psychotropic agents, categories such as antidepressants or antipsychotics have obvious value and remain commonly used. Certainly, it is well known that the antidepressants are useful for a range of disorders other than depression, yet the term is a convenient reference to several classes of medication. The specific kinds of antidepressants and antipsychotics are often classified in terms of chemical structure or neurochemical effects.

From the perspective of comparative clinical psychopharmacology, such classification will likely be problematic. The important cognitive components of depression make it a disorder that seems particularly relevant to an understanding of humans and other primate species. The term "antidepressants" would thus seem to hold relatively less value when applied to animal behavior disorders, when depression per se is not recognized in these animals.

For a medication class having a specific neurochemical effect, is it possible to arrive at a name that reflects its behavioral effect in a variety of species? For example, the selective serotonin reuptake inhibitors seem to alter the assessment of harm in a range of preclinical and clinical paradigms (31). It might be hypothesized that this group of agents is therefore therapeutic for conditions where harm may be underestimated (e.g., aggression) or overestimated (e.g., excessive grooming). However, most such characterizations are likely to be inaccurate or incomplete: inaccurate, because most neurochemicals play a role in a variety of different behaviors, and incomplete, because even drugs seeming to have a specific action, such as the GABA-ergic agents, may vary significantly in their effects on different species.

At this stage, then, it may be best for comparative clinical psychopharmacology to employ a categorization of psychotropic agents based primarily on neurochemical effects and secondarily on behavioral effects. Psychotropic agents of importance to a comparative clinical psychopharmacology include: 1) dopaminergic agents, 2) noradrenergic/serotonergic agents, 3) GABA-ergic agents, 4) anticonvulsants, and 5) hormonal agents.

DOPAMINERGIC AGENTS

Dopamine neurons in the midbrain project to several areas, including the cortex and the limbic system (mesocorticolimbic neurons). Dopamine neurons are believed to regulate and allow integrative functions in the areas onto which they project (32). Dopamine projections of the striatum may be involved in filtering signals relating to basic biologic drives (limbic area) and sensorimotor processing (cortex), which are then synchronized and translated into behavior via the pallidal and pontine motor nuclei (32). Stimulation of dopamine neurons results in an increased facilitation of such response sequencing, but a parallel decrease in variation or adaptability with consequent stereotypy (33).

Dopamine blockers can be divided into two categories: the classic neuroleptics, which act primarily on the dopamine system, and the newer atypical neuroleptics, which function as both dopamine blockers and serotonin antagonists. Classic neuroleptics include the phenothiazines (e.g., chlorpromazine, acepromazine), the butyrophenones (e.g., haloperidol), and the thioxanthenes (e.g., thiothixene). Recently introduced atypical neuroleptics include clozapine, risperidone, and olanzapine.

Possible clinical effects of dopamine blockers include 1) increasing sedation, 2) decreasing aggression, 3) decreasing stereotypies. In humans, the classic neuroleptics are associated with the development of tardive dyskinesia and are therefore typically reserved for the treatment of psychotic disorders. In animals, these agents may have a role in calming agitated subjects, such as dogs with noise/thunder phobias (34). Further work needs to be undertaken, however, to establish which stereotypies (e.g., psychogenic alopecia (8)) and other behavior disorders respond to these agents.

A number of drugs act to facilitate dopaminergic neurotransmission. Psychostimulants such as methylphenidate displace dopamine and norepinephrine from presynaptic binding sites. Certain antidepressants, such as the monoamine oxidase inhibitors and bupropion, also act to increase dopaminergic activity. In humans, the psychostimulants may act paradoxically to calm hyperactive subjects, though they may increase stereotypic behaviors. Stimulants may have a similar paradoxical effect on hyperactivity in dogs (35). In addition, psychostimulants are used to treat narcolepsy in humans and animals (34).

NORADRENERGIC/SEROTONERGIC AGENTS

Several theories have been posited to explain noradrenergic function (36). An early idea was that the locus coeruleus (LC) was involved in brain-alarm systems, increasing an individual's attention and vigilance (37). Moreover, the LC has been described as resulting in focused rather than automatic functioning (38). Thus, in threatening or demanding situations, the noradrenergic system seems to play a role in focusing attention onto salient events (36).

Likewise, several theories have been put forward to explain serotonergic function in different species (39). Soubrie (31), for example, has argued that serotonin plays a role in the behavioral facilitation system that mobilizes an animal's active engagement with the environment, as well as playing a role in the behavioral inhibition system that arrests ongoing behavior. Decrease in serotonergic transmission leads to an inability to adopt passive or waiting attitudes or to accept situations that necessitate or create strong inhibitory tendencies. More generally, Jacobs and Fornal (39) argue that serotonin facilitates gross motor output and inhibits sensory information processing.

Noradrenergic/serotonergic reuptake blockers can be divided into the older tricyclic antidepressants, which work on the serotonergic and noradrenergic system (as well as having anticholinergic effects), and the newer agents, which include the selective serotonin reuptake inhibitors (SSRIs; e.g., fluoxetine), the nonselective serotonin reuptake inhibitors (NSRIs; e.g., venlafaxine), and agents that are both serotonin reuptake inhibitors and serotonin antagonists (e.g., nefazodone). The tricyclics can be divided into the (older) tertiary amine and the (newer) secondary amine tricylics, or into predominantly serotonergic (e.g., clomipramine) and predominantly noradrenergic (e.g., desipramine) agents.

Noradrenergic/serotonergic reuptake blockers have been used to decrease separation anxiety (40). SSRIs also have this effect, and in addition they may be effective for 1) decreasing aggression, 2) reducing a range of stereotypies (3), and 3) treating phobic/anxiety disorders (17).

Apart from the noradrenergic/serotonergic reuptake blockers, several other agents facilitate neurotransmission in these systems. Noradrenergic agonists of note include yohimbine, an alpha-2 antagonist. In humans, yohimbine increases anxiety levels but facilitates sexual functioning, so that it may have a role to play in the treatment of certain sexual disorders. Serotonergic agonists are exemplified by 5-HT_{1A} agonists such as buspirone. Clinical uses of the $5\text{-}HT_{1A}$ agonists include 1) reduction of anxiety, 2) treatment of aggression, and 3) management of elimination disorders in cats (16).

Finally, a number of agents act to reduce noradrenergic or serotonergic neurotransmission. Clonidine acts as an alpha-2 autoreceptor agonist, thereby blunting adrenergic transmission; behavioral effects therefore include sedation. Beta blockers act as beta-adrenergic receptors to competitively antagonize the beta effects of norepinephrine and epinephrine; these agents reduce the peripheral concomitants of anxiety. Clonidine and the beta blockers have been minimally studied in animal behavior disorders.

GABA-ERGIC AGENTS

Gamma-aminobutyric acid (GABA) is the principal inhibitory neurotransmitter system of the human brain. Benzodiazepines are agents that bind to receptors situated on the same membrane complex as the GABA receptor and act to potentiate GABA-ergic inhibition. These benzodiazepine receptors are particularly dense in the limbic system.

Benzodiazepines generally result in 1) increased sedation and 2) decreased anxiety. These agents are typically used in nonpathological subjects to cause sedation. They may have a role in the treatment of phobic/anxiety disorders. One clinical advantage of these agents is their rapid onset of action; however, chronic administration leads to physical dependence.

ANTICONVULSANTS

Lithium has long been used as a mood stabilizer, particularly in human patients with manic-depressive or bipolar disorder. More recently, the anticonvulsants valproate and carbamazepine have been found to be effective in this disorder; they are also useful in the treatment of certain kinds of impulsive disorders, such as borderline personality disorder. The anticonvulants' mechanism of action in these disorders is presently open to speculation, as they have an array of neurochemical effects. One important hypothesis suggests that valproate and carbamazepine work via reduction of brain kindling.

In animals, anticonvulsants may be useful in treating seizure-like behavior disorders, such as tail-chasing in dogs (41) or episodic aggression (22). Anticonvulsants have not been studied in most animal behavior disorders.

HORMONAL AGENTS

A variety of agents can be used to supplement, increase, or decrease testosterone, estrogen, and progesterone levels. Such agents typically lead to alterations in sexual activity and interspecies aggression. In humans, the use of hormonal agents for psychiatric disorders is restricted to postmenopausal hormone replacement therapy, treatment of late luteal dysphoric disorder, and, less frequently, to the treatment of paraphilias. In animals, surgical modification of hormonal activity is commonly used to alter sexual activity and aggression. Hormonal agents are available that would effect similar changes.

Basic Questions in Comparative Clinical Psychopharmacology

The field of comparative clinical psychopharmacology is young. A number of basic questions need to be better studied in order to consolidate this arena of investigation. These include pharmacodynamic (i.e., what the drug does to the body), pharmacokinetic (i.e., what the body does to the drug), and methodologic issues.

1. *What kinds of doses are necessary to effect changes in animal behavioral disorders?*

Interspecies pharmacokinetic differences may necessitate important differences in dosing strategies. Lack of attention to such issues can result in inadequate treatment. For example, depressed patients who are rapid metabolizers of tricyclics require higher doses of these agents in order to respond favorably.

A typical clinical rule is to administer the highest dose of an agent that can be tolerated by the person or animal. However, given the lack of subjective data in veterinary practice, the objective measures for such a rule need to be better ascertained. Specifically, studies of drug levels may need to be undertaken in animals receiving psychotropic medications for behavior disorders.

2. *How much time is necessary to effect changes in animal behavior disorders?*

Again, the importance of this pharmacodynamic question is emphasized by findings in human studies, which show that in a number of disorders treatment must continue for several weeks before there will be a quantifiable therapeutic outcome. For example, in depression, a 4- to 6-week trial of medication is required before clinical changes can be ascertained. In obsessive-compulsive disorder, lag time for clinical improvement may be 10 to 12 weeks.

Much less information is available for the treatment of animal behavior disorders. Anecdotal experience suggests that pharmacotherapeutic response times may be quicker in some animals for some disorders than the response times usually seen in humans. Nevertheless, a conservative approach, in which the veterinarian emphasizes that response may not be immediate and continues treatment over several weeks, would seem warranted at present (42).

3. *How can symptom change be measured reliably in animal behavior disorders?*

Scales for measuring symptomatic change have been developed only recently. Reliability and validity studies of such scales have been a crucial first methodologic step in the effort to advance clinical trials of psychopharmacologic agents. Typically, the statistical analysis of such clinical trials is dependent on changes in scale measures.

In humans, symptom scales have the advantage of including both subjective and objective items. In animals, of course, symptom scales are restricted to objective items. Few such measures have been standardized by those interested in animal psychopharmacology, and a great deal of further work must be done in order to provide reliable and valid scales for the field.

4. *What kinds of designs are necessary for clinical trials in animal behavior disorders?*

In human psychopharmacology, the gold standard is a randomized, double-blind, placebo-controlled trial. While it has been argued by some researchers that even this design allows participants to ascertain whether they are on an active ingredient, the high placebo response in many psychiatric conditions makes the open clinical trial a preliminary investigation.

It might be argued that in animal psychopharmacology, given the objectivity with which symptoms can be measured, placebo-controlled trials are less necessary. While there is possibly some truth to this argument, a placebo response of up to 30% in animal psychopharmacology has been noted (see Appendix). The position in animal psychopharmacology is perhaps similar to that in child psychopharmacology—the attitude of the child's parent (or animal's owner) regarding medication may play an important role in determining reported outcome.

Conceptualizing Brain and Mind

Behaviorism has been a major conceptual underpinning of past work on animal behavior disorders. Many clinicians have viewed symptoms as conditioned behaviors and have based their treatments on the classic principles of positive and negative reinforcement. The neurobiologic underpinnings of learning are typically ignored by researchers working in this tradition. Further, the mind—whether animal or human—is viewed as a "black box," with the focus of all theory and research resting solely on observable stimuli and responses.

Although psychiatry has also been influenced by behaviorism, a variety of other influences have helped shape the field. While psychoanalysis was once a predominant paradigm, today medical and cognitive science are more crucial influences. In effect, psychiatry has undergone a "remedicalization," in which mental illnesses are conceptualized as specific medical disorders and in which neurobiologic etiology and intervention are central. In addition, cognitive models of the mind as a symbol processor or even as a parallel processor are playing increasingly important roles in the theory and practice of psychotherapy.

Nevertheless, the cognitive revolution, in which behaviorist models in psychology were replaced by computational ones, has also had an impact on the study of animal behavior. Increasingly, there is talk of "animal minds" (43). If it is permissible to talk about computer "memory" and "processing," then a discourse on human and even animal symbol manipulation or parallel processing is a short step away.

The question arises, then, of how to integrate behavioral and medical/cognitive science in comparative clinical psychopharmacology. At a practical level, we must consider using different kinds of intervention (behavioral therapy, psychotropic agents) serially or in combination. At a theoretical level, we must determine how best to conceptualize the integration of brain and psyche. For example, consider a dog with separation anxiety: A behavioral regime might be instituted to condition the animal to become more comfortable with the stress of separation, and a pharmacologic regime might be instituted to change the threshold for anxiety at separation. One of the most interesting recent studies on human anxiety disorder indicates that in obsessive-compulsive disorder, both behavioral therapy and pharmacotherapy resulted in similar normalization of brain dysfunction on functional imaging (44). While similar studies have not yet been done in animals, an extrapolation of the human work might lead to the hypothesis that separation anxiety in animals is mediated by a specific neurobiologic system that can be altered by either behavioral or pharmacologic intervention.

Comparative clinical psychopharmacology should remain aware of such data. The mind can be understood as an emergent property of the brain. While analysis of the mind is certainly important in higher animals, it also may be useful in understanding behavior disorders in lower animals. However, such an analysis does not preclude neurobiologic data—alterations to the mind are accompanied by changes in its neurobiology, and changes in neurobiology are accompanied by changes in the mind.

Conclusion

A search for precise convergences in the clinical psychopharmacology of different species will undoubtedly be quixotic. The differences in both brain and mind in humans and other animal species make direct extrapolation of data impossible in many cases. Certainly, for disorders that primarily involve complex dysfunctions of cognition, such divergences will make it particularly difficult to establish a wide-ranging comparative clinical psychopharmacology.

Still, convergences between animals and humans may be more likely for some behavior disorders than others. There is increasing evidence, for example, that grooming disorders in animals have analogues in humans. In order to investigate fully such convergences, the methodologies of current neurobiology, including psychopharmacologic challenges, brain imaging, and postmortem analysis, will need to be employed (45).

Indeed, it seems clear that we have much to learn by investigating clinical psychopharmacology from a comparative perspective. In particular, such an investigation may shed light on our understanding of nosologic questions, psychotropic mechanisms, and other significant issues within contemporary psychopharmacology. Such work will therefore benefit not only animals suffering from behavioral disorders but also humans with psychiatric disorders.

Acknowledgment: Dr. Stein is supported by a grant from the Medical Research Council of South Africa.

References

1. Bloom FE, Kupfer DJ. Psychopharmacology: the fourth generation of progress. New York: Raven, 1995.
2. Houpt KA, Wolski TR. Domestic animal behavior for veterinarians and animal scientists. Ames, IA: Iowa State University Press, 1982.
3. Dodman NH, Moon A, Stein DJ. Animal models of obsessive-compulsive disorder. In: Hollander E, Stein DJ, eds. Obsessive-compulsive disorders: etiology, diagnosis, treatment. New York: Marcel Decker, 1997.
4. Stein DJ. Philosophy and the DSM-III. Compr Psychiatry 1991;32:404–415.
5. McGrave EA. Diagnostic criteria for separation anxiety in the dog. Vet Clin North Am Small Anim Pract 1991;21:247–255.
6. Rapoport JL, Ryland DH, Kriete M. Drug treatment of canine acral lick: an animal model of obsessive-compulsive disorder. Arch Gen Psychiatry 1992;48:517–521.
7. Stein DJ, Shoulberg N, Helton K, Hollander E. The neuroethological model of obsessive-compulsive disorder. Compr Psychiatry 1992;33:274–281.
8. Willemse T. The effect of dopamine antagonists on psychogenic alopecia in cats. Presented at the Second World Congress of Veterinary Dermatology, Montreal, Canada, May 13–16, 1992.
9. Dodman NH, Shuster L, White SD, et al. Use of narcotic agonists to modify stereotypic self-licking, self-chewing, and scratching behavior in dogs. J Am Vet Med Assoc 1988;193:815–819.
10. Klein DF. A proposed definition of mental illness. In: Spitzer RL, Klein DF, eds. Critical issues in psychiatric diagnosis. New York: Raven, 1978.
11. Stein DJ, Bouwer C. Blushing and social phobia: a neuroethological speculation. Med Hypotheses, 1997 (in press).
12. Odendaal JSJ. A diagnostic classification of problem behaviour in dogs and cats. 1997 (in press).
13. Kiley-Worthington M. Stereotypes in horses. Equine Pract 1983;5:34–40.

14. Fox MW. Psychopathology in man and lower animals. J Am Vet Med Assoc 1971a;159: 66–77.
15. Markowitz H, Stevens VJ. Behavior of captive wild animals. Chicago: Nelson-Hall, 1978.
16. Hart BL, Eckstein RA, Powell KL, Dodman NH. Effectiveness of buspirone on urine spraying and inappropriate urination in cats. J Am Vet Med Assoc 1993;203:254–258.
17. Stein DJ, Borchelt P, Hollander E. Pharmacotherapy of naturally occurring anxiety symptoms in dogs. Res Commun Psychol Psychiatry Behav 1994b;19:39–48.
18. Harlow HF, Harlow MK. Psychopathology in monkeys. In: Kimmel H, ed. Experimental psychopathology in monkeys. New York: Academic, 1971.
19. Panskepp J, Meeker R, Bean NJ. The neurochemical control of crying. Pharmacol Biochem Behav 1980;12:437–443.
20. Moyer KE. Kinds of aggression and their physiological basis. Comm Behav Biol 1968;2: 65–87.
21. Reis D. Brain monoamines in aggression and sleep. Clin Neurosurg 1971;18:471–502.
22. Dodman NH, Miczek KA, Knowles K, et al. Phenobarbital-responsive episodic dyscontrol (rage) in dogs. J Am Vet Med Assoc 1992;201:1580–1583.
23. Thomson WR, Melzack R. Early environment. Sci Am 1956;194:30–42.
24. Scott JP. Critical periods in the development of social behavior in dogs. In: Kazda S, Denenberg V. The postnatal development of the phenotype. Prague: Academia, 1970.
25. Fox MW. Integrative development of brain and behavior in the dog. Chicago: University of Chicago Press, 1971.
26. Mitler MM, Soave O, Dement WC. Narcolepsy in seven dogs. J Am Vet Med Assoc 1976;168:1036–1038.
27. Knecht CD, Oliver JE, Redding R, et al. Narcolepsy in a dog and a cat. J Am Vet Med Assoc 1973;162:1052–1053.
28. Iorio LC, Eisenstein N, Brody PE, Barnett A. Effects of selected drugs on spontaneously occurring abnormal behavior in beagles. Pharmacol Biochem Behav 1982;18:379–382.
29. Tancer ME, Stein MB, Bessette BB, Uhde TW. Behavioral effects of chronic imipramine treatment in genetically nervous pointer dogs. Physiol Behav 1990;48:179–181.
30. Adamec RE. Anxious personality in the cat: its ontogeny and physiology. In: Carroll BJ, Barrett JE, eds. Psychopathology and the brain. New York: Raven, 1991:153–168.
31. Soubrie P. Reconciling the role of central serotonin neurones in human and animal behavior. Behav Brain Sci 1986;9:319–364.
32. Le Moal M. Mesocorticolimbic dopaminergic neurons: functional and regulatory roles. In: Bloom FE, Kupfer DJ, eds. Psychopharmacology: the fourth generation of progress. New York: Raven, 1995.
33. Lyon M, Robbins TW. The action of central nervous system stimulus drugs: a general theory concerning amphetamine effects. In: Essman W, Valzelli L, eds. Current developments in psychopharmacology, vol 2. New York: Spectrum Publications, 1975.
34. Hart BL. Canine behavior: collected columns from canine practice journal. Santa Barbara, CA: Veterinary Practice, 1980.
35. Hart BL, Hart LA. Psychoactive drugs and behavioral therapy. In: Hart BL, Hart LA, eds. Canine and feline behavioral therapy. Philadelphia: Lea & Febiger, 1985:249–264.
36. Robbins TW, Everitt BJ. Central norepinephrine neurons and behavior. In: Bloom FE, Kupfer DJ, eds. Psychopharmacology: the fourth generation of progress. New York: Raven, 1995.
37. Aston-Jones G, Chiang C, Alexinsky T. Discharge of noradrenergic locus coeruleus neurons in behaving rats and monkeys suggests a role in vigilance. Prog Brain Res 1991;88:501–520.
38. Cole BJ, Robbins TW. Forebrain norepinephrine: role in controlled information processing in the rat. Neuropsychopharmacology 1992;7:129–141.
39. Jacobs BJ, Fornal CA. Serotonin and behavior: a general hypothesis. In: Bloom FE, Kupfer DJ, eds. Psychopharmacology: the fourth generation of progress. New York: Raven, 1995.

40. Dodman NH. The dog who loved too much: tales, treatments, and the psychology of dogs. New York: Bantam, 1996.

41. Dodman NH, Knowles KE, Shuster L, et al. Behavioral changes associated with suspected complex partial seizures in bull terriers. J Am Vet Med Assoc 1996;208:688–691.

42. Moon-Fanelli AA, Dodman NH. Phenomenology, development and pharmacotherapy of compulsive tail chasing behavior in bull terriers and related breeds: an open trial of clomipramine and fluoxetine. 1997 (in press).

43. Griffin DR. Animal minds. Chicago: University of Chicago Press, 1994.

44. Baxter LR, Schwartz JM, Bergman KS, et al. Caudate glucose metabolic rate changes with both drug and behavior therapy for OCD. Arch Gen Psychiatry 1992;49:681–689.

45. Stein DJ, Dodman NH, Borchelt P, Hollander E. Behavioral disorders in veterinary practice: relevance to psychiatry. Compr Psychiatry 1994b;35:275–285.

1 AGGRESSION

Neurochemical Bases of Aggression

Klaus A. Miczek
Berend Olivier

Ideally, pharmacotherapy for excessive aggressive behavior is based on adequate neurochemical information about the sites and mechanisms of the therapeutic agents. Indeed, fascinating developments in cloning receptors for neurotransmitters and neuromodulators such as dopamine, serotonin, neuropeptides, and neurosteroids hold promise for new therapeutic agents. Unfortunately, these biochemical advances in the molecular identification of targets for intervention are not matched by an increased understanding of their functional significance in general, nor with regard to the complex neurobiologic mechanisms mediating different kinds of aggressive behavior. In order to select the most reliable and robust findings in the neurobiology of aggressive behavior, it appears advisable first to characterize the kinds of aggressive behavior and the animal species on which the findings are based.

Perspectives on Aggression

By far, most neurochemical data on aggressive behavior stem from laboratory rodents that have been bred to be placid. In order to engender aggressive behavior under controlled conditions that allow for neurochemical measurements, several experimental protocols or "models" have been developed (1). These experimental protocols focus on different types of aggressive behavior, and it has become apparent that each type of aggressive behavior derives from clearly differentiated neurobiologic mechanisms. The research methodologies for studying aggressive behavior in placid laboratory animals reflect scientific traditions that conceptualize, in distinctly different ways, the distal and proximal antecedents, the events immediately triggering aggressive acts, and the consequences of these acts.

The experimental research from the authors' laboratory was supported by USPHS research grants AA 05122 and DA 02632.

BIOMEDICAL PERSPECTIVE

Clinical concerns led to the biomedical designation of *aggression as a disease*. Neurologic and psychiatric diseases in humans, ranging from mental retardation, attention deficit disorder, organic mental syndromes, schizophrenia, delusional disorder, brief reactive psychosis, mood disorders, anxiety disorder, dissociative disorders, impulse control disorders, adjustment disorder, and personality disorders, as well as *seizures*, brain *traumas*, and various toxic insults, have all been associated with aggressive outbursts. Thus far, the American Psychiatric Association has not considered aggressive behavior itself a separate diagnostic category, but aggression does constitute a major problem in a variety of psychiatric conditions, and the same applies to veterinary medicine.

SOCIAL SCIENCE PERSPECTIVE

In the social sciences, aggressive behavior is studied as an *antisocial behavior*, as contrasted with prosocial activities; that is, aggressive behavior is considered mainly the product of adverse living conditions, impaired socialization, inappropriate role models, learning to resolve conflicts via confrontation, and lack of access to resources. These influences are particularly significant early in life, presumably during "critical periods" of development. Social scientists focus on such types of aggression as those induced by preventing access to rewarding contingencies (*frustration-induced aggression*), reactions to noxious, aversive events (*pain-induced aggression*), and impoverished living conditions (*isolation-induced aggression*). When the lack of any aggressive behavior is considered normative, then the objective of intervention is the suppression of these behaviors by appropriate arrangement of environmental conditions and modification of aggressive behavior by managing the contingencies for this behavior.

ETHOLOGIC PERSPECTIVE

In the ethologic tradition, students of animal behavior view aggressive behavior as part of the *social and reproductive strategy* for a given species. The type, intensity, frequency, and ritualization of aggressive behavior characterize individuals as being members of a species that is either adapted to live dispersed or in a socially cohesive group. Most data on the neurobiology of aggressive behavior stem primarily from laboratory rats that descend from colonially organized *Rattus norvegicus*. Additional information comes from laboratory mice (*Mus musculus*) whose feral ancestors mark, patrol, and defend territories from which they exclude other adult males, and some data derive from domestic cats, fish, and avian and invertebrate species. Ethologists focus on types of aggression that function to establish and maintain social relations (*dominance* or *rival aggression*), to exclude other adult species members from the territory (*territorial aggression*), or to protect offspring (*maternal aggression*). Intervention strategies seek to modify the social milieu of the individual and to remove the provocative events for these types of aggression.

The study of aggressive behavior in lower animal species builds on the premise that these behavior patterns have evolved (2). Yet, it is debatable whether a linear *scala naturae* applies to the evolution of social systems that extend from invertebrates to fish, birds, and mammals, including humans (3). Comparative studies reveal that the types of aggressive behavior become more diverse with increasing complexity of the species-specific social organization. This diversity is apparent in the more complex behavioral repertoire for aggressive acts, postures, displays and gestures, and by the intricate sequential and temporal structure of aggressive interactions at the mammalian level. The all-or-none signals or "releasers" for aggressive behavior in invertebrates or fish, as illustrated by pheromonal or visual releasers, become part of more elaborate multi-modal communication systems in mammals. The functions of aggressive acts also become more diverse in animal species with more complex social systems, ranging from basic defensive bites to elaborate agonistic displays that may signal the proximity of an ally, as illustrated in chimpanzees (4).

Aggressive acts belong to those behavioral and biologic functions that occur in an *episodic* fashion. A microanalysis of the temporal organization of aggressive behavior reveals "bursts" or epochs of rapidly succeeding aggressive acts, which are separated by long "gaps" between "bursts" (5), in addition to seasonal peaks and troughs and circadian rhythms in the occurrence of aggressive acts. Figure 1.1 depicts an event record of consecutive aggressive acts by a resident rat confronting an intruder, and in addition, summarizes more than 20,000 intervals between consecutive aggressive acts in a log-survivor plot. It is apparent that more than 85% of all aggressive acts are separated by very short intervals; i.e., they constitute aggressive "bursts," and the remaining intervals represent the "gaps" between aggressive bursts.

These behavioral considerations in terms of distal and proximal causes, triggering events, diversity in repertoire, sequential and temporal structure, and diverse functions have important implications for the neurobiologic processes mediating different types of aggressive behavior. Figure 1.2 depicts in schematic form the antecedents and consequences of aggressive "bursts," with particular attention to the time base that extends from multigenerational influences to momentary triggers. Furthermore, the feedback from the outcome of aggressive "bursts" on the antecedents for future occurrences of aggressive behavior is highlighted. Discrete neural circuits mediate different types of aggressive behavior, each involving at least minimal transmission from: 1) sensory organs that filter species-specific signals and releasers, 2) motor output for rapid action and prolonged postural displays that are patterned and sequenced in a species-

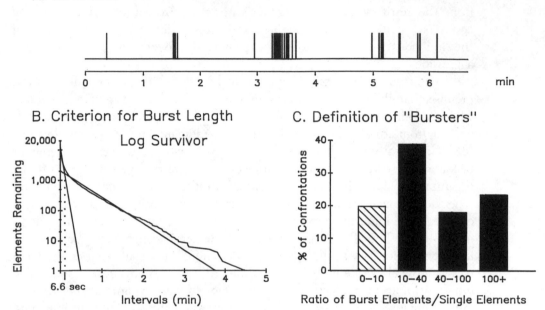

Figure 1.1.
Temporal analysis of aggressive behavior. **A**. The start and end times of all elements of aggressive behavior (i.e., pursuit, sideways threat, attack bite, aggressive posture) by a resident rat directed toward an intruder in real time during a selected confrontation. Each behavioral event is depicted as an upward deflection from the time line. **B**. Burst criterion. Log survivor plot of all intervals between consecutive occurrences of aggressive behavior as a function of interval size. Note the logarithmic scale on the y-axis. Regression lines are fitted against the steep and flat portions of the data curve. The intersection of the two regression lines defines the maximal interval size that is considered to be part of a "burst." The burst criterion in the present studies was 6.6 sec. **C**. Definition of "burster." The ratio between behavioral elements within an aggressive burst (i.e., within 6.6 sec or less since a previous aggressive element) to those elements outside of the burst criterion is called a "burster." Ratios that are smaller than 10 identify 77 out of 389 5-min confrontations with the least-clear burst characteristics. (Reproduced by permission from Miczek KA, Weerts EM, Tornatzky W, et al. Alcohol and "bursts" of aggressive behavior: ethological analysis of individual differences in rats. Psychopharmacology 1992;107:551–563.)

typical fashion, and 3) integrative elements for motivational, affective, and cognitive processes.

In invertebrates, fish, and birds, catecholamines, indolamines, and androgenic steroids are necessary for the display of attack and defensive behavior. At the mammalian level, these obligatory requirements shift to a modulatory influence of these amines and relative independence from androgenic steroids is seen for several types of aggressive behavior. Particularly when attack and

Aggression: Antecedents and Consequences

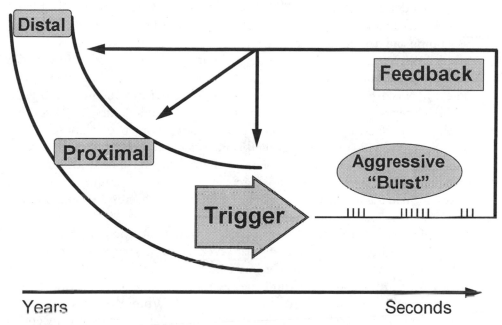

Figure 1.2.
Schematic representation of antecedent and consequent events to "bursts" of aggressive behavior. The timeline depicts how distal causes may predate the aggressive behavior by generations, proximal events by weeks and days, and how some events serve as immediate triggers of aggressive bursts. The consequences of aggressive behavior feed back to render future acts of aggression more or less likely.

defensive behavior have become established in the behavioral repertoire of a mammal, androgenic steroids and the monoamines are not all-or-none signals but modulators of these behaviors.

5-Hydroxytryptamine (5-HT; Serotonin)

In neurochemical research on aggression, the most intensively investigated neurotransmitter system comprises the serotonin-containing neurons that project from the *raphe* nuclei to the forebrain and those that project to the spinal cord, as well as the receptors upon which serotonin acts (6). At least two ascending projections can be differentiated anatomically: 1) thin, varicose serotonergic axons originating in the dorsal raphe, branching profusely and terminating diffusely in the striatum, thalamus, and cerebral cortex; and 2) the thick, nonvaricose axons, also called *basket axons*, originating in the median raphe and terminating in cerebral cortex and limbic structures such as the hippocampus (7). During the past two decades, peripheral "markers" of central serotonergic activity such as imipramine binding to blood platelets, the prolactin response to challenges with serotonergic agonists, and the lumbar CSF 5-hydroxyindoleacetic acid (5-HIAA) levels have been explored in highly aggressive patients and animals (7a). At present, it is unclear precisely how the ascending and descending serotonergic projections contribute to these peripheral markers of the functional state of brain serotonin (5-HT). Given the indirect, anatomically remote, and multiply determined nature of these measures, it would be premature to rely upon decreased imipramine binding to blood platelets, a blunted prolactin response to fenfluramine or buspirone challenge, or decreased 5-HIAA level in the CSF in order to diagnose aggression-prone individuals. Considering the anatomical complexities of the serotonin-containing neurons, it is impressive that peripheral indices of serotonin activity in blood or in CSF can detect any degree of significant variation between individuals with a history of certain types of aggressive behavior and those without such a history.

Of particular relevance to the potential pharmacotherapy of aggressive behavior are the discoveries of at least seven serotonin receptor families and subtypes (8). All of these receptors are metabotropic; i.e., they effect changes in a cascade of second and third messenger systems, except for the $5-HT_3$ receptor, which is a ligand-gated cation channel. While the classification of serotonin receptors undergoes periodic revision, actual cloning of the receptors has progressed to identify their molecular structure and relationship with each other. In the present intense growth phase of serotonin-receptor pharmacology, selective agonists and antagonists for the first four receptor families have emerged (9). Drugs targeting pre- and postsynaptic receptors and uptake sites for serotonin are beginning to reveal their utility in a wide range of physiologic and behavioral processes, and they may possibly have a role to play in modulating aggressive behavior.

NEUROCHEMICAL CORRELATES

In the 1960s and 1970s, assays of *whole brain* 5-HT or its major acidic metabolite 5-HIAA in male mice after isolated housing revealed either increases, decreases, or no change in the level of this amine or acid (10–12). A large percentage of outbred albino Swiss mice engage in aggressive behavior after being housed singly, but others become timid (13,14).

In the 1980s, assays of discrete brain areas revealed differential changes in limbic, striatal, and mesencephalic regions of aggressive animals, emphasizing the separate contributions of serotonin systems to the mediation of aggressive and defensive behavior patterns. For example, an increase in the ratio of 5-HT to 5-HIAA—an index of 5-HT turnover—was found in the *amygdala* of male mice that attacked an intruder for the first time (15). In the carnivorous mink, 5-HIAA levels were increased in the amygdala and *hypothalamus* when the animal was sated and less likely to prey (16). By contrast, hypothalamic, limbic, and mesencephalic regions of Syrian hamsters and laboratory mice revealed no changes in either 5-HT or 5-HIAA after prolonged fighting (17,18). Substantial decreases in 5-HT levels in the *raphe nuclei* and *striatum* as well as in *hippocampal* 5-HIAA were seen in laboratory rats that reacted to electric shock with defensive postures and acts, whereas the firing rate of raphe neurons increases in tree shrews that are threatened and defend themselves (19,20). The early evidence from post mortem tissue assays prompts several conclusions: 1) serotonin activity in terminal regions such as the hippocampus and amygdaloid complex differs from that in raphe nuclei in individuals who are aggressive and defensive; 2) increases in 5-HT turnover and metabolite level may result from aggressive behavior, suggesting demand-regulating modulation of 5-HT neuronal activity; and 3) aggressive and defensive acts are associated with opposite changes in 5-HT activity in raphe cells vs. terminal fields, pointing to potentially inhibitory, permissive, and facilitatory functions.

Nearly three decades of research in various animal species and human patient populations have been devoted to delineate the association of the major serotonin metabolite 5-HIAA with aggressive behavior. Ever since the early report on wholebrain measures of low 5-HIAA in isolated aggressive mice (21), considerable evidence in biological psychiatry has accrued for low levels of CSF 5-HIAA in 1) violent suicide attempters; 2) in individuals with either a life history of aggression or high Rohrschach ratings of hostility who are preoccupied by violent thoughts; 3) individuals with high outwardly directed hostility, adult criminal behavior, or in youngsters who are cruel toward animals; and 4) in recidivists for fire-setting and homicidal acts. While there are some notable exceptions in human and nonhuman primate studies, the inverse correlation between CSF 5-HIAA levels and the history of aggressive behavior has been found repeatedly during the past two decades. A particularly important characteristic of individuals with low CSF 5-HIAA appears to be the impulsive nature of their aggressive behavior, which led to the proposal that loss of "*impulse control* rather than aggressiveness or violence as such" is linked to a deficiency in brain serotonin (22).

The introduction of in vivo microdialysis methodology has allowed continuous monitoring of extracellular concentrations of 5-HT in limbic and cortical regions of individual animals that have a history of repeated aggressive behavior and are about to initiate an aggressive confrontation, engage in a burst of aggressive acts, and then terminate aggressive behavior. In the prefrontal cortex of aggressive rats, decreased 5-HT release follows, rather than precedes, the aggressive confrontation (23). By contrast, 5-HT in the nucleus accumbens of aggressive rats is hardly affected by the anticipation, execution, or termination of an intense aggressive behavior. These dynamic changes in cortical 5-HT during and, particularly, following aggressive behavior contrast with the retrospective analysis of single postmortem assay data or single CSF values. Therefore, the interpretation of a deficiency in 5-HT activity as a causal factor in aggressive behavior on the basis of correlational data appears premature.

NEUROTOXINS AND LESIONS

Experimental deficiencies in brain 5-HT represent the most direct test of the link between 5-HT and aggressive behavior (24). Early electrolytic lesion studies of the serotonin-containing cell bodies in the raphe nuclei provided the first evidence that placid laboratory rats made serotonin-deficient became more irritable, reacted with exaggerated defensive responses to mild provocations, and started to kill mice. Neurochemically more selective targeting of serotonin neurons was achieved with cytotoxic agents such as 5,7-dihydroxytryptamine (5,7-DHT). The neurotoxic lesion produced by these agents can produce increased defensive reactions and biting in nonaggressive rats. Removing L-tryptophan, serotonin's dietary precursor, produces less attack and threat behavior in isolated mice but can increase defensive reactions and increases the likelihood that a laboratory rat will kill a mouse.

It is important to note that even severe depletion of brain 5-HT does not necessitate increased defensive and killing responses. Even severe neurotoxic insults to 5-HT neurons will not induce a rat to kill a mouse if it has been habituated to the potential prey (25). These observations indicate that intact brain 5-HT systems are not sufficient to inhibit aggressive and defensive acts in an all-or-none fashion but are subject to modulation by social learning (Fig. 1.3). Carnivores such as cats, ferrets, or grasshopper mice (*Onychomys leucogaster*) actually stop killing after inhibition of 5-HT synthesis (26). Moreover, the emerging evidence favors the conclusion that species vary substantially in terms of inhibition or disinhibition of aggressive acts by brain serotonin systems.

RECEPTORS

The most promising evidence for pharmacotherapeutic management of aggressive behavior is derived from the developments in 5-HT receptor pharmacology. During the 1980s, eltoprazine, a piperazine derivative, was developed as a prototypic "serenic," primarily on the basis of its demonstrated efficacy as a treatment that decreased offensive aggressive behavior in mice, rats, pigs, and monkeys in the absence of any marked deleterious side effects in these species (27). The site and mechanism of action for eltoprazine's anti-aggressive effects were thought to be the $5\text{-HT}_{1A/1B}$ receptor subtypes where this drug acted as high-affinity agonist. However, in the absence of specific antagonists for these receptor subtypes, it was difficult to establish unambiguously either the 5-HT_{1A} or the 5-HT_{1B} receptor subtype as a critical target site. Moreover, the 5-HT_{1B}

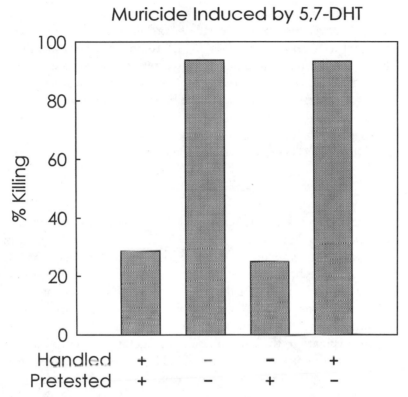

Figure 1.3.
Percentage of rats killing mice following 5,7-dihydroxytryptamine (5,7-DHT) injection in three experiments that exposed the rat to the mouse prior to the 5,7-DHT treatment and involved handling or that did not include these manipulations. (Reproduced by permission from Marks PC, O'Brien M, Paxinos G. 5,7-DHT-induced muricide: inhibition as a result of preoperative exposure of rats to mice. Brain Research 1977;135:383–388.)

receptors are absent in primates, thus reducing the pharmaceutical interest in developing this class of substances.

In late 1993, evidence was presented that mice with a "knock-out" mutation of a gene for 5-HT$_{1B}$ receptors fought incessantly (28). These mice appeared to sleep, eat, drink, copulate, move about, regulate their temperature, and respond to pain without detectable deficiency, rendering their high incidence of aggressive behavior as a specific phenotypical consequence of this genetic modification. Despite the considerable limitations of the molecular "knock-out" technique, the 5-HT$_{1B}$ knock-out mice are prompting the development of more subtle, anatomically discrete, inducible, and reversible ways of modifying 5-HT receptor subtypes in order to effect selective changes in aggressive behavior.

After synthesis, storage, and release, 5-HT is removed from the synaptic cleft by transport back into the presynaptic nerve terminal. Inhibition of the transporter mechanism prolongs the action of 5-HT at postsynaptic neurons, and the development of selective serotonin reuptake inhibitors (SSRIs) has emerged as a beneficial option in the treatment of certain mood and eating disorders. Fluoxetine and fluvoxamine, two SSRIs, suppress defensive and biting reactions as well as territorial aggression in rodents (29,30). In addition to modulating aggressive and defensive behavior, serotonin affects a wide range of behavioral and physiological functions, and it is not surprising that the behavioral specificity of the anti-aggressive effects of SSRIs, particularly if given chronically, has been a matter of some concern.

Catecholamines

Classically, increased sympathetic and adrenal activity was recognized as characterizing the "fight-flight" response (31). Many types of aggressive behavior and other intense emotional behavior patterns are accompanied by greatly increased catecholaminergic activity in autonomically innervated organs such as the heart. Increases in the catecholamine synthesis rate–limiting enzyme tyrosine hydroxylase, in epinephrine and norepinephrine, and their acidic metabolites are detectable in various peripheral fluid compartments of individuals who are in the early phase of an aggressive confrontation and who are actually in the process of fighting (32,33). Peripheral indices of catecholaminergic activity, however, are remote from the neural mechanisms that mediate aggressive behavior. For example, the blood levels of monoamine oxidase (MAO) correlate weakly, if at all, with CNS levels of MAO (34).

NOREPINEPHRINE

Direct evidence for a role of brain noradrenergic activity in the mediation of aggressive behavior started to emerge when brain tissue assay data became available from animals that had just fought. Early measurements indicated increased wholebrain norepinephrine (NE) in isolated aggressive mice (11,35), whereas estimates of NE turnover relating the acidic metabolite to the parent amine showed inconsistent effects. Increases in forebrain, diencephalic, and mesencephalic NE turnover were found in rats and cats that displayed biting and defensive responses (12,36). An early subcellular study showed that synaptosomal uptake of cortical NE increased in mice after episodes of intense fighting (37), and increases in NE in frontal cortex characterize strains of mice that are aggressive (38). In striatum and olfactory tubercle, NE levels actually decrease in mice after fighting (39). In hamsters, no comparable changes in cortical or mesencephalic NE levels, synthesis, or metabolism were detected (17). The widely distributed projections to all forebrain and cortical regions by noradrenergic neurons may be traced to their origin in the locus coeruleus, and single unit activity in coeruleal noradrenergic cells increases greatly in monkeys that are threatened (40).

The postmortem neurochemical assay data on NE should prompt in vivo microdialysis studies that monitor noradrenergic activity prior to an aggressive confrontation, during the actual fighting, and after the termination of the episode. Such information will be necessary in order to learn about the relative significance of noradrenergic activity in cortical, limbic vs. brain-stem regions, and to distinguish NE release that is related to events antecedent to an aggressive act from those that are its consequences. These data would enable testing the proposed roles of brain noradrenergic activity in selective attention, general arousal, and specific fear or anxiety functions (41).

Noradrenergic receptor research in aggressive individuals is derived from the discovery of beneficial effects of beta-adrenergic receptor blockers in certain violent patients (42). In institutionalized psychiatric patients and in several laboratory rodents, beta-blockers given in a dose range that does not compromise motor functions were confirmed to be effective in reducing aggressive behavior. During the last decade, the prototypic beta-blockers propranolol and pindolol also were found to show high affinity for 5-HT$_{1A}$ receptors, and the antagonistic action of these drugs at these sites may be related to their therapeutic effects in the management of aggressive behavior.

DOPAMINE

Even several decades after the introduction of neuroleptics, it remains unclear how and where in the brain these frequently used pharmacotherapies in the management of aggressive human patients produce their antiaggressive effects. Typical neuroleptic drugs bind with high affinity and selectivity to D2 dopamine (DA) receptors, located postsynaptically. The major DA systems in the brain are anatomically discretely organized, and these systems apparently serve different functions. Three major DA fiber pathways ascend from the midbrain to discrete terminal fields in forebrain structures; the nigrostriatal DA system originates in the *substantia nigra pars compacta* and projects to the *caudate n.* and *putamen*; DA cells in the *ventral tegmental area* give rise to the *mesolimbic* and *mesocortical* pathways, the former terminating in the *olfactory tubercle* and *ventral striatal* region, including the core and shell of the n. accumbens, and the latter in the *prefrontal cerebral cortex*. Neuroendocrine control is exerted by the short *tuberoinfundibular* DA pathway that orignates in the *arcuate n.* and terminates in the *median eminence*. The discrete anatomic organization of the DA systems contrasts with the more diffuse projections of the noradrenergic neuronal systems, and this neuroanatomical difference among the two major catecholamines appears to be functionally relevant.

Early neurochemical studies pointed to increases in DA and indices of DA synthesis and turnover in the wholebrain of laboratory mice that had just fought (11). Anatomically more specific postmortem analyses revealed that DA levels and turnover were increased in the n. accumbens, striatum, frontal cortex, and hypothalamus of aggressive mice (15,38,43). Defensive reactions by rats and mice lead to increased DA uptake and turnover in several limbic and cortical structures (44–46).

The most persuasive evidence for the role of forebrain DA systems in aggressive behavior has been obtained from on-line monitoring of DA in limbic and cortical termination areas via in vivo microdialysis (23,47). When confronted with an intruder, a resident rat pursues, threatens, and attacks the intruder. The resident's aggressive behavior persists, even when the intruder is protected by a screen. Sampling from n. accumbens and medial prefrontal cortex in resident rats indicates that extracellular DA increases, presumably reflecting increased release, in n. accumbens and in the medial prefrontal cortex following exhibition of aggressive behavior, but not during the initiation or execution of aggressive acts. These findings extend previous postmortem studies of limbic DA that focused on a single measurement at a specific time point after the relevant behavior had already occurred. They also prompt a new interpretation of these data, in that there appears to be a feedback relationship between aggressive acts and mesocorticolimbic DA activity.

The site of action for the most frequently used antiaggressive drugs is the D_2 dopamine receptor. Molecular studies have identified two families of dopamine receptors: 1) the D_1 family, comprising D_1 and D_5 receptors; and 2) the D_2 family, comprising D_2, D_3, and D_4 receptors. The pharmacology of the D_1 and D_2 receptors is most fully established in terms of selective agonists and antagonists; that of the D_3 receptors is currently being evaluated, whereas the D_4 and D_5 selective agents have yet to emerge. On the basis of studies with laboratory rodents and primates, it has become evident that the suppression of aggressive behavior by the typical D_2 receptor–blocking drugs is part of a behaviorally pervasive suppression of many types of active behavior. Ever since their introduction several decades ago, phenothiazines and butyrophenones were found to be effective in decreasing aggressive behavior in many animal species and human patient populations, but at the same time were found to lack behavioral specificity in their antiaggressive effects (1). The behavioral "cost," in the form of compromised conditioned performance measurements, to obtain the "benefit" of antiaggressive effects was recently illustrated in an experimental protocol in which mice were treated with SCH23390 and raclopride—D_1 and D_2 receptor subtype selective antagonists; decreased operant responding was seen after administration of doses that were actually lower than those necessary to achieve significant antiaggressive effects (48). The other DA receptor subtype selective agents' significance for the pharmacotherapy of aggressive behavior awaits future assessment.

Clozapine, the first of a new class of so-called atypical antipsychotic agents, has significant affinity for D_4, and also D_3 and D_2 receptor subtypes, as well as for muscarinic, alpha-adrenergic, and serotonergic receptors. There is evidence that clozapine has significant antiaggressive effects in laboratory mice and human schizophrenic patients (49,50). Similar effects may be expected to characterize other atypical antipsychotics. Which of the receptor actions of these atypical antipsychotics is responsible for their antiaggressive effects remains to be determined. The key advantage of the atypical antipsychotic drugs is the lower risk of side effects, particularly tardive dyskinesia, with long-term use. In a small proportion of schizophrenic patients, chronic clozapine use may lead to agranulocytosis requiring repeated blood sampling and careful monitoring. This latter problem does not appear to be of significance with the newly introduced olanzapine.

Glutamate and GABA

The recent discovery of several receptor subtypes has prompted intensive neuropharmacological research of GABA (gamma-aminobutyric acid) and excitatory amino acids (EAA), such as glutamate, beyond their long-established role in convulsive disorders. Activation and blockade of GABA and EAA receptor subtypes have been found to modify cognitive and affective processes (51). Particularly, glutamate action on either N-methyl-D-aspartate (NMDA), AMPA, or kainate receptor subtypes and their isoforms has been investigated for its role in anxiety and neuroadaptive and neurodegenerative processes, including learning and memory (52).

NMDA RECEPTOR

The NMDA receptor comprises: 1) a recognition site to which glutamate and NMDA bind; 2) a strychnine-insensitive site to which glycine binds; 3) a channel-binding site for phencyclidine-like agents that is voltage- and use-dependent; 4) a further channel site for magnesium; 5) an extracellular zinc site; and 6) a site that selectively binds polyamines. The NMDA receptor-linked channel controls the flow of sodium and calcium, and their influx increases cellular excitation (53).

While early neurochemical assay data from brains of singly housed aggressive laboratory mice showed decreases in N-acetyl-L-aspartic acid, the most consistent evidence for a significant role of the NMDA receptor in aggressive and defensive behavior derives from microinjection studies. Aspartate or glutamate microinjections into the periaqueductal grey (PAG) region of rats or cats evoked strong defensive reactions, mimicking those in response to an attacking opponent (54,55). Blockade of NMDA receptors with AP-7, injected either systemically or directly into the PAG, suppressed the facilitatory effects of electrical stimulation of the amygdala on hypothalamically evoked affective-defensive responses in cats (56). It appears that the midbrain NMDA receptors in the mesencephalic PAG region play a key role in the mediation of defensive reactions, with agonists facilitating and antagonists inhibiting these responses.

At present, the only available evidence for a role of the strychnine-insensitive glycine site on this receptor complex derives from observations in laboratory mice with the partial agonist D-cycloserine. Oral dosing with D-cycloserine resulted in decreased aggressive behavior and increased social interactions (57).

Most evidence for involvement of the NMDA receptor complex in aggressive and social behavior derives from studies with phencyclidine (PCP), which blocks the ion channel noncompetitively. These studies document profound changes in social and aggressive behavior in laboratory rodents, cats, dogs, and primates (1). In socially inexperienced isolated mice, single PCP doses may increase some aspects of aggressive behavior (6,58,59). However, most often PCP dose-dependently disrupts social and aggressive behavior in various animal species, and increases submissive displays in macaque monkeys (60,61). As already suggested by informal reports from hallucinogen-abusing humans, PCP effects in animals result in erratic exaggerations of either aggression or submission, or complete withdrawal from social intercourse. If it were possible to assess the functional state of the NMDA receptor complex prior to any drug treatment (e.g., by PET scan), the most likely PCP effects on aggression might become predictable.

GABA$_A$-BENZODIAZEPINE RECEPTOR

About one third of all synaptic transmission in the brain involves GABA, primarily in short inhibitory interneurons. GABA's hyperpolarizing action at the postsynaptic neuronal membrane may be responsible for this transmitter's inhibitory function at the physiologic and behavioral level, including the proposed inhibition of aggressive behavior (62). GABA levels in limbic and striatal structures are lower in mice and rats that display aggressive behavior (63). Spanish fighting bulls show lower GABA content in the striatum and hypothalamus than nonaggressive Frisian bulls (64). GABA and muscimol binding in limbic areas is increased in aggressive rats and hamsters (65). At present, the changes in receptor binding and levels in limbic structures suggest a mediating role for GABA in aggressive and defensive behavior, and experimental manipulations that target particularly the GABA$_A$ receptor confirm the significance of this neural mechanism.

The GABA$_A$ receptor has a pentameric structure and the alpha, beta, and gamma subunits have been cloned (66,67). This chloride-channel receptor complex contains a high-affinity site for GABA, and modulatory sites for benzodiazepines, barbiturates, progestin neurosteroids, picrotoxin, and possibly alcohol (68).

Benzodiazepine Agonists

Benzodiazepines, which are allosteric modulators of the GABA$_A$–benzodiazepine receptor complex; barbiturates; and alcohol share anxiolytic, amnesic, hypnotic, sedative, anticonvulsant, and ataxic effects. Further evidence linking these substances and GABA$_A$ receptors comes from studies showing that pharmacologic blockade of the benzodiazepine site on the GABA$_A$–benzodiazepine receptor complex can antagonize several of the physiologic, behavioral, and neurochemical effects of these drugs. In terms of aggression, mice that were selectively bred for high levels of aggressive behavior showed less GABA-dependent chloride uptake into cortical neurons, lower benzodiazepine receptor binding in cortical and limbic structures, and more aggression-reducing effects of chlordiazepoxide treatment than nonaggressive mice (69).

In the first decade of benzodiazepine research, these prototypic anxiolytic drugs were shown to reduce aggressive behavior, often due to their sedative and motor incoordinating properties at intermediate to higher doses in many animal species. This evidence supported the characterization of benzodiazepines as antiaggressive drugs which could "tame" even feral animals ranging from mink, to cats, to monkeys (70,71). Subsequently, benzodiazepines, barbiturates, alcohol, and, most recently, neurosteroids such as allopregnanolone and alphaxolone were found to share biphasic effects on aggressive behavior, with higher doses decreasing the frequency of threats and attacks and lower doses increasing these behaviors (72,73). However, some benzodiazepines such as alprazolam or oxazepam—two des-chloro-phenyl derivatives—seem to be more selective in their reduction in defensive and escape activities and also in their antiaggressive effects in mice (74).

Benzodiazepine Receptor Antagonists

The prototypic benzodiazepine receptor antagonist flumazenil binds to fewer cortical and limbic sites in selectively bred aggressive mice than in selectively bred nonaggressive mice; and muscimol-activated chloride flux in cortical tissue of highly aggressive mice is less than that for nonaggressive mice (69). Pharmacologically, flumazenil may suppress social interactions but has no robust effect on aggressive behavior in laboratory rats and monkeys (75). Benzodiazepine antagonists, flumazenil and ZK93426 (a beta-carboline derivative), selectively prevented the aggression-heightening effects of lower alcohol doses, without having an effect on the aggression-decreasing and sedative effects of higher alcohol doses in laboratory rats and squirrel monkeys (76).

Partial Benzodiazepine Agonists

The benzodiazepine receptor partial inverse agonist Ro15–4513, introduced in the mid-1980s, has been studied for its prevention or reversal of the physiologic and behavioral effects of alcohol. Alcohol's sedative, ataxic, muscle relaxant, and hypnotic effects were demonstrated to be at least partially and transiently reduced by Ro15–4513 (77). Pretreatment with benzodiazepine receptor inverse agonists reduces the enhancing effects of alcohol on behavior that is suppressed by bright light or electric shock in laboratory rodents. However, in attempts to antagonize the aggression-heightening effects of alcohol in squirrel monkeys, Ro15–4513 pretreatment produced tremors and seizures (78). The risk of inducing epileptogenic activity in a significant proportion of individuals renders benzodiazepine receptor partial inverse agonists such as Ro15–4513 unusable, and the entire strategy as problematic for eventual clinical development.

NEUROSTEROIDS

In addition to their classic genomic action, certain C21 steroids can affect the GABA$_A$ receptor complex. Some of these GABA$_A$-active steroids have been found to be allosteric positive modulators of the GABA$_A$ receptor complex in vitro, while others are negative modulators. Among the most well documented of the positive modulators is the naturally occurring metabolite of progesterone, allopregnanolone (5α-pregnan-3α-ol-20-one) (79,80).

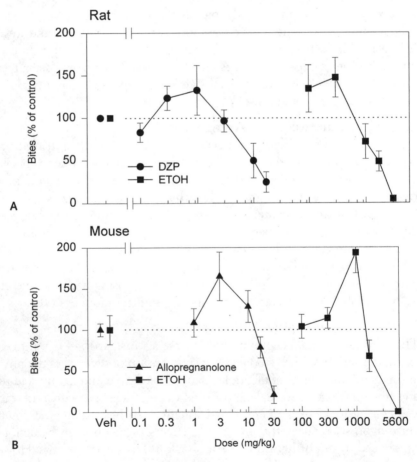

Figure 1.4.
Changes in the frequency of attack bites, expressed as percent of control (100% = control; dashed horizontal line), as a function of dose for diazepam (DZP), and ethanol (ETOH) in resident rats confronting an intruder (**A**), and allopregnanolone and ETOH in resident mice confronting an intruder (**B**). Vertical lines in the data points indicate ± 1 SEM. (Reproduced by permission from Miczek KA, DeBold JF, van Erp AMM, Tornatzky W. Alcohol, GABA$_A$ = benzodiazepine receptor complex and aggression. In: Galanter M, ed. Recent developments in alcoholism: alcoholism and violence, vol. 13. New York: Plenum, 1997:139–171.)

Functionally, steroids like allopregnanolone and alphaxalone have also been shown to share physiologic and behavioral effects with other positive modulators of GABA$_A$, such as benzodiazepines, barbiturates, and ethanol. In laboratory rats, they have anxiolytic, anticonvulsant, anesthetic, and analgesic actions (81–83). However, unlike ethanol and benzodiazepines, the effects of GABA$_A$-active steroids on aggression remain to be delineated. Recent evidence shows that acute administration of allopregnanolone to male mice has biphasic effects on aggression that are quite similar to those of ethanol (84). As shown in Figure 1.4, lower doses of allopregnanolone and alphaxolone increased the frequency of the salient components of aggressive behavior in male mice, while these substances reduced aggressive behavior at still higher doses. Such biphasic dose-effect curves are also very similar in pattern to the behavioral responses to ethanol and to diazepam (Figure 1.4). The close similarity in the dose-effect curves of these drugs extends the hypothesis that their shared effects on the GABA$_A$ receptor complex underlie their actions on aggression (85). Allopregnanolone is not the only neuroactive steroid with effects on aggression. Others have found that a negative modulator of GABA$_A$, dehydroepiandrosterone, inhibits aggression in either male or female mice toward lactating females (86).

Peptides

OPIOID PEPTIDES

Shortly after the discovery of enkephalins and endorphins in the brain, their major role in social affiliation and attachment was postulated (87). In support of this proposal, opioid receptor antagonists such as naloxone and naltrexone were found to enhance distress vocalizations in young chicks, rodents, guinea pigs, and dogs that were separated from their littermates.

Experiences with intense social conflict resulted in altered met-enkephalin and dynorphin levels and in receptor occupancy in mesencephalic and hypothalamic structures of gerbils and mice, particularly in the loser of the confrontation (88–90). Functionally, the most notable change after an aggressive confrontation was the opioid-like analgesia in the defeated mouse, which was reversed by receptor antagonists acting on mu (OP$_3$) and sigma (OP$_1$), but not kappa (OP$_2$) subtypes in the hypothalamic region and in the PAG area (91–93). The significant role of enkephalins acting on mu receptors in defensive reactions has also been demonstrated in cats. When defensive hissing is evoked by electrical stimulation of hypothalamic and PAG sites, microinjection with the met-enkephalin analog DAME (D-Ala2-Met5-Enkephalinamide) suppresses defense, and opiate receptor blockade increases this response (94). Further support for a significant role of opioid peptides and their receptors in defense may be derived from studies in mice and rats that show enhanced defensive reactions (95–97).

The evidence for opioid peptides in the mediation of offensive aggressive behavior is considerably less strong than that for defensive and defeat responses. Withdrawal from long-term treatment with opiates results in increased aggressive behavior in laboratory rats and mice (98,99). The opioid receptor antagonists naloxone and naltrexone have been found to decrease attacks by male and female mice, and there are interesting observations that these drugs suppress self-injurious behavior in children (100). Whether receptor antagonists with increased selectivity for opioid receptor subtypes will result in agents with pharmacotherapeutic potential for aggressive behavior remains to be demonstrated.

Vasopressin

Monogamous biparental prairie voles (*Microtus ochrogaster*) display intense aggression toward unfamiliar intruders in order to defend their mate, nest, and territory. Monogamous voles have a distinctive distribution of neural receptors for arginine-vasopressin (AVP), which differs from that for polygamous voles; AVP-containing neurons are sexually dimorphic in their innervation of brain targets (101). Functionally, AVP neural pathways have been found to play a significant role in the recognition of a specific social partner (i.e., social memory), in the defense of the territory, and in the establishment and maintenance of social affiliative behavior (102,103).

When male voles were treated with a vasopressin-1a receptor antagonist prior to mating with a sexual partner, they did not develop a preference for the mate, nor did they develop aggressive behavior in defense of the mate. Conversely, AVP infusion into the cerebral ventricles engendered aggressive behavior and partner preference (104). Similarly, intrahypothalamic microinfusions of AVP in hamsters and AVP injections into the amygdala and septum of castrated rats shorten the latency to attack, and vasopressin receptor antagonists into the hypothalamus decrease aggressive behavior. The androgen-dependence of AVP effects has been demonstrated by diminishing AVP receptor binding and aggressive behavior in hamsters through castration (105). It has been suggested that the inhibitory action of SSRIs (*vide supra*) may be due to the inhibition of brain vasopressin (106).

Summary

The multiple phylogenetic and ontogenetic causes of different types of aggressive behavior appear to be based on distinctive neurobiologic mechanisms. The reciprocal relationship between neurochemical processes and aggression is illustrated by the marked changes in mesocorticolimbic DA, cortical 5-HT and GABA, mesencephalic opioid, and vasopressin peptide systems in animals that engage in episodes of attack behavior when compared with those who defend and submit in social confrontations. Classically, catecholaminergic activation in the sympathetic branch of the autonomic nervous system defines the flight-fight syndrome, and increased noradrenergic forebrain activity characterizes individuals during social confrontations. Increased activity in the prefrontal cortex and the ventral striatum by mesencephalic dopaminergic neurons is prominent in animals during and after social confrontations, and neural sensitization may ensue, possibly involving immediate early gene expression, as reflected in augmented responses to dopaminergic drugs.

The role of brain serotonin systems and their receptors in different types of aggressive behavior is gradually being delineated. In human psychopathology, most individuals with antisocial personality disorder who engage in impulsive violent acts are characterized by lower CSF 5-HIAA values and a blunted prolactin response to 5-HT agonist challenge. The diagnostic value of such measurements relying upon indices of 5-HT function that are peripheral to the corticolimbic terminals remains problematic. In vivo microdialysis data in rodents suggest that decreases in cortical 5-HT follow rather than precede aggressive episodes. The currently known 15 serotonin receptor subtypes as well as the uptake transporter molecules are beginning to be investigated for pharmacologic intervention, and the $5-HT_1$ receptor family has emerged as a promising target for antiaggressive agents.

Drug action on NMDA and $GABA_A$ receptor subtypes has yielded marked modulatory influences on several types of aggressive behavior. The $GABA_A$–benzodiazepine receptor complex is a major site that differentiates highly aggressive animals from less aggressive individuals. Additionally, this site is mainly involved in the potentiation or the reversal of alcohol's aggression-heightening effects by benzodiazepine agonists or antagonists, respectively.

It has become apparent that behavior in social conflict alters peptide activity in the brain, among the most significant being the opioid peptides, corticotrophin releasing hormone (CRH), and vasopressin. The development of selective receptor agonists and antagonists for opioid and vasopressin receptor subtypes has begun to demonstrate effective modulation of affiliative, maternal, aggressive, defensive, and submissive behavior patterns.

References

1. Miczek KA. The psychopharmacology of aggression. In: Iversen LL, Iversen SD, Snyder SH, eds. Handbook of psychopharmacology, vol. 19: New directions in behavioral pharmacology. New York: Plenum, 1987:183–328.
2. Scott JP. Aggression. Chicago: University of Chicago Press, 1958.
3. Wilson EO. Sociobiology. Cambridge: Belknap Press, 1974.
4. De Waal FBM, Hoekstra JA. Contexts and predictability of aggression in chimpanzees. Anim Behav 1966;28:929–937.
5. Miczek KA, Weerts EM, Tornatzky W, et al. Alcohol and "bursts" of aggressive behavior: ethological analysis of individual differences in rats. Psychopharmacology 1992;107:551–563.

6. Miczek KA, Haney M, Tidey J, et al. Neurochemistry and pharmacotherapeutic management of violence and aggression. In: Reiss AJ, Miczek KA, Roth JA, eds. Understanding and preventing violence: biobehavioral influences on violence, vol. 2. Washington, DC: National Academy Press, 1994:244–514.

7. Mamounas LA, Molliver ME. Evidence for dual serotonergic projections to neocortex: axons from the dorsal and median raphe nuclei are differentially vulnerable to the neurotoxin p-chloroamphetamine (PCA). Exp Neurol 1988;102:23–36.

7a. Volavka J. Neurobiology of violence. Washington, DC: American Psychiatric Association Press, 1995.

8. Hoyer D, Martin GR. Classification and nomenclature of 5-HT receptors: a comment on current issues. Behav Brain Res 1996;73:263–268.

9. Olivier B, Mos J. New 5-HT (serotonin) compounds. In: Hollander E, Zohar J, Marazzati D, Olivier B, eds. Obsessive compulsive disorder. Chichester, NY: John Wiley & Sons, 1994:277–290.

10. Garattini S, Giacalone E, Valzelli L. Isolation, aggressiveness and brain 5-hydroxytryptamine turnover. J Pharm Pharmacol 1967;19:338–339.

11. Modigh K. Effects of isolation and fighting in mice on the rate of synthesis of noradrenaline, dopamine and 5-hydroxytryptamine in the brain. Psychopharmacology 1973;33:1–17.

12. Salama AI, Goldberg ME. Temporary increase in forebrain norepinephrine turnover in mouse-killing rats. Eur J Pharmacol 1973;21:372–374.

13. Yen CY, Stanger RL, Millman N. Ataractic suppression of isolation-induced aggressive behavior. Arch Int Pharmacodyn Ther 1959;123:179–185.

14. Krsiak M. Isolation-induced timidity in mice as a measure of anxiolytic activity of drugs. Activit Nervosa Sup 1974;16:241–242.

15. Haney M, Noda K, Kream R, Miczek KA. Regional 5-HT and dopamine activity: sensitivity to amphetamine and aggressive behavior in mice. Aggressive Behav 1990;16:259–270.

16. Nikulina EM, Popova NK. Predatory aggression in the mink (Mustela vison): roles of serotonin and food satiation. Aggressive Behav 1988;14:77–84.

17. Payne AP, Andrews MJ, Wilson CA. Housing, fighting and biogenic amines in the midbrain and hypothalamus of the golden hamster. In: Miczek KA, Kruk M, Olivier B, eds. Ethopharmacological aggression research. New York: Alan R. Liss, 1984:227–247.

18. Hadfield MG, Milio C. Isolation-induced fighting in mice and regional brain monoamine utilization. Behav Brain Res 1988;31:93–96.

19. Walletschek H, Raab A. Spontaneous activity of dorsal raphe neurons during defensive and offensive encounters in the tree-shrew. Physiol Behav 1982;28:697–705.

20. Lee EHY, Lin HH, Yin HM. Differential influences of different stressors upon midbrain raphe neurons in rats. Neurosci Lett 1987;80:115–119.

21. Valzelli L, Garattini S. Behavioral changes and 5-hydroxytryptamine turnover in animals. Adv Pharmacol 1968;6B:249–260.

22. Linnoila M, De Jong J, Virkkunen M. Family history of alcoholism in violent offenders and impulsive fire setters. Arch Gen Psychiatry 1989;46:613–616.

23. Van Erp AMM, Miczek KA. Prefrontal cortex dopamine and serotonin: microdialysis during aggression and alcohol self-administration in rats. Soc Neurosc Abst 1996;22:161.

24. Miczek KA, Donat P. Brain 5-HT systems and inhibition of aggressive behavior. In: Bevan P, Cools A, Archer T, eds. Behavioral pharmacology of 5-HT. Hillsdale, NJ: Lawrence Erlbaum Associates, 1989:117–144.

25. Marks PC, O'Brien M, Paxinos G. 5,7-DHT-induced muricide: inhibition as a result of preoperative exposure of rats to mice. Brain Res 1977;135:383–388.

26. McCarty RC, Whitesides GH, Tomosky TK. Effects of p-chlorophenylalanine on the predatory behavior of Onychomys torridus. Pharmacol Biochem Behav 1976;4:217–220.

27. Olivier B, Mos J, Rasmussen D. Behavioural pharmacology of the serenic, eltoprazine. Drug Metabol Drug Interact 1990;8:31–83.

28. Saudou F, Amara DA, Dierich A, et al. Enhanced aggressive behavior in mice lacking 5-HT1B receptor. Science 1994;265:1875–1878.

29. Olivier B, Mos J, de Koning P, Mak M. Serenics. Prog Drug Res 1994;42:167–302.

30. Fuller RW. Fluoxetine effects on serotonin function and aggressive behavior. In: Ferris CF, Grisso T, eds. Understanding aggressive behavior in children, Vol. 794. New York: New York Academy of Sciences, 1996:90–97.

31. Cannon WB. Organization of physiolical homeostasis. Physiol Rev 1929;9:399–431.

32. Lamprecht F, Eichelman B, Thoa NB, et al. Rat fighting behavior: serum dopamine-B-hydroxylase and hypothalamic tyrosine hydroxylase. Science 1972;177:1214–1215.

33. Stoddard SL, Bergdall VK, Townsend DW, Levin BE. Plasma catecholamines associated with hypothalamically-elicited defense behavior. Physiol Behav 1986;36:867–873.

34. Asberg M, Schalling D, Traskman-Bendz L, Wagner A. Psychobiology of suicide, impulsivity, and related phenomena. In: Meltzer HY, ed. Psychopharmacology: the third generation of progress. New York: Plenum, 1987:655–668.

35. Welch BL, Welch AS. Effect of grouping on the level of brain norepinephrine in white Swiss mice. Life Sci 1965;4:1011–1018.

36. Reis DJ, Fuxe K. Brain norepinephrine: evidence that neuronal release is essential for sham rage behavior following brainstem transection in cat. Proc Natl Acad Sci USA 1964;64:108–112.

37. Hendley ED, Moisset B, Welch BL. Catecholamine uptake in cerebral cortex: adaptive change induced by fighting. Science 1973;180:1050–1052.

38. Tizabi Y, Thoa NB, Maengwyn-Davies GD, et al. Behavioral correlation of catecholamine concentration and turnover in discrete brain areas of three strains of mice. Brain Res 1979;166:199–205.

39. Tizabi Y, Massari VJ, Jacobowitz DM. Isolation induced aggression and catecholamine variations in discrete brain areas of the mouse. Brain Res Bull 1980;5:81–86.

40. Redmond DE Jr, Huang YH. New evidence for a locus coeruleus-norepinephrine connection with anxiety. Life Sci 1979;25:2149–2162.

41. Robbins TW, Everitt BJ, Cole BJ, et al. Functional hypotheses of the coeruleocortical noradrenergic projection: a review of recent experimentation and theory. Physiol Psychol 1985;13:127–150.

42. Elliott FA. Propanolol for the control of belligerent behavior following acute brain damage. Annu Neurol 1977;1:489–491.

43. Hutchins DA, Pearson JDM, Sharman DF. Striatal metabolism of dopamine in mice made aggressive by isolation. J Neurochem 1975;24:1151–1154.

44. Mos J, Van Valkenburg CFM. Specific effect of social stress and aggression on regional dopamine metabolism in rat brain. Neurosci Lett 1979;15:325–327.

45. Dantzer R, Guilloneau D, Mormede P, et al. Influence of shock-induced fighting and social factors on dopamine turnover in cortical and limbic areas in the rat. Pharmacol Biochem Behav 1984;20:331–334.

46. Puglisi-Allegra S, Cabib S. Effects of defeat experiences on dopamine metabolism in different brain areas of the mouse. Aggressive Behav 1990;16:271–284.

47. Van Erp AMM, Miczek KA. Alcohol self-administration and aggression in rats: dopamine and serotonin in n. accumbens. Soc Neurosci Abst 1995;19:1702.

48. Miczek KA, Tornatzky W. Ethopharmacology of aggression: impact on autonomic and mesocorticolimbic activity. In: Ferris C, Grisso T, eds. Understanding aggressive behavior in children. Ann NY Acad Sci 1996;794:60–77.

49. Garmendia L, Sanchez JR, Azpiroz A, et al. Clozapine: strong antiaggressive effects with minimal motor impairment. Physiol Behav 1991;51:51–54.

50. Ratey JJ, Gordon A. The psychopharmacology of aggression: toward a new day. Psychopharmacol Bull 1993;29:65–73.

51. Winslow JT, Insel TR. The infant rat separation paradigm: a novel test for novel anxiolytics. Trends Pharmacol Sci 1991;12:402–404.

52. Nakanishi S. Molecular diversity of glutamate receptors and implications for brain function. Science 1992;258:597–603.

53. Watkins JC, Krogsgaard-Larsen P, Honore T. Structure-activity relationships in the development of excitatory amino acid receptor agonists and competitive antagonists. Trends Pharmacol Sci 1990;11:25–33.

54. Bandler R, Carrive P. Integrated defence reaction elicited by excitatory amino acid microinjection in the midbrain periaqueductal grey region of the unrestrained cat. Brain Res 1988;439:95–106.

55. Depaulis A, Vergnes M, Bandler R. Midbrain cell bodies mediating defensive reactions in the rat. In: Brain PF, Parmigiani S, Blanchard RJ, Mainardi D, eds. Fear and defence, vol. 8. London: Harwood Academic, 1988:179–199.

56. Siegel A, Schubert K, Shaikh MB. Neurochemical mechanisms underlying amygdaloid modulation of aggressive behavior in the cat. Aggressive Behav 1995;21:49–62.

57. McAllister KH. D-Cycloserine enhances social behaviour in individually-housed mice in the resident-intruder test. Psychopharmacology 1994;116:317–325.

58. Burkhalter JE, Balster RL. The effects of phencyclidine on isolation-induced aggression in mice. Psychol Rep 1979;45:571–576.

59. Wilmot CA, Vander Wende C, Spoerlein MT. The effects of phencyclidine on fighting in differentially housed mice. Pharmacol Biochem Behav 1987;28:341–346.

60. Tyler CB, Miczek KA. Effects of phencyclidine on aggressive behavior in mice. Pharmacol Biochem Behav 1982;17:503–510.

61. Schlemmer RF, Young JE, Davis JM. Stimulant-induced disruption of non-human primate social behavior and the psychopharmacology of schizophrenia. J Psychopharmacol 1996;10:64–76.

62. Mandel P, Ciesielski L, Maitre M, et al. Inhibitory amino acids, aggressiveness, and convulsions. In: De Feudis FV, Mandel P, eds. Amino acid neurotransmitters. New York: Raven, 1981:1–9.

63. Mandel P, Mack G, Kempf E. Molecular basis of some models of aggressive behavior. In: Sandler M, ed. Psychopharmacology of aggression. New York: Raven, 1979:95–110.

64. Muñoz-Blanco J, Yusta B, Cordoba F. Differential distribution of neurotransmitter amino acids from the limbic system of aggressive and non-aggressive bull strains. Pharmacol Biochem Behav 1986;25:71–75.

65. Potegal M, Perumal AS, Barkai AI, et al. GABA binding in the brains of aggressive and non-aggressive female hamsters. Brain Res 1982;247:315–324.

66. Haefely WE. The gabaA-benzodiazepine receptor complex and anxiety. In: Sartorius N, Andreoli V, Cassano G, et al, eds. Anxiety: psychobiological and clinical perspectives. New York: Hemisphere, 1990:23–36.

67. Luddens H, Korpi ER. Biological function of GABAA/Benzodiazepine receptor heterogeneity. J Psychiatr Res 1995;29:77–94.

68. Grant KA. Emerging neurochemical concepts in the actions of ethanol at ligand-gated ion channels. Behav Pharmacol 1994;5:383–404.

69. Weerts EM, Miller LG, Hood KE, Miczek KA. Increased GABAA-dependent chloride uptake in mice selectively bred for low aggressive behavior. Psychopharmacology 1992;108:196–204.

70. Heuschele WP. Chlordiazepoxide for calming zoo animals. J Am Vet Med Assoc 1961;139:996–998.

71. Bauen A, Possanza GJ. The mink as a psychopharmacological model. Arch Int Pharmacodyn Ther 1970;186:133–136.

72. Miczek KA, O'Donnell JM. Alcohol and chlordiazepoxide increase suppressed aggression in mice. Psychopharmacology 1980;69:39–44.
73. Miczek KA, Weerts EM, DeBold JF. Alcohol, benzodiazepine-GABA$_A$ receptor complex and aggression: ethological analysis of individual differences in rodents and primates. J Stud Alcohol 1993;11(suppl):170–179.
74. Krsiak M, Sulcova A. Differential effects of six structurally related benzodiazepines on some ethological measures of timidity, aggression and locomotion in mice. Psychopharmacology 1990;101:396–402.
75. File SE, Pellow S. Intrinsic actions of the benzodiazepine receptor antagonist Ro 15-1788. Psychopharmacology 1986;88:1–11.
76. Weerts EM, Tornatzky W, Miczek KA. Prevention of the proaggressive effects of alcohol by benzodiazepine receptor antagonists in rats and in squirrel monkeys. Psychopharmacology 1993;111:144–152.
77. Bonetti EP, Burkard WP, Gabl M, Mohler H. The partial inverse benzodiazepine agonist Ro 15-4513 antagonizes acute alcohol effects in mice and rats. Br J Pharmacol 1985;86(suppl):463–467.
78. Miczek KA, Weerts EM. Seizures in drug-treated animals. Science 1987;235:1127.
79. Majewska MD, Harrison NL, Schwartz RD, et al. Steroid hormone metabolites are barbiturate-like modulators of the GABA receptor. Science 1986;232:1004–1007.
80. Gee KW, Bolger MB, Brinton RE, et al. Steroid modulation of the chloride ionophore in rat brain: structure-activity requirements, regional difference and mechanism of action. J Pharmacol Exp Ther 1988;246:803–812.
81. Seeman P. The membrane actions of anesthetics and tranquilizers. Pharmacol Rev 1972;24:583–655.
82. Crawley JN, Glowa JR, Majewska MD, Paul SM. Anxiolytic activity of an endogenous adrenal steroid. Brain Res 1986;398:382–385.
83. Wieland S, Lan NC, Mirasedeghi S, Gee KW. Anxiolytic activity of the progesterone metabolite 5alpha-pregnan-3alpha-ol-20-one. Brain Res 1991;565:263–268.
84. DeBold JF, Barros H, So S, Miczek KA. The effects of allopregnanolone and alcohol on intramale aggression in mice. Alcohol Clin Exp Res 1995;19:11A.
85. Miczek KA, DeBold JF, van Erp AMM, Tornatzky W. Alcohol, GABA$_A$-benzodiazepine receptor complex, and aggression. In: Galanter M, ed. Recent developments in alcoholism: alcoholism and violence, vol. 13. New York: Plenum, 1997:139–171.
86. Young J, Corpechot C, Haug M, et al. Suppressive effects of dehydroepiandrosterone and 3-b-methyl-androst-5-en-17-one on attack towards lactating female intruders by castrated male mice. 2. Brain neurosteroids. Biochem Biophys Res Commun 1991;174:892–897.
87. Panksepp J, Herman B, Conner R, et al. The biology of social attachments: opiates alleviate separation distress. Biol Psychiatry 1978;13:607–618.
88. Miczek KA, Thompson ML. Analgesia resulting from defeat in a social confrontation: the role of endogenous opioids in brain. In: Bandler R, ed. Modulation of sensorimotor activity during altered behavioural states. New York: Alan R. Liss, 1984:431–456.
89. Raab A, Seizinger BR, Herz A. Continuous social defeat induces an increase of endogenous opioids in discrete brain areas of the Mongolian gerbil. Peptides 1985;6:387–391.
90. Külling P, Frischknecht H-R, Pasi A, et al. Social conflict-induced changes in nociception and beta-endorphin–like immunoreactivity in pituitary and discrete brain areas of C57BL/6 and DBA/2 mice. Brain Res 1988;450:237–246.
91. Miczek KA, Thompson ML, Shuster L. Opioid-like analgesia in defeated mice. Science 1982;215:1520–1522.
92. Miczek KA, Thompson ML, Shuster L. Naloxone injections into periaqueductal grey area and arcuate nucleus block analgesia in defeated mice. Psychopharmacology 1985;87:39–42.

93. Miczek KA, Thompson ML, Shuster L. Analgesia following defeat in an aggressive encounter: development of tolerance and changes in opioid receptors. In: Kelly DD, ed. Stress-induced analgesia. Ann NY Acad Sci 1986;467:14–29.

94. Shaikh MB, Shaikh AB, Siegel A. Opioid peptides within the midbrain periaqueductal gray suppress affective defense behavior in the cat. Peptides 1988;9:999–1004.

95. Rodgers RJ. Differential effects of naloxone and diprenorphine on defensive behavior in rats. Neuropharmacology 1982;21:1291–1294.

96. Tazi A, Dantzer R, Mormede P, Le Moal M. Effects of post-trial administration of naloxone and beta-endorphin on shock-induced fighting in rats. Behav Neural Biol 1983;39:192–202.

97. Haney M, Miczek KA. Delta opioid receptors: reflexive, defensive and vocal affective responses in female rats. Psychopharmacology 1995;121:204–212.

98. Gianutsos G, Lal H. Narcotic analgesics and aggression. In: Valzelli L, Ban T, Freyhan FA, Pichot P, eds. Modern problems of pharmacopsychiatry: psychopharmacology of aggression, vol. 13. New York: Karger, 1978:114–138.

99. Kantak KM, Miczek KA. Aggression during morphine withdrawal: effects of method of withdrawal, fighting experience and social role. Psychopharmacology 1986;90:451–456.

100. Herman BH, Hammock MK, Arthur-Smith A, et al. Naltrexone decreases self-injurious behavior. Ann Neurol 1987;22:550–552.

101. Insel TR, Shapiro LE. Oxytocin receptors and maternal behavior. In: Pederson CA, Caldwell JD, Jirikowski, Insel TR, eds. Oxytocin in Maternal, Sexual, and Social Behaviors. New York: The New York Academy of Sciences, 1992:122–141.

102. Ferris CF, Albers HE, Wesolowski SM, et al. Vasopressin injected into the hypothalamus triggers a stereotypic behavior in golden hamsters. Science 1984;224:521–523.

103. Le Moal M, Dantzer R, Michaud B, Koob GF. Centrally injected arginine vasopressin (AVP) facilitates social memory in rats. Neurosci Lett 1987;77:353–359.

104. Winslow JT, Hastings N, Carter CS, et al. A role for central vasopressin in pair bonding in monogamous prairie voles. Nature 1993;365:545–548.

105. Delville Y, Ferris CF. Sexual differences in vasopressin receptor binding within the ventrolateral hypothalamus in golden hamsters. Brain Res 1995;681:91–96.

106. Ferris CF. Serotonin diminishes aggression by suppressing the activity of the vasopressin system. In: Ferris CF, Grisso T, eds. Understanding aggressive behavior in children, vol. 794. New York: New York Academy of Sciences, 1996:98–103.

107. Miczek KA, Haney M. Psychomotor stimulant effects of d-amphetamine, MDMA and PCP: aggressive and schedule-controlled behavior in mice. Psychopharmacology 1994;115:358–365.

Pharmacologic Treatment of Aggression in Veterinary Patients

2

Nicholas H. Dodman

Despite connotations that aggression in humans represents a disturbed or psychopathologic state, most forms of aggressive behavior in animals are species-typical behaviors that confer survival benefits to individuals and social groups. Although the neurophysiologic mechanisms underlying aggression are hard-wired, involving discrete neural mechanisms, aggressive behavior per se is the end product of an intricate interaction between innate and learning mechanisms. In nature, aggression is often employed either to protect valued resources (including food, space, progeny, and mates) or as a self-defensive measure. Aggression of this type can be viewed as a cohesive force, functioning to maintain the integrity and dynamics of a group, or as a dispersive force designed to repel would-be infiltrators or intruders. Predatory aggression is another type of aggression that has entirely different causation and function.

Because of the numerous circumstances that can elicit aggression, several different classification systems have been developed to standardize scientific and clinical communication on the subject. None of the taxonomies is entirely satisfactory or universally applicable to physiologic, pharmacologic, and clinical discussions, however. The most widely employed clinical categorization of aggression is based on an operational definition popularized by Moyer (1). Moyer classified aggression into seven main categories, including instrumental (dominance), fear-induced, and territorial aggression. An alternative classification, suggested by Reis (2), is more useful when it comes to designing pharmacologic treatment strategies. Reis considered all forms of aggression to be of two main types: affective and predatory. Affective aggression is characterized by autonomic arousal, threats, and physical aggression elicited in response to perceived threats and challenges. Affective aggression may be subdivided

For clarity of presentation, dosages of pharmacologic agents used to treat aggression were omitted from the text. Instead, information regarding dose rates of pharmaceuticals commonly employed in domestic small animals (dogs and cats) is provided in Table 2.1 at the end of this chapter.

into offensive and defensive subtypes, depending upon the motivation for the aggressive behavior (3). Although the neural circuits involved in affective defense behavior have been studied extensively (4), there have been no substantive physiologic studies of affective offense behavior due to the difficulties in establishing a reliable animal model (Miczek KA, personal communication, 1995). From a therapeutic perspective, it may be unnecessary to make such a distinction, as both responses involve heightened arousal and agonistic behavior and may involve similar neural mechanisms. O'Farrell (5) considers all nonpredatory canine aggressive behavior to be related to dominance. A recent classification of conditions leading to human aggressive behavior also implies that types of aggression associated with heightened arousal might reasonably be considered together, at least with regard to therapy (6).

Predatory aggression, the function of which is to incapacitate and kill prey animals, is associated with minimal autonomic arousal and no elaborate behavioral display (7). The neural circuits involved in predatory aggression have been studied extensively in the laboratory and are distinct from those involved in affective aggression (8,9).

Affective Aggression

OFFENSIVE FORMS

Dominance-related and territorial aggression are offensive forms of aggression aimed at preservation of self, status, and/or resources. Intermale and maternal aggression have similar motivation, but in these offensive behaviors the competitive or protective drive is amplified by the changes in the prevailing hormonal milieu. The reduction of intermale aggression reported following castration of male dogs, augmentation of aggressive behavior following ovariohysterectomy in bitches (10), and estrus-linked increased aggression exemplify the modifying effect of hormones on aggressive behavior. The fact that not all aggressive male dogs show a decrease in aggressive behavior following castration is evidence supporting an innate or a learned component to the behavior.

DEFENSIVE FORMS

Fear-, pain-, and stress-induced aggression are defensive forms of aggression. However, even if aggression is motivated by fear or some other aversive experience, the ultimate expression of the behavior elicited has dominant characteristics inasmuch as it is designed to control surrounding events. In defensive aggression, the threshold for agonistic behavior is lowered by the release of catecholamines (11).

TREATMENT OPTIONS

Because of fundamental similarities underlying the two subtypes of affective aggression, it is possible to generalize about the applicability of pharmacologic treatment options. For example, as dynamic changes in central serotonin level are thought to be involved in the establishment and maintenance of dominant attitudes and behavior (12,13), stabilization of serotonin levels using a serotonin reuptake inhibitor (SRI) should produce a decrement in this type of aggressive behavior and, in general, this is what is observed (14,15). When hormonal influences are considered to be magnifying underlying dominance-related (affective) aggression, it is often possible to decrease the aggressive response to confrontations by changing the internal hormonal milieu. This can be accomplished surgically by castration or by administering hormones with antiaggressive properties (e.g., synthetic progesterone-like substances). Lastly, when fear, pain, or stress escalate aggression through the release of catecholamines, it is possible to raise the threshold for aggression by means of adrenergic and dopaminergic antagonists (16).

The facilitatory or inhibitory roles of various neurotransmitters in affective aggression is illustrated schematically in Figure 2.1.

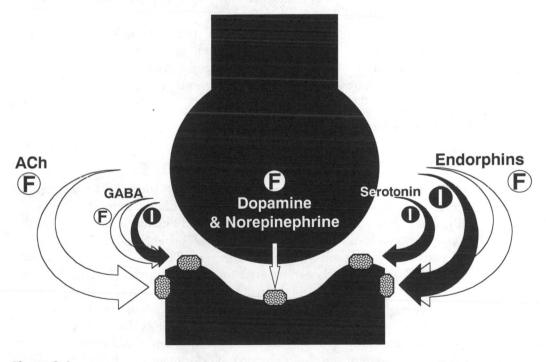

Figure 2.1.
The facilitatory or inhibitory roles of various neurotransmitters in affective aggression. F = faciliatory, I = inhibitory.

Serotonergic Manipulations in Affective Aggression

Arguably, treatment designed to enhance central serotonergic activity should produce a decrease in affective aggressive behavior, possibly by decreasing the threshold to aggression-triggering stimuli or by decreasing the propensity to engage in sudden aggressive outbursts (17,18). Evidence to support the role of serotonin as a modulator of aggression is building:

1. Animals showing certain aggressive behaviors have reduced indices of serotonergic activity, e.g., decreased prolactin response to fenfluramine challenge (19), and below normal levels of CSF 5-hydroxyindoleacetic acid (5-HIAA) (20,21).
2. There is genetic evidence that impaired synthesis or metabolism of serotonin leads to increased impulsivity and aggression (22–25).
3. Serotonergic mechanisms have been shown to operate in the acquisition and maintenance of dominance in primates. Engaging in and winning dominance-related struggles in vervet monkeys generates high blood levels of serotonin, so serotonin dynamics seem to be involved in this response. Monkeys treated with SRIs do not need to engage in as many dominance struggles to maintain their social position in a group, thus becoming less aggressive and engaging in more affiliative behaviors (12,13).
4. SRIs and direct acting serotonin receptor agonists have been demonstrated to reduce aggression in a variety of species (14,15,26).
5. Reduced serotonergic availability seems to be associated with increased aggression across several diagnostic categories (27,28).

Treatment of Aggression with Serotonergic Agents

SEROTONIN REUPTAKE INHIBITORS

Several SRIs have begun to find a place in veterinary medicine for a variety of applications, including the treatment of anxiety (29), compulsive behaviors (30), and aggression (15,31). Clomipramine and fluoxetine are probably the most widely employed drugs of this type, though other SRIs, such as sertraline and paroxetine, are probably equally effective. The primary pharmacologic action of SRIs is to block a transporter mechanism in the presynaptic membrane, consequently inhibiting the reuptake of serotonin (32). The specificity of the various SRIs for serotonin receptors varies. Clomipramine, a tricyclic compound that is less specific for serotonin uptake sites than other SRIs, has significant catecholaminergic, antihistaminic, and anticholinergic activity in addition to its potent serotonin reuptake blocking activity (33). Other SRIs, referred to as *selective* serotonin reuptake inhibitors (SSRIs), have greater specificity for serotonergic sites. Intuitively, it may seem that SSRIs would be more appropriate for the treatment of aggression because of their selectivity for serotonergic systems and because they are associated with fewer side effects. It is possible, however, that the side actions of other less specific serotonergic drugs may sometimes complement treatment. For example, it has been shown that chronic administration of clomipramine prevents the increase of norepinephrine (NE) induced by chronic stress (34). This would be a desirable attribute in the treatment of stress-linked affective aggression and suggests that tricylic antidepressants may be of value in the treatment of some forms of affective aggression. The results of one experimental study appear to counter this prediction, as rodents treated with classic tricyclic antidepressants showed enhancement of foot shock-induced aggression (Eichelman B, personal communication, 1993). This model, however, engenders chiefly defensive reactions. It is clear that more clinical studies are required to investigate the relative efficacy of SSRIs and other less selective 5-HT reuptake inhibitors in the treatment of affective aggression.

Although the anticompulsive effects of SRIs may take several weeks to become apparent, antiaggressive effects are sometimes seen much sooner. In a study designed to evaluate the efficacy of fluoxetine in the treatment of dominance-related aggression in dogs, one of nine dogs ceased all aggressive behavior immediately following the initiation of treatment (15). The other dogs in this study showed a more gradual decrease in aggressive behavior over a period of 4 weeks. The authors have also observed a rapid decrease (c. 2 days) in affective aggressive behavior in cats treated with clomipramine and fluoxetine.

Side Effects

Side effects of SRIs can be predicted from their pharmacologic properties. Clomipramine, for example, has potent anticholinergic properties and its most frequent side effects in humans (i.e., dry mouth, constipation, and excessive sweating) are attributable to this property. Central nervous and cardiovascular problems are also encountered in human patients, as are sexual dysfunction, sleep disturbances, and other less common side effects (33). Clomipramine has the potential for causing seizures, though the incidence of this disconcerting side effect is low (33). In dogs treated with clomipramine, sedation, hyporexia, constipation, and, in one case, a seizure-like disturbance (involving spontaneous hysteria, vocalization, and salivation) have been reported to the authors. The seizure-like complication was successfully managed by reducing the dose of clomipramine to one half of the usual dose (i.e., 2 mg/kg q12h) following the incident. In a published series of five dogs treated with clomipramine to alleviate signs of anxiety, the only side effects reported were transient mild sedation in one dog and dose-dependant agitation in another (29). In general, the side effects of clomipramine in dogs appear to be dose-related and transient. In cats treated with clomipramine, the author has observed other complications, such as delayed micturition, localized alopecia, lacrimation, thirst, and galactorrhea (possibly related to prolactin release). Some cats also became withdrawn and antisocial.

SSRIs, like fluoxetine, have weak affinity for binding to multiple neuroceptors and because of this are virtually devoid of cholinergic and cardio-vascular side effects (35). In people treated with fluoxetine, dysphorias, dizzi-ness, and insomnia are reasonably frequent side effects, depending upon the dose and dosing regimen, and neurologic side effects, including seizures, are a possibility (35). The principal side effects reported in study dogs receiving fluoxetine at 1 mg/kg were mild sedation (2 [20%] of 10) and hyporhexia (2 [20%] of 10) during weeks 2 and 3 of a 4 week treatment program (15). This conforms to what we have observed in other dogs treated at our clinic. One cat receiving fluoxetine had a seizure-like disturbance during treatment so the medication was discontinued.

Despite the potential side effects of SRIs and SSRIs, these medications are still relatively safe. The maximum non-lethal dose of fluoxetine in cats and dogs is 50 mg/kg and 100 mg/kg, respectively (33). This is approximately 50 times the usual clinical daily dose. In addition, SRIs are well tolerated in the majority of patients. This is welcome news to the owners of aggressive dogs, cats, and horses, as SRIs provide a valuable addition to the treatment armamentarium.

SEROTONIN RECEPTOR AGONISTS

Serenics

In the 1980s a group of serotonin (5-HT1) receptor agonists was developed specifically to inhibit aggressive behavior without other significant behavioral or somatic side effects (36,37). These so-called *smart drugs*, which specifically targeted the receptor and produced minimal side effects, were termed the *serenics*. Of the group, eltoprazine showed the most promise and was entered into human clinical trials in 1990. A promising illustration of the veterinary potential of eltoprazine was provided by the demonstration that eltoprazine virtually eliminated fighting to establish a social hierarchy in young pigs (36). Other relevant veterinary research was lacking, although the phar-macokinetics of eltoprazine were studied in the dog (38). Summarizing some of the results of this study, peak plasma levels were measured 1.5 to 1.9 hours after oral administration; half-life was about 2.4 hours; and bioavailability was 67% ± 20%.

In 1991 we had the opportunity to treat two aggressive dogs with eltoprazine and received reports from the owners of a substantial reduction in the dogs' aggressive behavior. Unfortunately, the reduction in aggression was associated with an apparent increase in anxiety. Both dogs began to pant excessively and withdrew from social situations while under treatment with higher doses of eltoprazine (1 mg/kg tid). One of the dogs refused to go downstairs during treatment with eltoprazine and became extremely anxious when attempts were made to coerce it. These side effects were minimized when the dose of eltoprazine was reduced to 0.25–0.5 mg/kg tid, but their occurrence suggested to us that eltoprazine's antiaggressive properties, in dogs at least, may be attributable to an anxiogenic effect. Others also were suspicious of anxiogenic mechanisms as underlying the antiaggressive effects of serenics, and these earlier contentions have now been substantiated (40).

Recently Solvay Duphar, Weesp, Netherlands, the manufacturers of eltoprazine, have ceased further human clinical trials and have no plans to proceed with the development of this or other serenic compounds.

Buspirone

The most well-known and frequently prescribed serotonin receptor agonist is buspirone. Buspirone is an azaspirodecanedione compound, which was approved by the U.S. Food and Drug Administration (FDA) in 1986 for the treatment of anxiety in humans (41). Because of its specific anxiolytic activity, lack of sedative-hypnotic and anticonvulsant effects, minimal interaction with CNS depressants and absence of potential for physical dependence or withdrawal, the term *anxioselective* was coined to describe the action of buspirone and related compounds (42). Like eltoprazine, buspirone is an agonist at 5-HT1A receptors (43), but is also a dopamine D2 receptor antagonist (44). Buspirone has been reported to have antiaggressive effects in animals (45–48). Its antiaggressive effect was originally believed to be secondary to its anxiolytic properties (6); however, Ratey, Miller, and Parks (49) report an uncoupling of the antianxiety and antiaggressive effects of the drug related to dosage. This is not to say that buspirone's anxiolytic properties can never contribute to its antiaggressive effects. It is still thought that when aggression covaries with anxiety, anxiolytics may decrease aggressive behavior by decreasing anxiety (50). The exact mechanism of buspirone's action in an individual case is not always clear, as it depends to some extent on the dose employed (49), patient factors (51), and the chronicity of treatment (43). At the onset of treatment, buspirone decreases 5-HT release by binding to 5-HT autoreceptors. This might be anticipated to increase aggressive behavior in the short term. An increase in aggression and agitation has been reported in some cats (52) and in humans (47) following the institution of buspirone therapy. Eventually the 5-HT autoreceptor is thought to desensitize, so that 5-HT neurons resume normal firing and postsynaptic mechanisms prevail (43). This has been shown to reduce aggression in the long term (47).

The author is unaware of any organized veterinary trials of buspirone in the treatment of aggression in pet animals. At Tufts University School of Veterinary Medicine, we have used buspirone in selected clinical cases of aggression for about 5 years. Although it appeared initially that buspirone was a reliable treatment for territorial aggression in cats, subsequently the results of treatment of feline intraspecific aggression with buspirone have been variable.

Currently we believe that it may be best to treat the cat that is the chief recipient of aggression with buspirone, and to treat the aggressor with an SRI or not at all. In dogs, we have had some success with buspirone in treating anxiety-related aggression, but formal studies are required to consolidate these early clinical impressions.

Treatment of Aggression by Manipulation of the Catecholamines

DOPAMINE ANTAGONISTS

This heterogeneous group of compounds is sometimes referred to collectively as *neuroleptics* (literally, "nerve-paralyzing" agents) after early investigators erroneously attributed the immobility produced in rodents to a peripheral effect. Subsequently, terms like *tranquilizer* (tranquilus = calmer), *ataractic* (a = without, taraktos = disturbed), *sedative* (sedare = to sleep), and *antipsychotic* were used to describe this group of drugs. There are three main types of neuroleptics: 1) low potency, 2) high potency, and 3) atypical.

The low potency group includes many of the classic phenothiazine neuroleptics. The prototypic phenothiazine is chlorpromazine, a drug that revolutionized the treatment of human psychoses and some aspects of veterinary practice. A more potent phenothiazine derivative, acepromazine, largely superseded chlorpromazine, in the United States at least; however, these two drugs have such similar actions that extrapolations from one to the other are valid. Phenothiazines are far from "smart" drugs, in that they lack specificity and have numerous side effects related to their ancillary actions. Although dopamine blockade accounts for the principal sedating and "taming" actions of phenothiazines, these drugs also possess anticholinergic, antihistaminic, and adrenolytic properties (53). In addition, phenothiazines lower the threshold for seizures and should be avoided in seizure-prone patients (54).

The chief disadvantage of phenothiazines in treating clinical aggression is their lack of specificity. Doses that decrease aggression cause a parallel reduction in social and exploratory behavior, and in alertness and locomotion in general (9). Although this may not be a concern in the short-term management of aggression and may even be a desirable feature, it is a disadvantage when it comes to chronic treatment of aggression. Tardive dyskinesia and other extrapyramidal side effects complicate the long-term use of phenothiazines and most other neuroleptics in human patients (55). Despite these caveats and concerns, phenothiazines like chlorpromazine, acepromazine, and piperacetazine have been recommended for the treatment of aggressive syndromes in dogs and cats (56).

Theoretically, high-potency neuroleptics, including some phenothiazines (e.g., fluphenazine) and butyrophenones (e.g., droperidol and haloperidol), would appear to be better agents for the control of aggressive behavior in clinical patients because they are less sedating; however, they do carry an increased risk of generating extrapyramidal syndromes (57). Although extrapyramidal effects apparently are uncommon in veterinary medicine, they do occur. A Parkinson-like syndrome has been reported following the administration of fluphenazine to a horse (58), and we have observed head bobbing in Doberman Pinschers after the administration of droperidol or pimozide. The only potent neuroleptic that has received much attention for the management of aggression in veterinary patients is the butyrophenone derivative, azaperone. An injectable preparation of azaperone was marketed in Britain under the trade name Suicalm, and in the United States as Stresnil (Janssen Pharmaceutical, Inc., Titusville, NJ) for the control of fighting in newly mixed groups of pigs. The antiaggressive effect of azaperone in pigs is brief, merely postponing the hierarchy fights, and no economic or commercial advantage accrues from its use (36,59).

We have prescribed haloperidol for the treatment of dominance-related aggression in dogs and have had few, if any, favorable results. In one case of "sibling rivalry" between two dogs (managed remotely by an owner/veterinarian), the effect of haloperidol, 0.5 mg/kg sid PO, given to both dogs, was to make them more sedate and to display increased affection to the owner, but aggression between the dogs remained unchanged.

The advent of atypical antipsychotic drugs, like clozapine, has ushered in a new era of hope for the treatment of human psychosis because of their relative freedom from extrapyramidal side effects (60). Clozapine has a profile of pharmacologic action substantially different from other antipsychotics, as it acts as an antagonist at D3 receptors and, in addition, has serotonergic properties (61). Although an earlier experimental study in mice rejected a *specific* antiaggressive effect attributable to clozapine (62), more recently clozapine has been demonstrated to have strong antiaggressive effects at doses below those producing motor impairment (63).

Clinically, clozapine has been found effective in the management of severely aggressive psychiatric patients (64,65). One serious adverse effect of clozapine is that it can produce agranulocytosis in humans, but according to the manufacturer, this complication does not occur in dogs. Seizures, however, are a potential complication of treatment, particularly when higher dosages are employed. Other side effects, including tremor, increased exploration, dystony, and hypersalivation, are additional causes for concern (66). We have used clozapine in the treatment of some aggressive dogs. The preliminary results have been disappointing, with no dramatic reductions in aggressive behavior reported. Hypersalivation was a complication of treatment in some dogs, occurring for a short while after dose increases were made. Clozapine analogs under investigation have fewer side effects than the parent molecule, including a complete absence of hypersalivation (67), and may prove useful in the future.

Beta-Adrenergic Antagonists

Catecholamines, which are integrally involved in fight-flight responses, have been shown to lower the threshold for aggressive behavior (11). Beta-2 but not beta-1 adrenoreceptors are important in this response (68). That catecholamine antagonists decrease affective aggression has been validated many times in laboratory and clinical settings (9,69). Although beta-adrenergic antagonists have been recommended for veterinary treatment of aggression (70), there have been no formal trials to verify their efficacy. The authors have clinical experience in using propranolol to treat fear-related aggression in dogs and have received reports of an estimated 0 to 30% decrease in the aggressive behavior. Unfortunately, the half-life of propranolol is short in dogs (0.77–2 hours), so a long-acting preparation (Inderal LA Wyeth-Ayerst, Philadelphia, PA) may be more appropriate in this species.

Most beta-blockers have both central and peripheral actions. Peripherally, beta-blockers block the beta-adrenergic effects of epinephrine and norepinephrine on cardiac, bronchial, intestinal, and vascular muscle; though perhaps more relevant to their antiaggressive action, they also block beta-adrenergic innervation of muscle spindles (69). As well as blocking beta-adrenergic receptors peripherally and centrally, beta-blockers act as antagonists at central 5-HT1 receptors (71,72). Both central and peripheral effects may contribute to the antiaggressive effects of these agents, and a debate continues about the relative contribution of each site of action. This may seem a somewhat esoteric controversy, but it does have direct relevance to the selection of a particular beta-blocker in preference to another. If central sites of action are important, more lipid-soluble agents, like propranolol and pindolol, may be preferable to less lipid-soluble compounds, like nadolol and atenolol, as they cross the blood-brain barrier with greater ease. Evidence supporting a central action of beta-blockers in aggression comes from the observation that beta-blockers that fail to cross the blood-brain barrier in significant quantities do not reduce aggression in some laboratory animal models (9). Conversely, nadolol, which has low lipid solubility, was found an effective treatment for aggression in one human clinical trial (69). The latter report attributed the antiaggressive effect of nadolol to antagonism of beta-adrenergic mechanisms responsible for maintaining tone at muscle spindles. Unfortunately, nadolol does cross the blood-brain barrier to some extent, so these results are difficult to interpret.

Assuming that the antiaggressive effects of beta-blockers involve at least some central component, another issue concerns the relative importance of serotonergic versus beta-adrenergic blocking potential. If serotonergic mechanisms are primarily involved, then pindolol would be a more effective antiaggressive drug than propranolol because it binds more strongly to 5-HT1 receptors (73). We have occasionally employed pindolol to treat canine aggression and have not yet been able to establish it as any more effective than propranolol, though formal studies comparing the two drugs are lacking. It is worth noting that pindolol is considerably more expensive than propranolol and may be associated with troublesome side effects. One dog receiving pindolol developed temporary urinary incontinence and another became extremely anxious. Since pindolol is a mixed agonist-antagonist, it is possible that the effects of urinary incontinence and anxiety were due to pindolol's agonist action at beta-adrenergic receptors and 5-HT1 receptors, respectively.

Beta-blockers have antiaggressive effects at doses well below those that impair locomotion and, in this respect, they are relatively specific treatments for the aggression (9). They can be anticipated to reduce aggression in several different contexts (9); however, their effectiveness in any particular situation cannot be guaranteed. Barring pindolol, beta-blockers are normally associated with few if any behavioral side effects, though cardiovascular changes of bradycardia and hypotension are inevitable accompaniments of effective therapy. Bronchoconstriction makes asthma a contraindication for the use of beta-1 blockers in humans; however, reactive airway disease is less common in animals.

LITHIUM

Several studies in humans have demonstrated that lithium carbonate may have value in treating aggression (74). Lithium disturbs sodium transport across cell membranes, inhibits the recycling of inositol phosphate second messengers, and has a variety of effects on neurotransmitters and their release (75,76). One of the effects of lithium is to decrease the turnover of norepinephrine and dopamine, but it also appears to enhance the action of serotonin and to augment the synthesis of acetylcholine (76).

In human psychiatry, lithium has been used to treat bipolar disorders and depression, although it has also been employed to treat aggression (77,78). To date, lithium is the only agent that has been shown in a blind placebo-controlled study to decrease impulsive aggressive behavior in individuals with antisocial personality disorder (79). Lithium has also been used successfully to treat aggressive behavior in a dog (80) but, other than this single case report, veterinary information on the use of lithium for the treatment of aggression is lacking. Unfortunately, lithium is relatively toxic and has the potential for producing numerous short-term side effects and some rare but serious long-term side effects (81). In addition, the therapeutic window for lithium, in terms of blood levels that are effective yet nontoxic, is narrow, and blood lithium levels should be monitored carefully when treatment is initiated. In humans, blood levels above 1.5 mEq/L generally result in lithium toxicity, whereas levels below 0.9 mEq/L are often ineffective (81). Although lithium is well absorbed from the gastrointestinal tract, its passage across the blood-brain barrier is slow and its half life is long (20–24 hr in humans), making titration of the dose to achieve the desired effect difficult.

STIMULANTS

Stimulants, such as amphetamines, methylphenidate, and pemoline, are only appropriate for the treatment of aggression when aggression is a component of attention-deficit hyperactivity disorder (ADHD). Nonserotonergic antidepressants (Certain tricyclics, bupropion, monoamine oxidase inhibitors) are also beneficial in ADHD, probably because of their catecholaminergic effects (82). ADHD, with or without associated aggression, is a well-described syndrome in human medicine (83) but has not yet been properly documented in veterinary medicine. The response of people with ADHD to treatment with stimulants appears paradoxical in that the treatment calms. Some hyperactive, aggressive dogs respond similarly and are presumed to have an equivalent condition (84,85). This phenomenon illustrates the qualitative opposite effects of amphetamine in a hyperactive neural system, that is, the law of initial value. Although a single low-dose amphetamine challenge can be employed to diagnose ADHD in dogs (86), some veterinarians prefer to gauge the condition in the field by assessing the animal's response to a short course of one of the stimulants (87). Unaffected dogs respond to stimulants with an increase in motor activity, heart rate, and respiratory rate. The response of dogs with ADHD is the opposite.

GABA-ERGIC DRUGS

The gamma-aminobutyric acid (GABA)/benzodiazepine/chloride receptor complex is intimately involved in the modulation of aggressive and social behavior (88). Low doses of GABA agonists, such as diazepam and chlordiazepoxide, may increase aggression, whereas moderate to high doses more often suppress it (89). The increase in aggression sometimes seen with benzodiazepines has been termed "paradoxical" and is one of the chief factors complicating the use of these drugs in the treatment of clinical aggression. Other disadvantages of benzodiazepines as therapeutic agents in aggression treatment include their lack of specificity, numerous side effects, and addiction potential. Sedation and ataxia often accompany the early phase of treatment with benzodiazepines, although this effect is transient, lasting just a few days or a week. Hyperphagia and associated weight gain are two other undesirable side effects of benzodiazepine treatment. Recently, acute fulminating hepatic failure has been associated with the use of diazepam in cats (90). Tolerance to the antiaggressive effects of benzodiazepines can occur, and withdrawal reactions with heightened aggression are also possible following sudden termination of long-term therapy (9).

ANTICONVULSANTS

Anticonvulsants comprise a mixed group of compounds that share the common capacity of raising the seizure threshold by stabilizing neuronal membranes. Some of the more widely used compounds include:

> Barbiturates (e.g., phenobarbital)
> Hydantoins (e.g., diphenylhydantoin)
> Succinimides (e.g., ethosuximide)
> Benzodiazepines (e.g., diazepam, chlorazepate, clonazepam)
> Miscellaneous (e.g., primidone, valproic acid, carbamazepine)

Seizure activity sometimes directly promotes aggressive behavior (16,91,92). This pathologic form of aggression is best treated with anticonvulsants and/or specific treatments designed to eliminate the underlying disease process (see Chap. 3). The most obvious example of seizure-related aggression occurs postictally in association with generalized, tonic-clonic seizures (formerly known as grand mal seizures). Less frequently diagnosed are partial seizures affecting the temporal lobe of the brain (93). Such partial seizures do not cause loss of consciousness but may affect mood or distort perception, leading to rage, extreme fear, predatory, or compulsive behavior (16,94). Both dogs and cats show aggressive behavior related to partial seizure activity (91–95). Treatment with phenobarbital is sometimes effective (94), but other anticonvulsants, alone or in combination, may be more appropriate for control of such seizures (96). Agents that may be more effective for the treatment of aggression linked to partial seizures include valproate, carbamazepine, and lamotrigine (96,97). In human medicine, valproic acid and carbamazepine are agents of choice, but in dogs, and possibly cats, these drugs may be metabolized too quickly for effective blood concentrations to be maintained without frequent dosing (98).

Recently it has been recognized that anticonvulsants have nonspecific antiaggressive effects, possibly as a result of stabilization of limbic neuronal discharges or by enhancement of serotonin (79). There is a report of the successful use of carbamazepine for the treatment of aggression in cats where seizures were not thought to underlie the aggression (99). That anticonvulsants reduce aggression in animals in which seizures are not involved has yet to be confirmed in multi-animal controlled studies. If certain types of affective aggression were found to respond to treatment with anticonvulsants, this would provide the clinician yet another approach for the management of refractory cases of aggression.

OPIOID ANTAGONISTS

The prototype opioid antagonist, naloxone, is available in injectable form for reversal of the effects of opiates in humans and animals. Naltrexone, another pure opioid antagonist, is marketed for treatment of alcoholism, and a related compound, nalmefene, has been investigated for the treatment of stereotypic self-scratching behavior in dogs (100). The role of opioid antagonists in the veterinary treatment of aggression has not yet been established, but extrapolations from laboratory animal research suggest their potential usefulness (101). For example, agonistic behavior can be significantly reduced in mice by pretreatment with opioid antagonists at doses that do not impair motor function (102). Also, some types of aggression in humans can be reduced by administering a single daily oral dose of naltrexone (103). The effect of opioid antagonists on aggressive behavior depends on the type of aggressive behavior being treated (88). Affective defense responses in cats are suppressed by opioids and enhanced by opioid antagonists (104). Offensive behavior, however, may be reduced by treatment with opioid antagonists (88). Our experiences with opioid antagonists for treating aggression in animals have been limited. We have found that high doses of opioid antagonists decrease aggression in horses, but treated horses also appear sedated (Dodman NH, Shuster L, unpublished data, 1983). Horses and cats exhibiting self-directed aggression also respond positively to treatment with opioid antagonists (105; Dodman N, Shuster L, unpublished data, 1995). A fearful cat we treated with naltrexone for psychogenic alopecia showed an increase in aggression toward a neighboring cat that it had previously avoided. In two dogs exhibiting sibling rivalry, high doses of naltrexone produced no change in aggressive behavior (Tribby M, personal communication, 1996).

Should opioid antagonists be conformed as valuable for the treatment of aggressive behavior in domestic animals, there are several points worth noting:

1. The half-life is short in animals so that frequent dosing would be necessary (100,106).
2. Bioavailability is low in most domestic species, necessitating high oral doses.
3. Side effects include hyporexia, sedation, and diarrhea.
4. High cost.
5. The taste of opioid antagonists is extremely bitter, causing problems with oral medication.

With these provisos in mind, it is nonetheless encouraging to have a new class of drugs to consider for the management of aggressive behavior in veterinary patients.

STEROIDS

Testosterone and estrogen appear to have proaggressive effects, which may involve serotonergic mechanisms (107,108); however, their elimination by gonadectomy is far from a panacea when it comes to reducing aggression (109).

Although orchiectomy increases brain serotonin levels in laboratory animals (110), typically male-type aggressive behavior usually persists to some extent in castrates because of perinatally determined, testosterone-mediated structural and functional organization within the CNS (56,111). Other types of aggression are minimally affected, if at all, by castration. Ovariohysterectomy in bitches may reduce estrus-linked aggression but may increase dominance-related aggressive behavior under certain conditions (10). An increase in pre-existing dominance aggression in young bitches following ovariohysterectomy may be attributable to loss of the stabilizing effect of progesterone. Progesterone and synthetic analogues (progestins) decrease aggression and have been recommended as antiaggressive agents in dogs and cats (56,112). The primary site of action of progestins was thought to be the intracellular T-tubules within the CNS, but more recently an anesthetic-like cell membrane stabilizing effect seems to better account for their action (113).

High-dose progestin therapy, though effective at reducing aggression, is associated with unacceptable and life-threatening side effects and should probably be avoided. An increase in appetite, weight gain, lethargy, gynecomastia, Addisonian changes, acromegaly, and diabetes mellitus are possible side effects of progestin therapy (56). The use of low-dose, short-term therapy with progestins reduces the severity of side effects. If low doses, of perhaps one tenth of the usual recommended dose, are found effective for the treatment of aggression, this will change the current perspective on progestins, permitting their consideration as valid treatments for behavior problems of an aggressive nature.

Predatory Aggression

This adaptive behavior is hard-wired in the CNS of all predatory species, including the dog and cat. As it involves minimal affective and autonomic change, there are some who do not consider it to be a form of "aggression" in the popular sense of the word, but more a survival-oriented component of maintenance behavior. However, if the definition of aggression is considered to encompass all behavior intended to harm another living being, then predatory aggression qualifies for consideration here. Appropriately directed predatory aggression is not a behavior about which behaviorists are frequently consulted. Owners normally accept the fact that their cat brings home dead rodents or that their dog chases squirrels. Problems arise when predatory behavior is directed toward humans or other inappropriate targets. The term "predatory aggression" has been used to describe some aggressive behaviors in children. Items that cluster together to identify this type of aggression in children include: 1) hiding aggressive acts, 2) planning aggressive acts, 3) being very careful to protect the body when aggressive, and 4) stealing (114). Some of these characteristics may be relevant when interpreting aberrant forms of predatory behavior in animals.

CLINICAL PRESENTATIONS OF PREDATORY AGGRESSION

1. Dogs attacking other small animals, including cats.
2. Large dogs attacking small, rapidly moving smaller dogs.
3. Dogs chasing and nipping (or biting) groups of young children who are running and playing together.
4. Aggression of dogs toward infants.
5. According to some authorities, dogs' chasing cars, cyclists, skateboarders, joggers, and other moving things represents a form of predatory aggression (5).

In almost all of these instances, prevention and control are the cornerstones of treatment, as predatory behavior itself, being "hard-wired," is refractory to most nonpharmacologic behavior modification therapy. However, predatory aggression, like other forms of aggression, involves discrete brain regions and neurotransmitter systems and can be manipulated should this be deemed necessary and appropriate. One of the principal neurotransmitters involved in the propagation of predatory behavior is acetylcholine, which has a facilitatory effect (16). Serotonin and GABA have an inhibitory action on this type of aggressive behavior (16,26). Theoretically, centrally acting anticholinergics, serotonergic agents, and GABA agonists (including benzodiazepines) should reduce the potential for this type of aggression.

CHOLINERGIC MANIPULATIONS AND PREDATORY AGGRESSIVE BEHAVIOR

One of the most striking reports emphasizing the role of acetylcholine in predatory behavior was published by Devinsky, Kernan, and Bear (115). These authors report the effects, on a cat and its owner, of exposure to high concentrations of a cholinesterase inhibitor from a commercial tick powder containing carbamate. The cat and its owner both developed behavior problems involving increased aggression that were reversed when exposure to the cholinesterase inhibitor was avoided. During the poisoning phase, the cat showed a marked increase in predatory behavior, leaving large numbers of dead birds and mice on the front lawn and bringing additional mice into the house "by the hour." Acetylcholine may also be involved in other types of aggression, as the cholinomimetic carbachol induces aggressive behavior in cats when injected into the amygdala (116). The corollary is that anticholinergic agents that cross the blood-brain barrier should reduce aggressive behavior. This extrapolation has yet to be confirmed clinically. Benztropine mesylate, an anticholinergic currently marketed as a human antiparkinson agent, is an anticholinergic agent that is worthy of consideration in this regard.

SEROTONERGIC INTERVENTION IN PREDATORY AGGRESSION

Eichelman and Barchas have reported that antidepressants reduce predatory aggression but increase affective aggression (117). In this report, the authors

Table 2.1. Drugs used to treat aggression

Drug	Dose rate	Route of administration	Dose interval	Potential side effects
Neuroleptics				
Acepromazine	1–2 mg/kg	PO	tid	Sedation
	0.05–0.10 mg/kg	IM or IV	prn	
Clozapine	Undetermined	PO	undetermined	Salivation, seizures
Serenics				
Eltoprazine	0.5–1.0 mg/kg	PO	tid	Panting, anxiety
Azapirones				
Buspirone	0.5–1.0 mg/kg	PO	bid or tid	Paradoxical response
Antidepressants				
Fluoxetine	1 mg/kg	PO	sid	Reduced appetite, drowsiness
Clomipramine	2.0–3.0 mg/kg	PO	bid	Anticholinergic effects, sedation
Beta-Blockers				
Propranolol	0.5–1.0 mg/kg	PO	tid	Bradycardia, hypotension
Pindolol	0.125–0.25 mg/kg	PO	bid	Anxiety
Antiepileptic drugs				
Phenobarbital	1–4 mg/kg	PO	bid	Sedation, hepatic dysfunction
Phenytoin	6–35 mg/kg	PO	tid	Hepatotoxicity
Valproic acid	15–200 mg/kg (dog)	PO	tid or qid	GI problems, hepatopathy
Diazepam	0.25–0.50 mg/kg	PO	bid or tid	Sedation, ataxia, hepatitis
Sustained-release diazepam (Valrelease)	0.25–0.5 mg/kg	PO	sid or bid	Sedation, ataxia, hepatitis
Clonazepam	1.5 mg/kg	PO	tid	Sedation
Benzodiazepines				
Diazepam	0.5–1.0 mg/kg	PO	bid or tid	Sedation, ataxia, hepatitis
Alprazolam	0.05–0.10 mg/kg	PO	tid	Sedation, paradoxical excitement
Stimulants				
Dextroamphetamine	0.5–1.0 mg/kg	PO	sid	Hyperactivity
Methylphenidate	0.25–0.50 mg/kg	PO	bid or tid	Hyperactivity
Progestins				
Medroxyprogesterone	5 mg/kg	IM	Single dose	Endocrine disturbances
Megestrol	2–5 mg/kg	PO	sid × 1–2 wk	Endocrine disturbances

were referring to the older tricyclic compounds, which have a mixed action, blocking the reuptake of both catecholamines and serotonin. It is probable that serotonin enhancement was responsible for the measured antipredatory effect while catecholaminergic mechanisms were operating to enhance affective aggression (79,118). In support of this, administration of the serotonin precursor 5-hydroxytryptophan blocks mouse killing, a form of predatory behavior in rats (119), while chronic pretreatment with antidepressants enhances apomorphine-induced, catecholaminergically driven aggressive behavior (120). Veterinary clinical information regarding the pharmacologic treatment of predatory aggression is in short supply, though we have had apparent success treating predatory aggression in dogs using amitriptyline and buspirone.

GABA AGONISTS AND PREDATORY AGGRESSION

GABA seems to play an inhibitory role with respect to predatory behavior. GABA injections into the olfactory bulbs of rats inhibit mouse killing (121). Theoretically, benzodiazepines, such as diazepam, alprazolam, and clorazepate, should be effective for the treatment of predatorily derived aggressive behaviors in dogs and cats, but at this time there is no published evidence to this effect.

References

1. Moyer KE. Kinds of aggression and their physiological basis. Communic Behav Biol (Part A) 1968;2:65–87.
2. Reis DJ. Central neurotransmitters in aggression. Res Publ Assoc Res Nerv Ment Dis 1974;52:119–148.
3. Blanchard RJ, Blanchard DC, Takahashi T, Kelley MJ. Attack and defensive behavior in the albino rat. Anim Behav 1977;25:622–634.
4. Bandler R. Identification of neuronal cell bodies mediating components of biting attack behavior in the cat: induction of jaw opening following microinjections of glutamate into hypothalamus. Brain Res 1982;245:192–197.
5. O'Farrell V. Manual of canine behavior. Brit Small Anim Vet Assoc. Glos, England: Cheltenham, 1986.
6. Ratey JJ, Leveroni CL. The treatment of clinical aggression: an integrative approach. Integra Psychol 1992;8:160–168.
7. Eichelman B. The biology and somatic experimental treatment of aggressive disorders. In: Berger PA, Brodie HKH, eds. The American handbook of psychiatry. New York: Basic Books, 1986:651–678.
8. Weiger WA, Bear DM. An approach to the neurology of aggression. J Psychiatr Res 1988;22:85–98.
9. Miczek KA. The psychopharmacology of aggression. In: Iversen LL, Iversen SD, Snyder SN, eds. Handbook of psychopharmacology, vol. 19. New York: Plenum, 1987:183–328.
10. O'Farrell V, Peachey E. Behavioral effects of ovariohysterectomy on bitches. J Small Anim Pract 1990;31:595–598.

11. Higley JD, Mehlman PT, Taub DM, et al. Cerebrospinal fluid monoamine and adrenal correlates of aggression in free-ranging rhesus monkeys. Arch Gen Psychiatry 1992;49:436–441.
12. Raleigh MJ, Nielsen DA, McGuire MT, et al. Behavioral and biochemical correlates of genotypic differences in vervet monkeys. Presented at the 33rd Annual Meeting of the American College of Neuropsychopharmacology, San Juan, Puerto Rico: December 1994:29. Abstract.
13. Raleigh MJ, McGuire MT, Brammer GL, et al. Serotonergic mechanisms promote dominance acquisition in adult vervet monkeys. Brain Res 1991;559:181–190.
14. Fuller RW. The influence of fluoxetine on aggressive behavior. Neuropsychopharmacology 1996;14:77–81.
15. Dodman NH, Donnelly R, Shuster L, et al. Use of fluoxetine to treat dominance aggression in dogs. J Am Vet Med Assoc 1996;209:1585–1587.
16. Eichelman B. Neurochemical and psychopharmacologic aspects of aggressive behavior. In: Meltzer HY, ed. Psychopharmacology: the third generation of progress. New York: Raven, 1987:697–704.
17. Porsolt RD. Serotonin: neurotransmitter "a la mode." Pharmacopsychiatry 1993;26:20–24.
18. Mann JJ. Violence and aggression. In: Bloom FE, Kupfer D, eds. Psychopharmacology: the fourth generation of progress. New York: Raven, 1995:1919–1928.
19. Kyes RC, Botchin MB, Kaplan JR, et al. Aggression and brain serotonergic responsivity: response to slides in male macaques. Physiol Behav 1995;57:205–208.
20. Mehlman PT, Higley JD, Faucher I, et al. Low CSF 5-HIAA concentrations and severe aggression and impaired impulse control in non-human primates. Am J Psychol 1994;151:1485–1491.
21. Miczek KA, Donat P. Brain 5-HT systems and inhibition of aggressive behavior. In: Bevan P, Cools A, Archer T, eds. Behavioral pharmacology of 5HT. Hillsdale, NJ: Lawrence Erlbaum Assoc, 1989:117–144.
22. Sandou F, Amara DA, Dierich A, et al. Enhanced aggressive behavior in mice lacking 5HT1B receptor. Science 1994;265:1875–1878.
23. Brunner HG, Nelsen M, Breakefield XO, et al. Abnormal behavior associated with a point mutation in the structural gene for monoamine oxidase A. Science 1993;262:578–580.
24. Nielsen DA, Goldman D, Virkunnen M, et al. Suicidality and 5-hydroxyindoleacetic acid concentration associated with a tryptophan hydroxylase polymorphism. Arch Gen Psychiatry 1994;51:34–38.
25. Nelson RJ, Demas GE, Huang PL, et al. Behavioral abnormalities in male mice lacking neuronal nitric oxide synthase. Nature 1995;378:383–386.
26. Olivier B, Mos J, van der Heyden J, et al. Serotonergic modulation of aggressive behavior. In: Olivier B, Mos J, Brain PF, eds. Ethopharmaco Analy of Agonistic Behav in Anim and Humans. Dordrecht, Netherlands: Martinus Nijhoff, 1987:162–186.
27. Siever LJ, Kahn RS, Lawlor BA, et al. Critical issues in defining the role of serotonin in psychiatric disorders. Pharmacol Rev 1991;43:509–525.
28. Mann JJ, Arango V, Underwood MD. Serotonin and suicidal behavior. Ann NY Acad Sci 1990;600:476–484.
29. Stein DJ, Borchelt P, Hollander E. Pharmacotherapy of naturally occurring anxiety symptoms in dogs. Res Commun Psychol Psychiatry Behav 1994;19:39–48.
30. Goldberger E, Rappoport JL. Canine acral lick dermatitis: response to the anti-obsessional drug clomipramine. J Am Anim Hosp Assoc 1991;27:179–182.
31. Overall KL. Animal behavior case of the month. J Am Vet Med Assoc 1995;206:629–632.
32. Harris MG, Benfield P. Fluoxetine: a review of its pharmacodynamic and pharmacokinetic properties, and therapeutic use in older patients with depressive illness. Drugs Aging 1995;6:64–84.

33. McTavish D, Benfield P. Clomipramine—an overview of its pharmacological properties and a review of its therapeutic use in obsessive compulsive disorder and panic disorder. Drugs 1990;39:136–153.

34. Adell A, Garcia-Marquez C, Armario A, et al. Chronic administration of clomipramine prevents the increase in serotonin and norepinephrine induced by chronic stress. Psychopharmacology 1989;99:22–26.

35. Sommi RW, Crismon ML, Bowden CL. Fluoxetine: a serotonin-specific second generation antidepressant. Pharmacotherapy 1987;7:1–15.

36. Olivier B, Van Dalen D, Hartog J. A new class of psychotropic drugs: serenics. Drugs Fut 1986;11:473–494.

37. Olivier B, Mos J. Serenics and aggression. Stress Med 1986;2:197–209.

38. Lammers R, van Harten J. Pharmacokinetics of eltoprazine in the dog. Drug Metabol Drug Interact 1990;8:141–148.

39. Kemble ED, Gibson BM, Rawleigh JM. Effects of eltoprazine hydrochloride on exploratory behavior and social attraction in mice. Pharmacol Biochem Behav 1991;38:759–776.

40. Rodgers RJ, Cole LC, Cobain MR, et al. Anxiogenic-like effects of fluprazine and eltoprazine in the mouse elevated plus-maze: profile comparisons with 8-OH-DPAT, CGS 12066B, TFMPP and mCPP. Behav Pharmacol 1992;3:621–634.

41. Tunnicliff G. Molecular basis of buspirone's anxiolytic action. Pharmacol Toxicol 1991;69:149–156.

42. Faludi G. Buspirone: a new possibility in the treatment of anxiety. Orv Hetil 1994;135:1807–1813.

43. de Montigny C. Is the serotonin system still a promising target for the future of pharmacotherapy of affective disorders? In: Neurobiology of affective disorders. Third Annual Bristol-Myers Squibb Symposium on Neuroscience Research, October 1991, Raven Health Care Communications, 22–25.

44. New, JS. The discovery and development of buspirone: a new approach to the treatment of anxiety. Med Res Rev 1990;10:283–326.

45. Tompkins EC, Clemento AJ, Taylor DP. Inhibition of aggressive behavior in Rhesus monkeys by buspirone. Res Commun Psychol Psychiatr Behav 1980;5:337–352.

46. Riblet LA, Taylor DP, Eison MS, et al. Pharmacology and neurochemistry of buspirone. J Clin Psychiatr 1982;43:11–16.

47. Stanislav SW, Fabre T, Crismon ML, et al. Buspirone's efficacy in organic-induced aggression. J Clin Psychopharm 1994;14:126–130.

48. McMillen BA, DaVanzo EA, Scott SM, et al. N-Aklyl-Substituted Aryl-piperazine drugs: relationship between affinity for serotonin receptors and inhibition of aggression. Drug Dev Res 1988;12:53–62.

49. Ratey JJ, Miller AC, Parks AW. The effects of buspirone on aggression, anxiety, impulsivity, and cognition in the dually diagnosed. Presented at the Mead-Johnson Visiting Faculty Presentation, Ft. Myers, FL, 1991.

50. Corrigan PW, Yudofsky SC, Silver JM. Pharmacological and behavioral treatments for aggressive psychiatric inpatients. Hosp Community Psychiatry 1993;44:125–133.

51. Stahl, SM. Serotonin neuroscience discoveries usher in a new era of novel drug therapies for psychiatry. Psychopharmacol Bull 1992;28:3–9.

52. Hart BL, Eckstein RA, Powell KL, Dodman NH. Effectiveness of buspirone on urine spraying and inappropriate urination in cats. J Am Vet Med Assoc 1993;203:254–258.

53. Booth NH. Psychotropic agents. In: Booth NH, McDonald LE, eds. Veterinary pharmacology and therapeutics, 6th ed. Ames, IA: Iowa State University Press, 1988:363–395.

54. Sheard MH. Psychopharmacology of aggression. In: Hippius H, Winokur G, eds. Clinical psychopharmacology. Amsterdam: Excerpta Medica, 1983:188–201.

55. Leventhal BL, Brodie HKH. The pharmacology of violence. In: Hamburg DA, Trudeau MB, eds. Biobehavioral aspects of aggression. New York: Liss, 1981:85–106.

56. Hart BL, Hart LL. Psychoactive drugs and behavioral therapy. In: Canine and feline behavioral therapy. Philadelphia. Lea & Febiger, 1985:249–262.

57. Poling A, Gadow KD, Cleary J. Neuroleptics. In: Drug therapy for behavior disorders. New York: Pergamon, 1990:49–73.

58. Brewer BD, Hines MT, Stewart JT. Fluphenazine induced parkinson-like syndrome in a horse. Equine Vet J 1990;22:136–137.

59. Blackshaw JK. The effect of pig pen design and the tranquilising drug, azapirone, on the growth and behaviour of weaned pigs. Aust Vet J 1981;57:272–275.

60. Claghorn J, Honigsfeld G, Abuzzahab S, et al. The risks and benefits of clozapine versus chlorpromazine. J Clin Psychopharmacol 1987;176:558–561.

61. Criswell HE, Mueller RA, Breese GA. Clozapine antagonism of D1 and D2 dopamine receptor-mediated behaviors. Eur J Pharmacol 1988;159:141–147.

62. McMillen BA, DaVanzo EA, Song AH, et al. Effects of classical and atypical antipsychotic drugs on isolation-induced aggression in male mice. Eur J Pharmacol 1989;160:149–153.

63. Garmendia L, Sanchez JR, Azpiroz A, et al. Clozapine: strong antiaggressive effects with minimal motor impairment. Physiol Behav 1992;51:51–54.

64. Ratey JJ, Leveroni C, Kilmer D, et al. The effects of clozapine on severely aggressive psychiatric inpatients in a state hospital. J Clin Psychiatry 1993;54:219–223.

65. Volavka J, Zito JM, Vitrai J, Czobar P. Clozapine effects on hostility and aggression in schizophrenia. J Clin Psychopharmacol 1993;13:287–289.

66. Bruhwyler J, Chleide E, Houbeau G, et al. Differentiation of haloperidol and clozapine using a complex operant schedule in the dog. Pharmacol Biochem Behav 1993;44:181–189.

67. Bruhwyler J, Liegeois JF, Chleide E, et al. Comparative study of typical neuroleptics, clozapine and newly synthesized clozapine analogues: correlations between neurochemistry and behavior. Behav Pharmacol 1992;3:567–579.

68. Matsumoto K, Ojima K, Ohta H, Watanabe H. Beta 2—but not beta 1—adrenoceptors are involved in desipramine enhancement of aggressive behavior in long-term isolated mice. Pharmacol Biochem Behav 1994;49:13–18.

69. Ratey JJ, Sorgi P, O'Driscoll MA, et al. Nadolol to treat aggression and psychiatric symptomatology in chronic psychiatric inpatients: a double-blind, placebo-controlled study. J Clin Psychiatry 1992;53:41–46.

70. Dodman NH, Shuster L. Pharmacologic approaches to managing behavior problems in small animals. Vet Med 1994;Oct:960–969.

71. Bell R, Hobson H. Effects of (-)-pindolol and SDZ 216–525 on social and agonistic behavior in mice. Pharmacol Biochem Behav 1993;46:873–880.

72. Frances H, Monier C, Debray M. Behavioral effect of beta-blocking drugs resulting from the stimulation or the blockade of serotonergic 5-HT 1B receptors. Pharmacol Biochem Behav 1994;48:965–969.

73. Hoyer D, Engel G, Kalkman HO. Molecular pharmacology of 5-HT 1, and 5HT-2 recognition sites in rat and pig brain membranes: radioligand binding studies with [3H]-5HT,[3H]8-OH-DPAT,(-) [125I]iodocyanopindolol, [3H]mesulergine and [3H]ketanserin. Eur J Pharmacol 1985;118:13–23.

74. Schiff HB, Sabin TD, Geller AL, Mark V. Lithium in aggressive behavior. Am J Psychiatry 1982;139:1346–1348.

75. Bernie R Olin, ed. Drug facts and comparisons. St Louis: Kluwer, 1992:1293.

76. Hollister LE. Antipsychotic agents and lithium. In: Katzung BG, ed. Basic and clinical pharmacology, 6th ed. Norwalk, CT: Appleton & Lange, 1995:432–447.

77. Campbell M, Small AM, Green WH, et al. Behavioral efficacy of haloperidol and lithium carbonate: a comparison in hospitalized aggressive children with conduct disorder. Arch Gen Psychiatry 1984;120:650–656.

78. Sheard MH. The effect of lithium and other ions on aggressive behavior. In: Valzelli EL, ed. Modern problems of pharmacopsychiatry. New York: Karger, 1978:53–68.

79. Coccaro EF, Siever LJ. The neuropsychopharmacology of personality disorders. In: Bloom FE, Kupfer DJ, eds. Psychopharmacology: the fourth generation of progress. New York: Raven, 1995:1567–1579.

80. Reisner I. Use of lithium for treatment of canine dominance-related aggression: a case study. Appl Anim Behav Sci 1994;39:190.

81. Poling A, Gadow KD, Cleary J. Antidepressants and lithium. In: Goldstein AP, Krasner L, Garfield SL, eds. Drug therapy for behavior disorders: an introduction. New York: Pergamon, 1991:108–129.

82. Wilens TE, Biederman J, Spencer TJ, Prince J. Pharmacotherapy of adult attention deficit/hyperactivity disorder. J Clin Psychopharmacol 1995;15:270–279.

83. Poling A, Gadow KD, Cleary J. Stimulants. In: Goldstein AP, Krasner L, Garfield SL, eds. Drug therapy for behavior disorders: an introduction. New York: Pergamon, 1991:90–107.

84. Corson SA, Corson EOL, Arnold LE, Knopp W. Animal models of violence and hyperkinesis. In: Serban G, Kling A, eds. Animal models of human psychobiology. New York: Plenum, 1976:111–139.

85. Campbell WE. Behavioral modification of hyperkinetic dogs. Mod Vet Prac 1973;54:49–52.

86. Ginsburg BE, Becker RE, Traitner A, Bareggi SR. A genetic taxonomy of hyperkinesis in the dog. Int J Dev Neurosci 1984;2:313–322.

87. Burghart W. Diagnosis and treatment of hyperactivity in the dog. Proceedings of the American Veterinary Medical Association Annual Meeting, San Francisco, July, 1994.

88. Miczek KA, Weerts E, Haney M. Neurobiological mechanisms controlling aggression: preclinical developments for pharmacotherapeutic interventions. Neurosci Biobehav Rev 1994;18:97–110.

89. DiMascio A. The effect of benzodiazepines on aggression. In: Garattini S, Mussini E, Randall RO, eds. The benzodiazepines. New York: Raven, 1973:433–440.

90. Hughes D, Moreau RE, Overall KL, Van Winkle TJ. Acute hepatic necrosis and liver failure associated with benzodiazepine therapy in 6 cats. Vet Emerg Critical Care 1996;6(1):13–20.

91. Dodman NH, Miczek KA, Knowles K, et al. Phenobarbital responsive episodic dyscontrol in dogs. J Am Vet Med Assoc 1992;201:1580–1583.

92. Dodman NH, Bronson R, Gliatto J. Tail chasing in a bull terrier. J Am Vet Med Assoc 1993;202:254–258.

93. De Lahunta A. Nonolfactory rhinencephalon: limbic system. In: Veterinary neuroanatomy and clinical neurology, 2nd ed. Philadelphia: Saunders, 1983:319–325.

94. Dodman NH, Knowles K, Shuster L, et al. Behavioral changes associated with suspected complex partial seizures in bull terriers. J Am Vet Med Assoc 1996;208:688–691.

95. Holzworth J. Feline hyperesthesia syndrome. In: Dyson J, ed. Diseases of the cat. Philadelphia: Saunders, 1986:654–655.

96. Anon. Drugs for epilepsy. Medical Lett Drugs Ther 1995;37.

97. Burstein AH. Lamotrigine. Pharmacotherapy 1995;15:129–143.

98. O'Brien D. Rational anticonvulsant therapy. Proceedings of the American Animal Hospital Association Meeting. Toronto, April, 1991:443–447.

99. Schwartz S. Carbamazepine in the control of aggressive behavior in cats. J Am Anim Hosp Assoc 1994;30:515–519.

100. Dodman NH, Shuster L, White SD, et al. Use of narcotic antagonists to modify stereotypic self-licking, self-chewing, and scratching behavior in dogs. J Am Vet Med Assoc 1988;193:815–819.

101. Winslow JT, Miczek KA. Naltroxone blocks amphetamine hyperactivity, but not disruption of social and agonistic behavior in mice and squirrel monkeys. Psychopharmacology, 1988:493–499.

102. Benton D, Brain PF. The role of opioid mechanisms in social interaction and attachment. In: Rodgers RJ, Cooper SJ, eds. Endorphins, opiates and behavioral processes. Chichester, England: John Wiley and Sons, 1988:217–235.

103. Sandman CA, Barron JL, Colman H. An orally administered opiate blocker, naltrexone, attenuates self injurious behavior. Am J Ment Retard 1990;95:93–102.

104. Siegel A, Pott CB. Neural substrates of aggression and flight in the cat. Prog Neurobiol 1988;31:261–283.

105. Dodman NH. Pharmacologic treatment of behavior problems in cats. Vet Int 1994;6: 13–20.

106. Dixon R, Hsiao J, Leadon D, Dodman NH. Nalmefene: pharmacokinetics of a new opioid antagonist which prevents crib-biting in the horse. Res Commun Sub Abuse 1992;13: 231–236.

107. Bonson KR, Johnson RG, Fiorella D, et al. Serotonergic control of androgen-induced dominance. Pharmacol Biochem Behav 1994;49:313–322.

108. Clarke AS, Barber DM. Anabolic-androgenic steroids and aggression in castrated male rats. Physiol Behav 1994;56:1107–1113.

109. Hart BL, Hart LA. Hormonal manipulation. In: Canine and feline behavioral therapy. Philadelphia: Lea & Febiger, 1985:231–248.

110. Van der Kar L, Levine J, Orden L. Serotonin in hypothalamic nuclei: increased after castration in male rats. Neuroendocrinology 1978;27:186–192.

111. Compaan JC, DeRuiter AJH, Koolhas JM, et al. Differential effects of neonatal testosterone treatment on aggression in two selection lines of mice. Physiol Behav 1991;51:7–10.

112. Hart BL. Progestin therapy for aggressive male behavior in male dogs. J Am Vet Med Assoc 1981;178:1070.

113. McEwen BS, Davis PG, Parsons B, Pfaff DW. The brain as a target for steroid hormone action. Ann Rev Neurosci 1979;2:65–112.

114. Campbell M, Kafantaris V, Cueva JE. An update on the use of lithium carbonate in aggressive children and adolescents with conduct disorder. Psychopharmacol Bull 1995;31:93–102.

115. Devinsky O, Kernan J, Bear DM. Aggressive behavior following exposure to cholinesterase inhibitors. J Neuropsychiatry Clin Neurosci 1992;4:189–194.

116. Rodgers RJ, Brown K. Amygdaloid function in the central cholinergic mediation of shock-induced aggression in the rat. Aggressive Behav 1976;2:131–152.

117. Eichelman B, Barchas J. Facilitated shock-induced aggression following anti-depressant medication in the rat. Pharmacol Biochem Behav 1975;3:601–604.

118. Zagrodzka J. Monoaminergic depletion and changes in aggressive behavior in cats and rats. Neuropsychopharmacology 1994;11:90.

119. Kulkarni AS. Muricidal block produced by 5-hydroxytryptophan and various drugs. Life Sci 1968;7:125–128.

120. Maj J, Mogilnicka E, Kordecka A. Chronic treatment with antidepressant drugs: potentiation of apomorphine-induced aggressive behavior in rats. Neurosci Lett 1979;13:337–341.

121. Mandel P, Mack G, Kempf E. Molecular basis of some models of aggressive behavior. In: Sandler M, ed. Psychopharmacology of aggressive behavior. New York: Raven, 1979:95–110.

Systemic Causes of Aggression and Their Treatment

3

Linda Aronson

Common wisdom demands that behavior problems be viewed in the context of the whole animal. That a dog hit by a car will show aggression toward those trying to help it is expected and is rightly seen as the dog's attempt to protect itself from further pain. In such instances the cause of the aggression is readily apparent; unfortunately, this is not always the case. Metabolic anomalies may cause behavioral responses contrary to those that intuition might suggest. Aggression can be the primary, and sometimes overwhelming, manifestation of a problem at the time of presentation, and as a result an underlying systemic cause for the behavior may not be sought.

In human medicine, there has also been much debate as to whether behavior problems are psychological or systemic in nature. It has been suggested in humans that true psychiatric problems are driven by nonmedical causes (e.g., social) and should be differentiated from mental illnesses resulting from disease of the CNS (1). It is probable that with the advent of more sophisticated imaging (e.g., computer assisted tomography [CT], magnetic resonance imaging [MRI], positron emission tomography [PET], single photon emission computed tomography [SPECT]) and other investigative tools (e.g., electroencephalogram [EEG], pharmacologic probes for biochemical imbalances), structural or metabolic causes could be determined for animals that have previously been viewed as strictly having behavior problems. However, given financial constraints and the fact that many of these problems appear to respond to conventional behavior therapy, the actual cause of the condition in animals may be moot.

Further muddying the issue, it is apparent that some of the conditions, previously viewed as "normal" animal behavior, which become problematic because they conflict with human needs and expectations, may in fact be the result of physiologic processes. For example, some conditions that produce aggression involve altered serotonergic tone. It has also been found that oppressive environments cause a long-lasting reduction in brain serotonergic activity and that this, in turn, produces an increase in aggressive behavior (2).

Likewise, social status can affect the serotonergic system, at least in the crayfish and probably in other crustaceans. It appears that dominant crayfish either have more excitatory serotonergic receptors or that the receptors have a lower response threshold, so that excitability of the lateral giant neuron is increased. In contrast, subordinate animals either have a predominance of inhibitory serotonergic receptors or those they have exhibit a higher serotonin threshold. As a result, the subordinate crayfish will flee, while the dominant crayfish will hold its ground and respond aggressively if necessary. The response changes with the animal's social status, however, and is not fixed for life (3).

It is probable that most "behavioral" aggression (i.e., that for which no clear-cut systemic cause can be demonstrated) is the result, at least in part, of stress, which is in and of itself a physiological condition. The possible exception to this would be some dominance aggression. The need to establish a hierarchy of dominance is, however, a programmed response in most species. In this chapter though, we will concentrate on particular systemic conditions which increase and/or randomize an animal's innate aggressive behavior.

Areas of the CNS Involved in Aggression Control

Three areas of the brain, the hypothalamus, limbic system, and frontal cortex, have been associated with aggression experimentally and in human and veterinary medicine. It has been suggested that the locus of CNS lesions leading to aggressive behavior could be inferred from the nature of the aggression (4). Brain-stem lesions produce aggression independent of history or environment; those in the limbic system produce aggression that depends on experience and is triggered by environmental stimuli; and cortical damage produces aggressive responses to trivial stimuli, which normally would be precluded by thought (i.e., comparison to past experience, probable outcome, etc.). Because "normal" aggression is frequently involved in obtaining and protecting food and mates, it is perhaps unsurprising that the same regions of the brain associated with the control of aggression are closely associated with the regulation of feeding and sexual behavior. Interestingly, "inappropriate" aggression is also frequently associated with eating and sexual triggers in domestic animals (5).

The need for a central aggression pathway has long been suggested (6). Animals use aggression to obtain food and mates, to defend offspring, self, and territory. Darwin reasoned that the aggressive posture assumed prior to attack came to be recognized by the soon-to-be victim, which could then either decide to fight, assume a submissive posture, or flee. In turn, Darwin believed, this awareness caused some animals to assume an aggressive posture in order to maintain their status, even though there was no intention to fight. This reasoning implies a sophisticated level of modulation of the neural pathway.

Kravitz (7) has demonstrated a system of opposing neurotransmitters in the lobster, such that serotonin causes the animal to assume a fighting stance while octopamine promotes a submissive posture. In mammals, it appears that the situation is not so simple and that there are multiple levels of control for aggressive behavior.

HYPOTHALAMUS

The hypothalamus is primarily associated with the autonomic nervous system. It receives sensory information on the internal functioning of the animal from osmoreceptors and chemoreceptors, and produces stereotypic reactions via the pituitary and motor centers in the brain stem. Bard (8) demonstrated that when the cortex and other structures rostral to the hypothalamus were ablated in cats, they periodically entered a state of "sham rage" with little or no provocation. The cats hissed, extended their claws, and demonstrated piloerection and pupillary dilation. If the brain was sectioned immediately caudal to the hypothalamus, sham rage could not be elicited. In the intact animal, stimulation of the lateral hypothalamic area enhanced predatory behavior (9). Carbachol, acetylcholine with physostigmine or neostigmine, and neostigmine injected into the lateral hypothalamus have been shown to increase this predatory behavior, whereas atropine injection blocks the aggressive response (10).

The ventromedial hypothalamus appears to exert an inhibitory effect on aggressive behavior. Stimulation produced a submissive posture (11), while ablation produced unprovoked attacks in previously friendly cats (12). Human patients with neoplasms that have destroyed the ventromedial hypothalamus bilaterally have attacked randomly. These attacks appear either to be unprovoked or may be triggered by hunger, and result in kicking, biting, scratching, and object throwing. At the time of the attack, patients appear unable to control their behavior, although they may express remorse and surprise later (13,14).

Ablation of pathways from the cortex to the hypothalamus may also produce uncontrolled aggression, as was seen in the case of a 10-year-old boy who had suffered congenital toxoplasmosis. He would bite other children, and although he warned them to stay away from him, did not claim any intention of injuring them. The biting behavior was suppressed by a cholinergic antagonist (15).

Anticholinesterase poisoning has also been shown to produce increased aggression in both humans and animals. In one case, application of carbaryl as an antiparasitic powder caused a cat to start killing large numbers of mice and birds, which it had not done before, and produced such aggression and argumentativeness in the owner that his long-time companion was forced to leave the house. The behavior of both pet and owner returned to normal within a week of termination of the use of the powder (16–19).

AMYGDALOID COMPLEX

The amygdaloid body is comprised of a number of nuclei and is located in the rostral portion of the temporal lobe. The amygdala has reciprocal connections to the hypothalamus via the ventral amygdalofugal pathway and the stria terminalis. Stimulation of the basolateral amygdala, which in turn increases activity in the ventromedial hypothalamus, tends to reduce aggressive behavior, while stimulation of the lateral or dorsal amygdala, which diminishes neural firing in the ventromedial hypothalamus, increases attack behavior (20). Unlike the hypothalamus, however, the amygdala receives major sensory input (visual, auditory, tactile, and gustatory) from the temporal neocortex. It also receives information directly from the olfactory bulbs and from polysensory convergence areas in the frontal and temporal lobes of the cortex. Within the amygdala, there are multiple interconnections permitting the coordination of the diverse sensory information. The amygdala appears to be involved in the recognition of objects, odors, sounds, tastes, and relating them to learned emotional sensations.

Bilateral removal of the temporal lobes in monkeys and cats, and even more limited lesions of areas of visual and tactile input, produces dramatic behavior changes. The animals constantly sniff and taste everything in their environment, as if they have lost all memory of previous encounters. They cannot distinguish food from nonfood, appropriate sex partners from inappropriate (i.e., same sex and interspecies copulations are attempted). These animals do not tend to relearn these associations, or, if they do, progress is slow and incomplete (21–24). The effects of bilateral amygdalectomy on behavior depend upon the animal's social status prior to ablation. Most animals become placid and much easier to handle; however, submissive animals show either no change in their level of aggression or became more aggressive. Objects that previously invoked fear or provoked attack no longer do so (25). In moments, the same object might elicit an aggressive posture, a submissive posture, and oral exploration.

Rabid animals have been reported to show indiscriminate eating behavior, biting at sticks, stones, and dirt, as well as hypersexuality in association with aggression (26,27). Animals displaying these behaviors have been found to have lesions primarily in the limbic system (28).

In humans, temporolimbic lesions have been reported as a result of viral encephalitis, head trauma, degenerative dementias such as Alzheimer's disease and Pick's disease, and accidental damage during surgery for intractable epilepsy. If the lesion is extensive, the patients respond in a manner similar to the monkeys. They express little response to any stimulus, losing both positive and negative feelings toward people they previously loved or hated. Aggressive responses cannot be evoked (29,30). Temporal lobe epilepsy is relatively common in both animals and humans. The amygdala appears to be particularly liable to seizure activity, which can lead to aggression (see Episodic

Dyscontrol [Rage] and Temporal Lobe Epilepsy under Systemic Causes of Aggression).

FRONTAL CORTEX

The frontal cortex receives afferents from the amygdala, thalamus, ascending reticular activating system, and other areas in the cortex. Efferents to the motor system produce complex learned movements. There are also efferents to the limbic system, hypothalamus, and basal ganglia. The frontal cortex appears to integrate the external environment and internal condition, and evaluates sensory stimuli on the basis of past experience. Frontal lobotomy has been performed in both humans and animals to alleviate aggressive behavior. In humans this has resulted in apathy and loss of personality and intellect. Lobotomy seemed to be more effective in reducing dog-to-dog aggression, as reported in a pack of malamutes, than in reducing the aggression of companion dogs and cats directed toward humans (31). Lobotomy has too many side effects to recommend it as a therapeutic method. More localized lesions in humans have shown that while lesions of the dorsofrontal convexity of the frontal lobe produce apathy, orbital lesions produce impulsive behavior and patients strike out at trivial stimuli in an apparently reflexive manner (32).

Systemic Causes of Aggression

Theoretically, all these areas of the brain are susceptible to injury from a variety of sources: head trauma, infection, aberrant parasitic migration, neoplastic or other space-occupying lesions, degenerative disease, malformation or vascular damage, altered neuronal activity (seizures), toxic challenge, and subtle changes in metabolic and neurotransmitter activity. Whether a particular condition manifests with aggression as the presenting complaint will depend upon the specific areas of the brain affected.

EPISODIC DYSCONTROL (RAGE) AND TEMPORAL LOBE EPILEPSY

Aggressive attacks resulting from partial epilepsy are episodic, as are tonic-clonic (formerly called in human medicine grand mal) epileptic seizures. The limbic structures of the brain involved in this response have the lowest threshold for "kindling," and are frequently the foci for abnormal electrical activity. In the case of generalized seizures, secondary foci are also liable to develop within the limbic system.

The surface-recorded EEG is a relatively crude tool for assessing neurophysiologic brain function. Abnormalities recorded over the temporal lobes may be the projections of activity in the limbic system or diencephalon, as well as the result of activity within the temporal lobes themselves. In humans, temporal lobe epilepsy (TLE) has been associated with two types of aggression: random ictal and postictal aggression and interictal aggression.

During seizures and in the immediate postictal period, patients may lash out with hands and feet or with objects. This aggression appears to be random and undirected. Interictal aggression can be induced by apparently trivial stimuli, and the threshold for anger appears to be reduced. Patients also may appear paranoid, or develop phobias, panic attacks, and bizarre sexual fetishes during the interictal period (33,34).

Both humans and animals with TLE exhibit in the dentate gyrus a characteristic sprouting of mossy fibers, which form recurrent excitatory synapses with other granule cells and thereby enhance the response to otherwise subthreshold stimuli. There is also an apparent increase in stimulation of gamma-aminobutyric acid (GABA) inhibitory interneurones. However, as neuronal activity increases, the mossy fibers release their stores of zinc ions, which reduce the GABA-induced inhibition and further enhance the spread of epileptic activity (35).

Increased temporal lobe spike activity has been associated with aggression in dogs (36,37). In animals in which mood changes are extreme, partial seizure activity resulting in episodic dyscontrol may mimic dominance aggression. Other behavior abnormalities may also be observed, including extreme fear, spinning/tail chasing, increased sensitivity to light and sound, hyperactivity, licking at paws and flanks, and snapping at nonexistent flies (38,39).

Episodic dyscontrol is usually first observed around puberty or in young adult dogs and generally increases in intensity with age. Aggression is usually described by owners as explosive and occurs in response to trivial or inapparent stimulation. Typically, the pupils dilate and the eyes glaze over. Salivation, vomiting, urination, and/or defecation may accompany the outbursts. The animal may appear lethargic and less responsive prior to an outburst, and will generally sleep and be unresponsive for long periods afterwards. Multiple, epileptiform spikes are typically recorded over the temporal lobe area, although the size and prominence of the canine zygomatic arch makes recording difficult in this region.

Episodic dyscontrol appears particularly common in certain breeds (Bull Terriers, Springer Spaniels, Cocker Spaniels) and, as with tonic-clonic seizures, appears to be inherited, in some cases at least (40). Tonic-clonic seizures are associated with increased aggression both during the seizure and in the postictal period; these too may be inherited in some breeds (41–43). Owners should be advised not to breed dogs with these conditions. The "rage syndrome" that has been described in Springer Spaniels is probably due to episodic dyscontrol. Beaver (44) has described a mental lapse syndrome that appears to result in similar displays of aggression, although the associated EEG patterns are somewhat different.

Treatment

Treatment of dogs with episodic dyscontrol is primarily aimed at controlling seizure activity. Phenobarbital (2–10 mg/kg PO q12 h) is probably the drug of first choice (37). As dogs develop tolerance to phenobarbital, it may be necessary to increase the dose. High plasma levels of phenobarbital may produce a temporary sedative effect, but this is generally short lived. In humans, anticonvulsants may increase aggression and cause hyperactivity in some patients (45). We have seen this in some veterinary patients but have found that reducing the phenobarbital dose and then increasing it gradually generally resolves the problem. Three tail-chasing Bull Terriers treated with phenobarbital by Dodman et al (38) subsequently had to be euthanatized when they developed severe aggression in conjunction with tail chasing. As this phenomenon has also been observed in untreated dogs, it probably reflects a progression in seizure activity rather than a response to phenobarbital.

Potassium bromide or sodium bromide may be given in conjunction with phenobarbital. An initial loading dose 350–600 mg/kg is divided into at least four doses given no less than 3 hours apart, followed by a maintenance dose of 30–120 mg/kg q24 h divided into two equal doses. Blood levels of 3.0 to 3.5 mg/mL in conjunction with phenobarbital, or 3.0 to 4.5 mg/mL alone are recommended for seizure control.

Diazepam is a useful anticonvulsant, but due to its short half-life and the rapid development of tolerance its use is more limited than that of phenobarbital. Rectally administered diazepam (0.5 mg/kg) has been used successfully to treat cluster seizures (46) and may be useful in the management of partial seizures, particularly for animals exhibiting preictal signs.

Valproate and carbamazepine are the current drugs of choice for control of human epilepsy. The latter also has mood-stabilizing properties and has been used to treat aggression resulting from schizophrenia and depression (47). Unfortunately, the half-life of both of these drugs is very short in dogs (valproic acid has a $t_{1/2}$ of 1.5–2.8 hours in dogs vs. 5–20 hours in humans). Canine doses of valproic acid of 30–200 mg/kg PO q8 h have been recommended, and it may be most useful as an adjunct to phenobarbital in the treatment of refractory cases. Like phenobarbital, valproic acid is hepatotoxic.

Phenytoin has been recommended for treatment of episodic dyscontrol in human patients (48). Phenytoin is poorly absorbed and has a short half-life in dogs, while in cats the long half-life makes overdosage more likely. Phenytoin is not recommended for use in cats, as they are liable to develop cerebellar ataxia. Phenytoin can also be used with phenobarbital; however, this combination enhances its hepatotoxic potential. The canine dose of phenytoin is 15–40 mg/kg PO q8 h. Dogs exhibiting episodic dyscontrol may also be dominant-aggressive, so that behavior modification aimed at treating dominance, while ineffective for controlling seizure activity, may be a helpful adjunct. Serotonin reuptake inhibitors may likewise produce some positive effects but do not

---

Case Study 3.1. Episodic dyscontrol

Signalment. A 45 lb, 6-year-old, intact female, Springer Spaniel.

Problem. Three aggressive attacks on her owners at approximately monthly intervals. These had resulted in serious bite wounds on two of the three occasions; the same would have occurred on the third had the dog not been restrained with a blanket by the male owner and removed to another part of the house. The dog was otherwise a wonderful pet and had shown no other signs of aggression or even dominant or fearful behavior. On each of the three occasions, the dog had vomited her breakfast and had developed a glassy look in her eyes. The owner described her as appearing disoriented during the attacks, and quiet for prolonged periods afterward. She showed no evidence of recognizing the owners when she attacked them.

Comments. While it is possible that the dog was guarding a valued resource (her vomited food), the owner's description of her behavior preceding, during, and after each episode suggest that she was actually exhibiting episodic dyscontrol (rage). The dog had also vomited earlier in her life and had made no attempt to protect the vomit.

Therapy. None was initiated. Given that there had only been three incidents and the owners now knew not to approach within 20 feet (the previous range of her attacks) when she vomited, we decided to observe and record any further episodes before initiating treatment with phenobarbital. In 6 months, there have been no more incidents. On one occasion, the dog vomited a small quantity of grass but exhibited no abnormal behavior at that time.

---

generally extinguish the aggressive behavior entirely. See Case Study 3.1 for an example of episodic dyscontrol.

FELINE HYPERESTHESIA SYNDROME

This condition has also been called "rolling skin" disease, neurodermatitis, neuritis, feline psychomotor epilepsy, and pruritic dermatitis of Siamese cats (49,50). While it may be more common in Siamese or Siamese crosses, it has been reported in a number of different purebreeds as well as domestic long and short hairs. The condition usually occurs in young cats between 1 and 5 years old and affects both sexes equally. There is no seasonal variation in its expression, although attacks occur more commonly in the evening or early morning hours.

Many of the associated behaviors occur in all cats, but in cats with feline hyperesthesia they are taken to extremes and interfere with normal activities. The skin over the lumbar region ripples, and the cat turns to look at its tail, which may be held stiffly erect. This escalates to growling at and attacking the tail to the point where such serious damage is inflicted that it may be necessary to amputate the tail; such action is not curative, as the cat may continue to attack the stump or tailhead. Some cats also attack the flank or pelvis. Cats are often restless, constantly wandering and pacing and frequently very vocal. This may be interrupted by periods of violent licking of the forelegs or chewing the claws. During attacks, the pupils are dilated, the eyes become glassy, and the cat may rush around attacking objects and people indiscriminantly. Alternatively, cats that are normally aggressive, may become unusually affectionate during bouts of feline hyperesthesia. Some affected cats appear nervous and have been described as either bewitched or hallucinating, and some may exhibit uncontrolled urination and/or defecation. Definite prodromal signs may precede frank seizures.

The frequency of attacks can vary from almost constant to relatively infrequent, and affected cats generally appear to be normal between episodes. Some cats show EEG abnormalities, including slow waves, dysrhythmias, and spike discharges. Others may be hyperthermic; however, there is no leukocytosis suggesting this may be due to increased muscular activity.

Hyperesthesia is also observed in cats suffering from pansteatitis resulting from vitamin E deficiency (51). Yellow pigment is deposited in fat cells, causing them to become inflamed and undergo necrosis. These changes in the subcutaneous fat layer cause the increased skin sensitivity. The condition is primarily seen in cats fed canned red-meat tuna, although even small amounts of certain fish can result in vitamin E deficiency. The problem should be ruled out when treating feline hyperesthesia. See Case Study 3.2 for an example of feline hyperesthesia.

Case Study 3.2. Feline hyperesthesia

Signalment. A 13 lb, 4.8-year-old, castrated male domestic short hair, inside-outside cat.

Problem. Spraying urine in house for approximately 1 year; past few months had begun to attack tip of tail visciously and had bitten through to the bone. The owner had noticed skin-rippling preceding the tail chasing. The cat would sometimes attack his flanks and chew on his claws. The owner noted a stiff, twitching tail, and hissing at tail preceding attacks. The cat's aggression was sometimes directed at owner if she intervened.

Previous therapy. Buspirone 5 mg PO q24 h had possibly reduced spraying slightly. (NB: This is far less than the recommended dose for this cat; recommended dose is 12–24 mg q12 h).

Therapy. Withdraw buspirone. Administer one-seventh of a 20 mg fluoxetine capsule q24 h, which was later increased to 5 mg fluoxetine q24 h.

Outcome. After an initial increase in spraying when buspirone was withdrawn, spraying diminished on fluoxetine and was eventually eliminated after the dose was increased. Tail chasing became more playful and less vicious. The owner also noticed that the cat was less likely to chase his tail if he was able to spend more time outside; the cat chased his tail more on wet or snowy days when he could not or did not want to go outside. Playing with a cat dancer-type toy reduced some of the aggressive attacks on the tail. After increasing the dose of fluoxetine, the owner reported that the tail chasing virtually disappeared, and when it did occur it was no longer preceded by skin-rippling but seemed to represent a play/grooming behavior only.

Treatment

Feline hyperesthesia has been treated as a partial seizure disorder and has been effectively treated with both phenobarbital (4–10 mg/kg PO q24h, divided q8h or q12h) and primidone (0.5–3.0 mg/kg PO q8h, q12h, or q24h as needed) (49,52). We have controlled some cases using serotonin reuptake inhibitors. Both clomipramine (1–2 mg/kg PO q24h) and fluoxetine (0.5 mg/kg PO q24h) seem to be effective.

Infectious Causes of Aggression

Viral, protozoal, bacterial, and fungal diseases, as well as certain parasites can produce diffuse or focal lesions within the brain. The signs associated with these conditions can include aggression when particular areas of the brain are affected.

VIRAL INFECTIONS

These are perhaps the most common infectious cause of aggression. Table 3.1 summarizes information on eight viruses that may produce aggression in affected animals (53–61). Unfortunately, there is little that can be done pharmacologically for most of these conditions.

BACTERIAL INFECTIONS

Bacteria may form abscesses in the brain, that is, areas of necrosis and suppuration. These are infrequently seen in small animals but are quite common in horses as a response to *Streptococcus equi*. In cattle, purulent sinusitis can result in abscesses caused by *Actinomyces pyogenes*, and infection with *Bacteroides* spp. has been reported. Dysfunction is usually slow in onset and results in unilateral compression of the cerebral cortex, with functional loss of one or both occipital lobes and resulting visual deficits. Only as the abscess further increases in size are aggression and other more general cortical signs seen. These may include head-tilt toward the side of the lesion, circling, head-pressing, mania or depression, convulsions, and coma.

Treatment

Surgery, in conjunction with appropriate antibiotic therapy, may be required to treat advanced cases (62). Gram stains of CSF smears are used to determine which antibiotic to use. Penetrance of the blood-brain barrier must also be considered, and doses of antibiotic may need to be higher than for nonbrain infections. Penicillin G produces CSF concentrations of only 10% of those found elsewhere in the body. At high doses (up to 100,000 IU/kg IVq4h), it may still prove effective against susceptible *Streptococcus* spp., particularly if administered in conjunction with probenecid. Ampicillin (150–200 mg/kg IV q8h) may also be effective. For gram-negative infections, third-generation

Table 3.1. Viral diseases which may cause aggression

Disease	Type	Species affected	Mode of transmission
Rabies	Rhabdovirus/Lyssavirus	Most (all?) mammals	Bite wounds primarily
Pseudorabies	Herpesvirus	Endemic in pigs; usually asymptomatic in adults; may be fatal in young. Also dogs, cats, cattle, sheep, goats	Carnivores: eat infected tissues Ruminants: oral, intranasal, subcutaneous, or intradermal infection
Feline immunodeficiency virus	Retrovirus/Lentivirus	Cats, especially older (than 5 years), males	Saliva from bite wounds; kittens in utero; postnatal from queen
Equine alphavirus encephalitis (Eastern, Western, Venezuelan encephalomyelitis)	Togaviridae	Horses	Insect vectors (mosquitoes, etc.); transmit from primary, avian reservoir
Malignant catarrhal fever	Herpesvirus	Cattle, deer	From sheep, wildebeests, or asymptomatic carriers in vicinity
Scrapie	Prion	Sheep and goats (similar disease in elk, mule deer, mink); incubation time 1–7 yr	Primarily oral, placenta of affected animals is infectious
Bovine spongiform encephalopathy (BSE)	Prion	Cattle	Attributed to feeding scrapie-infected sheep
Encephalomyelitis of cattle	Paramyxovirus	Cattle (Southern Germany and Switzerland	Inhalation
Infectious Canine Distemper Viral Encephalitis (CDVE)	Paramyxovirus	Dogs and wild canids also infects sea lions, lions, tigers, ferrets, and other Mustelidae (e.g. raccoons), Procyanidae and some Viveridae susceptible to distemper	Inhalation postvaccine

Compiled with data from references (26,53–61), and Fenner WR. Diseases of the brain. In Ettinger SJ, Feldmam EC (eds). Textbook of Veterinary Internal Medicine, diseases of the dog and cat, fourth edition. Philadelphia, PA, W.B. Saunders 1995:578–629.

cephalosporins (e.g., moxalactam, cefotaxime, ceftazidime) are probably the most effective drugs, but cost limits their use. Trimethoprim sulfonamide is useful in horses, but not in adult ruminants, due to digestion in the ruminoreticulum; the equine dose is 15–24 mg/kg IV q4–8 h.

Antibiotic therapy should be continued for 10–14 days. Animals should

Prevention	Therapy	Other associated behaviors	Comments
Vaccine	None	Pica, hypersexuality, intense pruritus leading to hair loss and deep ulcers	Aggression may be directed toward objects, humans, and/or other animals; may be a response to mild auditory or visual stimulation
Separate pigs from other species	None	Intense pruritus and self-mutilation; restlessness, salivation, and vocalization	Often presents as unexplained death
Confine cats to house	Azidothymidine, human recombinant alpha interferon, and phosphonylmexoxyethyl adenine have been suggested; rarely, if ever, attempted	Dementia, inappropriate elimination	Approximately 30% of affected cats have primarily neurologic signs
Vaccines; reduction of insect population, screens, spray	Good nursing care; diazepam, phenobarbital, or phenytoin for seizures; NSAIDs and corticosteroids may help	Hyperesthesia, hyperexcitability, constant chewing, pacing; may become frantic in response to mild auditory/tactile stimulation	Conscious proprioceptive deficits and cranial nerve damage are common. Residual deficits including abnormal social behavior are common, especially in EEE; VEE is a reportable disease in the U.S. Mortality: 57–90% EEE; 19–50% WEE (in VEE, usually animal dies before CNS signs are seen)
Keep cattle away from sheep and wildebeests; separate sick from healthy animals	None	Rage, obtundation, convulsions, continual chewing, pacing, bellowing	High mortality rate
Do not use contaminated pasture	Slaughter affected animals; quarantine or slaughter herd; do not use meat	Withdrawal from flock; intense pruritus; bite and lick flanks (sheep); cutaneous hypersensitivity (goats); nervousness	It is suggested that Creutzfeldt-Jakob disease (CJD) and kuru may be related to eating brains/eyes of affected sheep; injection of monkeys with brains of infected animals has produced disease indistinguishable from CJD; reportable in the U.S. and Canada
Slaughter	Slaughter	Apprehension, hyperesthesia, occasionally frenzied	Recent threefold increase in occurrence of CJD in Great Britain has been linked to consumption of meat from cattle with BSE (first recognized in 1986)
Slaughter		Salivation, hyperexcitability, bellowing, seizures	
Vaccine	Support fluid balance, antibiotics to prevent 2° bacterial infection, antipyretics, analgesics, anticonvulsants. Prognosis guarded.	Seizures, dementia, ataxia, severe personality changes	Young dogs (6–12 weeks), immature dogs (1–10 day post vaccination. Older dogs 1° white matter disease with cerebellar-vestibular signs

be observed closely for 3 weeks after therapy, as a recurrence of signs necessitates either increasing the dose or changing to a different antibiotic. Patients require: 1) supportive therapy, including sedation and other precautions to prevent self-injury; 2) fluid therapy; 3) analgesia if necessary; and, if they experience seizures, 4) either diazepam (0.01–0.40 mg/kg IV prn) or phenobarbital (20 mg/kg slowly IV in saline over 30 min once; then 2.2 mg/kg IV q24 h).

PROTOZOAL INFECTIONS

Toxoplasma gondii is a protozoan that can cause infection in most mammals, as well as fish, amphibians, and reptiles, although it is more common in dogs and cats. Cats, both domestic and otherwise, are the definitive hosts, and about 40% (range 0–100% depending on region) test seropositive for the protozoan. Carnivores usually acquire the disease in the form of bradyzoites encysted in an intermediate host, while herbivores obtain the disease via the fecal-oral route, after they eat sporulated oocysts excreted by cats. If a pregnant animal becomes infected, tachyzoites multiply in the placenta and are passed to the fetus; this form of infection is of particular concern in small ruminants and humans. While infection is common, disease is relatively rare, being most prevalent in immunosuppressed and young animals. In cats, any organ system can be affected, including the CNS; in other species, there may be a severe, often fatal, multisystemic disease, or one localized to the central or peripheral nervous system. Neurologic symptoms depend upon where the parasite becomes localized. In puppies, lower motor neuron disease is more common, while in adult dogs hyperexcitability, aggression, depression, tremors, paresis/paralysis, and seizures are seen more often.

Neosporum caninum is an intracellular protozoan that produces presenting signs similar to those of *T. gondii* and can be transmitted transplacentally in dogs and cats. Toxoplasmosis is diagnosed by serologic enzyme-linked immunosorbent assay (ELISA) testing, while definitive diagnosis of neosporosis requires demonstration of *Neospora* tachyzoites in tissue cysts or CSF.

Treatment

Clindamycin (12.5 mg/kg PO or IM q12 h) is the drug of choice to treat clinical toxoplasmosis. Clinical signs start to resolve in 24 to 48 hours after treatment is initiated. Clindamycin has been used to treat neosporosis, although it is not always effective. Toxoplasmosis is a zoonotic concern for patients suffering from AIDS and also for pregnant women, who may pass the infection to the fetus.

PARASITIC INFECTIONS

In dogs and cats, various parasites may localize in the CNS as part of an aberrant migration. The most common of these are *Dirofilaria immitis* and *Cuterebra*, although *Toxascaris*, *Ancylostoma*, *Taenia*, and *Angiostrongylus* may also do so. Clinical signs depend upon where the parasites localize, with signs being focal and progressive. There is no effective therapy.

In large animal species, aberrant migration is usually limited to the spinal cord. An exception is the invasion of the CNS of sheep, goats, cattle, horses, wild ruminants, and occasionally humans by an intermediate stage of the tapeworm *Taenia multiceps*, called *Coenuris cerebralis*. Members of the dog family are the primary hosts for the tapeworm, which herbivores acquire from fecal contamination of their pasture. The parasite reaches the CNS by way of the bloodstream. Large numbers of worms can cause an encephalitis, interfere with CSF drainage, or form cysts up to 5 cm in diameter. In advanced cases, the skull over the lesion enlarges and softens. Cysts can take 6 or 7 months to develop. There is no treatment for the disease.

In Africa (Kenya and Tanzania) and India, cerebral theleriosis is caused by the piroplasma parasites *Theileria annulata* and *Theileria parva* (63). These are transmitted by ticks, and infection is usually asymptomatic or characterized by lymphadenopathy, gangrene, and skin sloughing. CNS signs are seen predominantly in calves, which are sometimes aggressive. Diagnosis is difficult, as the parasite is only sporadically found in nervous tissue, although it may occasionally be found in blood smears. Mortality is high. Treatment may be attempted with primaquine or tetracycline (6 mg/kg IV q12 h).

FUNGAL INFECTIONS

Cryptococcus neoformans is the most ubiquitous mycotic organism; however, among the neurologic signs associated with the infection, aggression has not been reported.

Space-Occupying Lesions

Tumors, abscesses, and the cysts of coenuriasis are examples of space-occupying lesions. Granulomas, accumulations of inflammatory cells, and fibrotic tissue may also be formed in an attempt to remove or neutralize irritants such as fungi, protozoa, foreign bodies, or parasites. They may be solitary or multifocal and are slowly progressive. Adjacent tissue becomes edematous and inflamed.

GRANULOMATOUS MENINGOENCEPHALITIS (GME)

GME is an idiopathic, inflammatory disease of the CNS of dogs. It is characterized by large perivascular accumulations of mononuclear cells throughout the brain, spinal cord, and meninges, primarily affecting the white matter. These accumulations compress and invade the adjacent tissue. The disease may be focal, disseminated, or ocular. The focal form produces a space-occupying lesion. The disease occurs most often in small breed dogs, especially Poodles and Airedale Terriers. Affected dogs are usually young, but the age range for onset is about 1 to 10 years, with females being affected more often. Clinical signs depend upon the location of the lesion(s), but include seizures, aggression, and other behavior changes when the cerebrum is affected. The onset is often acute and signs are progressive over days or months. Antemortem diagnosis is difficult, but there is generally both an elevated white blood cell count (>1000 WBC/μL) and increased protein concentration in the CSF. Corticosteroids (prednisolone, 1–2 mg/kg PO q24h) may provide symptomatic relief, but there is no therapy for the primary disease. Clinical remission of greater than 1 year has been achieved, but signs recur if treatment is discontinued.

BRAIN TUMORS

As in GME, brain tumors produce clinical signs when the proliferating neoplastic tissue compresses and replaces normal brain parenchyma. Most tumors are of slow onset and produce focally progressive lesions. Secondary vascular damage may lead to ischemia and further tissue damage. Edema, inflammation, and hydrocephalus secondary to impaired CSF drainage are further complications. Metastatic brain tumors are rarely seen in veterinary medicine but may be solitary or multifocal and are generally peripherally located. Primary tumors are generally solitary, except for feline meningiomas. Animals with brain tumors are usually middle-aged or older, their clinical presentation reflecting the location of the tumor. Seizures are the most commonly observed symptom, occurring in approximately 50% of cases. Aggression in conjunction with neoplasms has not been noted in the veterinary literature, although one cat treated at our clinic presented for aggression that resulted from a cerebral tumor.

Nutritional Causes of Aggression

POLIOENCEPHALOMALACIA

This disease of ruminants is caused by abnormal thiamine metabolism. It can occur spontaneously or as a result of grain engorgement and is particularly prevalent in goats fed a sudden excess of carbohydrates. Signs may be acute or may develop over several days. Animals become anorexic, have diarrhea and muscle tremors, and may become obtunded or excited and aggressive, as well as showing other cerebral and vestibular signs. Mild stimulation produces tonic-clonic seizures. The animals may become recumbent and develop secondary brain-stem changes. Thiamine diphosphate is a coenzyme in the pathway whereby nervous tissue metabolizes glucose. The defect results in a lack of adenosine triphosphate (ATP), and the failure of ATP-dependent sodium and water pumps causes intraneuronal swelling, which in turn increases intracranial pressure and produces neuronal necrosis. Thiamine deficiency results in a reduction in reuptake of the neurotransmitters serotonin, aspartate, and glutamate.

Ruminants normally produce thiamine in their rumens. Reduction of ruminal thiamine can occur in a number of ways. The most common are due to bacterial thiaminases produced by certain bacteria or the ingestion of forage rich in thiaminases, such as bracken fern (*Pteridium aquilinum*) rhizomes. Impaired thiamine absorption, increased excretion, or decreased ruminal production are less frequent causes of the condition. Certain veterinary drugs (including piperazine, acepromazine, levamisole, and thiabendazole) metabolize to picolinium compounds that act as cosubstrates for thiaminase I, which is produced by *Bacillus thiaminolyticus* or *Clostridium sporogenes*. Thiaminases need a cosubstrate in order to cleave thiamine. Other drugs, such as amprolium (a coccidiostat used in poultry and calves), are inactive thiamine analogs, and prolonged feeding can result in polioencephalomalacia. Urea and molasses-enriched diets deplete thiamine precursors and will cause the condition, as will cobalt deficiency, excessive sulfate, or feeding thiamine-deficient milk to young animals. Sheep that graze excessively on Nardoo fern (*Marsilea drummondii*) are also susceptible, as the fern is thought to contain a form of thiaminase I.

Treatment

Treatment success depends on the severity of the condition. Unless irreversible damage has occurred, signs rapidly disappear when treatment is initiated. Thiamine antagonists must be removed both from feed and from the animal's system. In the meantime, thiamine may be administered (10 mg/kg IV, then 10 mg/kg IM q12h for 3 days). If there is no improvement, slaughter is recommended (64). If severely affected animals survive, they are irreversibly decorticate, often blind, and should be slaughtered without attempting treatment.

THIAMINE DEFICIENCY IN NONRUMINANTS

Horses and occasionally pigs that are fed plants containing a thiaminase may develop thiamine deficiency. Bracken fern and horsetail (*Equisetum arvense*) are not very palatable but remain toxic even when dried and fed as hay. Beets (*Beta vulgaris*) also contain thiaminases. As for cattle, treatment involves clearing the thiaminase from the animal's system and parenteral administration of thiamine hydrochloride. Horses should receive 100–1000 mg and swine, 5–100 mg IV, IM, or SQ, depending on the formulation (65).

Dogs, cats, and mink fed predominantly raw tuna, salmon, carp, or a variety of other fresh and saltwater fish are susceptible to thiamine deficiency, as these fish contain a thiaminase. Thiamine is widely available in most vegetables and legumes as well as in liver, kidney, heart, and muscle, so thiamine deficiency is otherwise unlikely. Onset is usually sudden and progressive, and the symptoms are similar to those seen in ruminants with polioen-cephalomalacia. If treated early, the animals recover completely; otherwise, the disease is fatal. Treatment consists of thiamine hydrochloride (dogs: 5–50 mg; cats: 1–20 mg IV, IM, or SQ, depending on formulation). This may be repeated q8h until signs regress. If the animal is then placed on a nutritionally balanced diet and is not anorexic, further thiamine supplementation may not be necessary. After the animal has recovered, 4 mg/kg for cats and 2 mg/kg for dogs may be given q24h for 3 weeks (65).

PROTEIN AND AGGRESSION

It has been suggested by several dog trainers that high protein levels contribute to aggressive behavior in dogs. Dodman et al (66) fed dogs diagnosed with dominant aggression, territorial aggression, and hyperactivity, diets with low (17%), medium (25%), and high (32%) protein levels. The 12 dogs in each behavior problem group were compared with a control group of dogs with no reported behavior problems. Dogs showing territorial aggression related to fear exhibited far fewer aggressive episodes on the low and medium protein diets. It was postulated that when dietary protein levels are low, more of the amino acid tryptophan crosses the blood-brain barrier, as there is less competition from other large neutral amino acids (the concentration of which is higher in high protein diets) for transportation. Tryptophan is converted into the neurotransmitter serotonin. It is also converted to several other neurally active metabolites along the kynurenine pathway, and one or more of these may be involved in the observed behavioral effect. It is possible that a more radical reduction in dietary protein levels would produce a reduction in dominance aggression and hyperactivity as well.

Toxins

LEUKOENCEPHALOMALACIA

This is a highly fatal disease of horses caused by ingestion of corn infected with the fungus *Fusarium moniliforme*. Other names for the disease include moldy corn disease and blind staggers. The condition has a sudden onset, and some animals die without showing any signs. In less acute cases, animals become aggressive, hyperexcitable, and may have seizures and show other cerebral signs. Animals may become comatose in 1 to 10 days. Focal lesions of the white matter of one or both cerebral cortices are found at necropsy, with lesions ranging from 0.5 cm in diameter to complete necrosis. The gyri are flattened, while the blood vessels tend to be engorged and may rupture. The cortex is soft and has a yellowish discoloration; cavitatory lesions may be filled with a gelatinous fluid (67,68). There is no effective treatment.

LEAD POISONING

It has recently been reported (69) that aggression, hyperactivity, and delinquent behavior in 11-year-old boys correlated with bone lead levels, and that these behavior problems existed even with lead levels below those previously considered toxic. Lead is toxic to all veterinary species; however, dogs and cattle are most likely to be affected, as they have greater access to lead. Lead can be ingested from a great number of sources. Animals exposed to lead also excrete it in their milk, and the young are more susceptible to the toxic effects than older animals. In most species, chronic lead exposure leads to gastrointestinal signs, which precede neurologic problems. However, ruminants generally only show neurologic signs. Behavioral signs include aggression, anxiety, hyperexcitability, increased vocalization, extreme fear, eye rolling, head pressing, and frenzied jumping and movement. Sheep and horses tend to show symptoms of muscular paralysis and spasms. Locomotive and autonomic disturbances are also observed. Lead readily crosses both the blood-brain and placental barriers. It also damages the blood-brain barrier, enabling other toxins to enter the brain. The behavioral signs of lead poisoning are thought to be due to inhibition of adenylcyclase and acetylcholinesterase (70,71). Lead also decreases cellular energy production and alters membrane calcium, sodium, and potassium ion distribution. Gross damage may include dilation or rupture of cerebral blood vessels; scattered areas of necrosis in the cerebral cortex, brain stem, and cerebellum; proliferation of cortical grey matter; gliosis; vacuolation; and fibrin deposition.

Treatment

It may be necessary to surgically remove solid lead objects from the gastrointestinal tract to prevent further exposure. A magnesium or sodium sulfate cathartic may be used if the lead is more diffuse. Systemic lead may be chelated with disodium calcium ethylenediamine tetraacetate (Caversenate). The resulting complex is soluble and is excreted in urine. For large animals, a 6.6% solution is given intravenously, at a dose of 73 mg/kg per 24 hours, which is divided into 2 to 3 daily doses or administered as part of a slow IV drip for 3 to 5 days. Only the lead in bone is chelated, and after a 2-day rest to allow redistribution of lead from the soft tissues, the therapy may be repeated. Small animals are given a 1% (10 mg/ml) solution diluted in saline or 5% dextrose. This may be administered subcutaneously at 27.5 mg/kg q6h or 50 mg/kg q12h for 5 days. After 5 days without treatment, another 5-day regimen may be given if necessary. Prolonged chelation may cause depletion of other body metals such as zinc and copper, and these may need to be supplemented (72). Succimer (*meso*-2,3-

dimercaptosuccinic acid), at a dose of 10 mg/kg PO q8h for 10 days, has proven very effective in treating canine lead poisoning (72).

ORGANOPHOSPHATE PESTICIDES

A variety of organophosphates are used as contact insecticides and acaricides, animal systemic/topical insecticides and parasiticides, plant systemic insecticides, soil nematocides, fungicides, herbicides and defoliants, and rodenticides. Animals can be exposed to these pesticides in many ways. Feeds can be contaminated either before or after harvest. Animal premises or the animals themselves may be sprayed, dusted, or painted with too much pesticide. Systemic parasitic compounds may be overdosed or have an additive or synergistic effect with other pesticides. Drinking water may also be contaminated. Species, breed, sex, age, and immune status all affect an animal's susceptibility to a particular organophosphate. Different products have different toxicities. While most organophosphates dissipate from the environment in 2 to 4 weeks, others may persist for more than 6 months. Acute toxicosis is due to irreversible inhibition of acetylcholinesterase (AChE). Behavioral, motor, and muscle stimulation are the predominant signs seen, and death may occur from respiratory failure. If an animal survives acute toxicosis, muscle weakness and ataxia may ensue. This is most prevalent in the rear limbs, but it may progress to such a point that the animal cannot elevate the head and neck enough to eat or drink.

Treatment

Many of the central and peripheral effects of organophosphates can be blocked by atropine sulfate (0.2–0.5 mg/kg, one-fourth given IV and the rest IM or SQ). This should be repeated every 3 to 6 hours as needed for 24 hours or more. Atropine levels are adequate if the animal has dilated pupils, stops salivating, and appears to be recovering. Overdosage can result in excitation, hypermotility, and signs of delirium. Because atropine does not affect the nicotinic cholinergic effects, the animal will continue to shiver and twitch. Unless these symptoms become severe, they are best left untreated, as antinicotinic agents would increase the risk of respiratory paralysis. If the animal is becoming paralyzed as a result of nicotinic stimulation, 2-pyridine aldoxime methiodide (2-PAM) may be administered. For small animals, the dose is 20–50 mg/kg given as a 10% solution IM or by slow IV injection. For large animals, the dose is 25–50 mg/kg given as a 20% solution IV over 6 minutes, or 100 mg/kg given by IV drip. 2-PAM does not work against all organophosphates, may work slowly against those still being absorbed, and in large amounts has anti-AChE activity, which could worsen the toxicosis.

Affected animals require oxygen if they become cyanotic. Any organophosphate still present should be washed from the skin. Mineral oil will reduce

Table 3.2. Other toxic causes of aggression

Toxic compound	Mode of action	Species affected	Other behavioral signs	Treatment
Zinc phosphide (rodenticide)	CNS stimulation	Dogs (other species only GI symptoms)	Aimless running, howling, snapping, snarling, seizures	Empty GI tract; lavage with 5% sodium bicarbonate; barbiturates for seizures
Salt poisoning	Water deprivation and/or excess salt intake; Na$^+$ overwhelm sodium transport pump and accumulate in CSF and neurons	All, especially swine and poultry	Hyperexcitability, stargazing, vocalization, seizures	1:1 Lactated Ringer's solution: 5% glucose solution, 40–80 mL/kg IV; furosemide, 1 mg/kg ±; dexamethasone, 0.4–0.8 mg/kg; q12h × 2–3 days; then small amounts ion-free water
Chlorinated hydrocarbon pesticides (e.g., DDT, aldrin, chlordane)	CNS stimulation by decreasing transmembrane resting potential and firing threshold	All	Abnormal postures, frenzied movements, seizures	Phenobarbital, 40 mg/kg; activated charcoal; remove source
Ergot alkaloids (*Claviceps purpurea* and *C. paspali*)	Chemically similar to serotonin; probably cause central neurotransmitter imbalance	All	Staggering, excess limb flexion, seizures	Remove contaminated feed; diazepam for seizures: cattle, 0.5–1.5 mg/kg IM or IV; horse (adult), 25–50 mg IV repeat in 30 mins if necessary, goats, 0.8 mg/kg IV; oral magnesium sulfate: cattle, 1–2 g/kg; horse, 500 g as 20% solution

Na$^+$ = sodium ions; DDT = dichlorodiphenyltrichloroethane.

absorption of any organophosphate still present in the intestinal tract. Supportive fluid therapy may be required. Labels should be carefully examined in any case in which organophosphate poisoning is suspected. Carbamates have similar uses to the organophosphates; they are also AChE inhibitors, and toxicosis can be treated in the same way.

OTHER TOXINS

These are summarized in Table 3.2 and represent less common causes of aggression.

Storage Diseases

MANNOSIDOSIS

Normal neurons are constantly degrading and resynthesizing glycolipids and glycoproteins. A defect in the enzyme alpha-mannosidase results in an autosomal recessive trait called α-mannosidosis. The undigested mannose and N-acetylglucosamine tetrasaccharides accumulate in the lysosomes, causing neuronal dysfunction. The disease is seen in Angus, Holstein, Simmental, Galloway, and Murray Grey cattle. Affected calves tend to grow more slowly than normal, but clinical signs are not apparent until 1 to 15 months of age. A mild ataxia of the pelvic limbs after exercise is generally the first indication of the disease. Cerebellar signs may also be observed. Aggression is very consistent for this storage disease. Signs become worse with stress. Generally cattle are recumbent within 3 to 4 months of onset, although they have been known to survive for 4 years. Although there is no treatment for the disease, blood tests that measure the concentration of acidic α-mannosidase in the blood are available and permit identification of heterozygote carriers (less than 30–40% the level of normal controls) of the disease.

Animals that chronically ingest leguminous plants of the genera *Astragalus*, *Oxytropis*, and *Swainsona* spp. (various locoweeds) develop very similar lesions, due to inhibition of lysosomal α-mannosidase (73). Although horses, cattle, goats, and sheep may all be affected, aggression is more likely to be seen in the horse. There is no proven therapy for locoweed poisoning, and animals remain affected for long periods after removal from the plants. Horses that recover tend to retain behavioral abnormalities and are extremely unpredictable.

FUCOSIDOSIS

An inherited deficiency of the enzyme α-L-fucosidase results in the accumulation of fucose-containing glycolipids, glycopeptides, and oligosaccharides in cells throughout the body. The disease has been reported in English Springer Spaniels as well as in human beings. Primary symptoms are neurologic and include confusion, inability to recognize the owner, and generalized seizures. Although fear is the predominant behavioral sign, this frequently leads to aggression when attempts are made to handle or physically restrain the dog. The disease is chronically progressive and invariably fatal. Alpha-L-fucosidase activity should be checked in all related animals. Homozygous affected dogs have less than 5% of the enzyme activity seen in homozygous normal animals, while heterozygous carrier levels are normally about 50% of those of normal dogs. However, as the distinction between normals and carriers is not clear-cut, it is recommended that no animal with subnormal levels be used for breeding. Affected dogs have been traced to a single common ancestor in the United Kingdom (74).

Encephalopathies

HEPATIC ENCEPHALOPATHY

Animals of all species with severe liver disease and/or portosystemic shunts may develop abnormal neurobehavioral signs. These are very variable among patients, but include disorientation, aggression, pacing, circling, head pressing, weakness, collapse, seizures, and coma. Onset can be abrupt or gradual: some animals have apparently normal intervals of behavior, while others remain lethargic and dull. High brain ammonia levels appear to be at least partly responsible for the syndrome, which is exacerbated by meat-rich diets. However, multiple factors are involved, and their interactions and sometimes synergistic effects cause the variability of signs observed. Plasma amino acid levels are altered, with an increase in aromatic amino acids (tyrosine and phenylalanine), and a decrease in short-branched chain amino acids (valine, leucine, isoleucine). In addition, endogenous benzodiazepine (BZD)-like substance levels increase in plasma and CSF. Endogenous BZDs bind to GABA receptors, and hyperpolarize cell membranes, making the cells less reactive (75). BZD antagonists such as flumazenil may relieve some of the symptoms of hepatic encephalopathy (76). In general, resolution of the underlying liver disease reverses the signs of encephalopathy. Carnivores fed soy and dairy protein-based diets show a diminution of symptoms. Gastrointestinal bleeding increases blood ammonia levels in patients with liver disease and worsens the severity of the encephalopathy, as do infection and inflammation, which increase catabolism.

Ruminants are particularly susceptible to excessive dietary urea, which is sometimes used as a source of protein in cattle ration formulations. In the rumen (or the cecum of horses), urea is cleaved to ammonia and carbon dioxide. Symptoms resemble those of hepatic encephalopathy.

FELINE ISCHEMIC ENCEPHALOPATHY

This is a peracute condition, affecting adult cats of either sex at any age. It appears to occur more frequently in the summer months. The symptoms are generally of unilateral cerebral disease and are quite variable. Some cats are severely obtunded with mild paresis and ataxia, while others may exhibit tonic-clonic seizures, severe aggression, dilated pupils, and blindness. Affected cats may circle toward the side of the lesion. Symptoms are nonprogressive, usually, but postural, gait, and behavioral abnormalities remain. Seizure activity may also continue. Cats are frequently euthanatized because of their aggression. At necropsy, lesions may be multifocal or involve up to two thirds of one cerebral hemisphere. Occasionally, bilateral cerebral damage has occurred, and brainstem lesions have also been seen. Most often, lesions are found in areas supplied by the middle cerebral artery but are not restricted to this region. No other organs are affected.

Treatment

Treatment can be attempted at onset with dexamethasone (2–4 mg/kg PO q8 h × 2 days, then a gradually tapered dose) and 20% mannitol (2 mg/kg IV at onset, and repeated 3 hours later). This treatment seeks to reduce the amount of tissue damage resulting from hemorrhage and tissue edema. Persistent seizures may be treated with phenobarbital (2 mg/kg PO q8–12 h). Once the condition has stabilized, prognosis is good (77,78).

SYSTEMIC LUPUS ERYTHEMATOSUS (SLE)

This autoimmune disease is seen primarily in dogs and is rarely seen in cats and large animals. Autoantibodies to nucleic acid are characteristic of the disease; there also may be antibodies to red blood cells, platelets, lymphocytes, immunoglobulin, and thyroglobulin. One or more organ systems can be affected, making presentation variable. Deposition of immune complexes causes vasculitis most frequently in the skin or kidneys; joints, muscles, and the heart may also be affected. In humans it is estimated that 40 to 90% of patients with SLE develop CNS *lupus*, a broad term for a number of neuropsychological problems, including severe headaches, memory loss, strokes (15–20%), seizures (5–25%), and psychosis (79,80). I have seen one case of SLE in a dog, which resulted in periods of apparent disorientation and aggression. The dog appeared unable to recognize members of its canine and human family and would bite them during these episodes.

One study has shown that antibody levels to double-stranded DNA in the serum of pet dogs living with human SLE patients was similar to that of dogs with SLE, and both groups showed the same abnormalities in serum protein electrophoresis patterns in contrast to a group of healthy dogs housed in a controlled environment (81). These findings suggest that exposure to common environmental factors or transmissible agents may have a role in producing SLE.

Treatment

CNS lupus seems to respond to glucocorticoid therapy. Prednisone (1 mg/kg PO q12 h) is given until signs of clinical remission are seen. The dose is then gradually tapered to an alternate-day schedule at a level that will keep the disease in remission. For severe cases or those failing to respond to prednisone alone, cyclophosphamide (2.5 mg/kg for dogs weighing <10 kg; 2 mg/kg if 10–35 kg; and 1.5 mg/kg if >35 kg) is given PO q24 h for 4 consecutive days each week. Cyclophosphamide should be discontinued 1 month after remission has occurred.

Congenital Malformations

LISSENCEPHALY

Lissencephaly is characterized by an almost smooth brain surface, due to the failure of gyri and sulci to form. The grey matter of the cerebral cortex is thickened (pachygria) due to abnormal cellular distribution. The condition appears to be the result of abnormal neuronal migration in utero. It is a rare condition, seen most often in Lhasa Apso dogs, but has also been reported in Wire Haired Fox Terriers and Irish Setters, where the predominant lesion has been cerebellar in nature. All or part of a litter or a single individual may be affected, and there appears to be a genetic component in these breeds. In humans, intrauterine hypoxia and perfusion failure have been suggested as causes of the condition. Seizures, intermittent blindness, abnormal gait, and postural reflexes are seen together with an inability to learn and what may be extreme aggression. In one case, a Lhasa Apso bitch was reported to appear unable to recognize the owners during aggressive episodes, and to be fearful and withdrawn most of the time (82). Standard therapy may be attempted for control of seizures, but euthanasia is usually recommended for affected dogs.

HYDROCEPHALUS

Hydrocephalus is the result of an increase in the volume of CSF. It can be congenital and may either be the result of genetic abnormality or viral exposure in utero. Injury, ischemia, infarction, or inflammation can all produce degeneration of cortical tissue, which is replaced by CSF. Neoplasia or inflammation may also result in hydrocephalus by causing obstruction of CSF flow through the ventricular system. Clinical signs of hydrocephalus are variable and may even be absent. When present, signs are referrable to abnormalities of the cerebral cortex, although cerebellar or brain-stem signs may be present. Aggression has been reported, often in conjunction with seizures (38,83).

Treatment

Treatment depends on the cause of the hydrocephalus. If the cause is obstructive, pressure can be relieved by tapping the ventricles, which produces symptomatic relief. A shunt may also be placed surgically, either into the jugular vein or the peritoneal cavity. Corticosteroids (dexamethasone 2–4 mg/kg) may produce temporary relief of symptoms by reducing inflammation.

Endocrine Causes of Aggression

THE THYROID AND AGGRESSION

Both hyperthyroid cats and hypothyroid dogs may present with aggression. In human medicine, aggression has been noted in hyperthyroid as well as hypothyroid patients, although it is more common in the former. In other species, the link has not been clearly demonstrated; however, aggression is quite common in elderly equids, particularly ponies. These animals often exhibit the long, wavy, retained haircoat and/or pot-bellied appearance associated with hypothyroidism and/or Cushing's disease. I have recently been treating a 16-year-old Appaloosa gelding with severe aggression directed toward other horses and a milder aggression directed toward handlers. His total serum thyroxine (T4) level was less than 0.6 μg/dL, testosterone levels were undetectable, and estrone sulfate level was 0.25 ng/mL. Treatment with levothyroxine sodium, 12 mg PO sid, has resulted in a mellowing of his behavior toward other horses, and he no longer tries to attack them under saddle.

THE THYROID AND FELINE AGGRESSION

Aggressive behavior is manifested in 20 to 25% of cats presenting with hyperthyroidism (84; Duddy JM, personal communication, 1996). The aggression resolves completely with treatment of the thyroid disorder. Hyperthyroidism is the most common endocrine disorder seen in cats and is usually the result of either hyperplasia or an adenoma of one or both glands. There is no sex or breed predisposition, but the majority of cats are at least 10 years old before they exhibit symptoms. Cats as young as 6 years old have been found to be affected. Almost all affected cats show evidence of weight loss, despite the presence of polyphagia in the majority of cases. There may also be digestive disturbances, an unkempt coat, and/or hair loss. Most are hyperactive, although a few are lethargic. These cats are easily stressed, and when stressed may become tachypneic and/or tachycardic (>240 beats/min). Other cardiac abnormalities may include hypertrophic cardiomyopathy, gallop rhythms, pulse deficits, diminished heart sounds, and murmurs.

Aggression is often expressed when attempts are made to restrain the cat. Irritability, reduction in time spent sleeping, ease of waking, and wool sucking are other behavioral abnormalities associated with hyperthyroidism.

Focal or generalized seizures have also been described, although they are apparently quite rare. Focal seizures may occur in response to light or sound stimulation and appear similar to precipitated focal motor seizures as described in hyperthyroid humans. Seizure activity is reduced or resolves completely with treatment of hyperthyroidism (85).

Approximately 95% of affected cats have a palpably enlarged thyroid. Diagnosis can usually be confirmed by an elevated baseline T4, although in some cases, this will be in the high-normal range. If so, the condition is established with either a triiodothyronine (T3) suppression test or thyrotropin-releasing hormone (TRH) stimulation test.

The mechanism by which hyperthyroidism results in aggression is not clear. Cerebral blood flow, glucose, and oxygen consumption increase. Hyperthyroidism decreases the activity of the CNS enzymes glutamate dehydrogenase and pyruvate dehydrogenase. It also has been shown to affect several neurotransmitter receptors and their concentrations in rat brains. Beta-adrenoreceptor concentration and dopaminergic neuronal activity in the striatum both increase, as does presynaptic alpha-2 adrenoreceptor activity. The concentrations of serotonin and 5-hydroxyindoleacetic acid (5-HIAA) in certain brain nuclei are consistently increased in hyperthyroid animals, while their concentrations are elevated in other nuclei in hypothyroid animals (86,87). The concentration of substance P in these nuclei is also affected by thyroid state, but the results are less consistent. Catecholamines and thyroid hormones are both synthesized from the amino acid tyrosine and have synergistic metabolic effects. By corollary, hyperactivity in hyperthyroid cats responds to treatment with beta-blockers.

Treatment

There are three established therapeutic protocols for treating hyperthyroid cats. The preferred method is to administer radioactive iodine. Peterson (88) has established a scoring system based on the severity of clinical signs, serum T4, and size of the thyroid tumor to estimate the dose of radioiodine; this technique has proved highly (94.2%) successful. Although subnormal T4 levels were quite common after treatment, only about 2% of the treated cats required supplemental levothyroxine (L-thyroxine) to relieve clinical signs of hypothyroidism. A further 2.5% had a relapse of their original condition. Because radioiodine treatment is expensive, is only available at a limited number of facilities, and requires prolonged hospitalization (7–25 days) of elderly animals while the radioactivity clears from their bodies, many owners opt for alternative therapy.

Surgical removal of one or both lobes of the thyroid is usually successful. Presurgically, methimazole is given at a dose of 5 mg PO q8h until the cat is euthyroid. Methimazole concentrates in thyroid tissue and inhibits the synthesis of thyroid hormones by interfering with the incorporation of iodine into the thyroglobulin. Propranolol (2.5–5.0 mg PO q8–12h) helps control tachycardia and arrhythmias in cats experiencing cardiac problems. Anesthetic induction with short-acting thiobarbiturates and maintenance with isoflurane is recommended to avoid cardiac complications. If all four of the parathyroid glands are removed inadvertently, hypocalcemia may occur postoperatively; if the external parathyroid glands are intact, usually this is only temporary. Signs of hypoparathyroidism are usually seen within 12 to 120 hours. Immediate therapy with 10% calcium gluconate, 0.5–1.0 mL/kg given IV slowly, will control muscle tremors and seizures. Once the cat has stabilized, oral calcium lactate and vitamin D therapy can be initiated. Laryngeal paralysis may occur if both the recurrent laryngeal nerves are damaged during surgery. Hypertrophy of remnant tissue (or of the other gland if only one is removed) can result in recurrence of the hyperthyroid state; alternately some cats become hypothyroid and require treatment with L-thyroxine sodium (initial dose 10–20 μg/kg PO q24h, adjusted based on clinical signs and serum T4 level).

Cats may also be treated with methimazole at an initial dose of 5 mg PO q8h. If serum T4 shows little or no change after 3 weeks, the dose should be increased by 5 mg every 3 weeks until there is an appropriate response (89). It may then be possible to cut back by increments of 2.5 to 5.0 mg to give the lowest effective dose. Some cats may do well with a single dose q24h (90). Once a therapeutic response has been achieved, serum T4 levels should be monitored at 3- to 6-month intervals. The bioavailability (45–98%), volume of distribution (0.12–0.84 L/kg) and half-life (2.3–10.2 hours) of methimazole are all extremely variable (91). There is a lag of 1 to 3 weeks between initial drug administration and significant change in serum T4, as methimazole does not affect the release or activity of thyroid hormones that have already been formed and stored. Treatment with propylthiouracil is not recommended due to the high incidence of adverse side effects.

THE THYROID AND CANINE AGGRESSION

While the majority of cats with hyperthyroidism become hyperactive, approximately 10% become obtunded, lethargic, and apathetic. A similar paradox occurs in an undetermined proportion of dogs with hypothyroidism, which become hyperactive and/or aggressive instead of presenting with lethargy and mental dullness. Hypothyroidism is the most commonly diagnosed endocrine disease in dogs, and the estimated incidence is from 1:156 to 1:500. A recent survey performed by the American Kennel Club showed that hypothyroidism was the number one health concern of breed clubs. The condition is found primarily in mid- to large-sized breeds and is usually detected in animals 3 years of age and older. There are definite breed propensities, and the condition is inherited. Typical signs of hypothyroidisim include weight gain, bilaterally symmetric alopecia, hyperpigmentation, poor dry hair coat, excessive hair loss, seborrhea and other skin conditions, anestrus in intact bitches, bradycardia, cold intolerance, and anemia. Hypothyroid dogs presenting with aggression and hyperactivity typically display few of these symptoms, are often younger, and may be in the early stages of thyroiditis. In some animals, the hair coat may be dull despite good quality food and grooming; the dog may tire faster than expected; and there may be skin lesions and a history of chronic ear infections and/or reproductive problems. The dog may be lethargic or hyperactive as well as aggressive. Aggression may be characterized as dominance- or fear-related and may be directed at people (owners and/or strangers) and/or other dogs (92).

Total serum T4 levels are compensated until there has been significant destruction of thyroid tissue. As free (unbound) T4 drops, the hypothalamus releases TRH, which stimulates pituitary secretion of TSH, with the remaining thyroid tissue increasing its T4 production. As the disease progresses, T3 levels are maintained as more T4 is converted to the active form of the hormone (T3). Total T4 (TT4) and free T4 (FT4) levels are artificially elevated by T4 autoantibodies (T4aa), while T3 autoantibodies (T3aa) depress total T3 (TT3) and elevate free T3 (FT3). As a result a simple TT4 assay may fail to detect thyroiditis, especially in its early stages. The TSH-stimulation test may not detect thyroiditis until 50 to 70% of the thyroid follicular tissue has been destroyed. For this reason, to diagnose hypothyroidism in our behavior patients, we prefer to rely on a thyroid panel measuring all six analytes (TT4, FT4, TT3, FT3, T4aa, T3aa). Another good indication of thyroid disease is an elevated serum cholesterol. Although this may result from diabetes mellitus, hyperadrenocorticism, nephrotic syndrome, cholestatic disorders, or dyslipoproteinemia, hypothyroidism is by far the most common cause.

The mechanism by which low thyroid levels result in aggression is unclear. Serotonin turnover has been shown to increase in hypothyroid rats (93), and it is possible that some forms of aggression in dogs result from either low or unstable levels of serotonin in the brain. The brain's sensitivity to the neurotransmitter dopamine has also been demonstrated to be increased by hypothyroidism (94). Finally, cortisol clearance is reduced in hypothyroid animals, putting them in a constant state of stress. Elevated glucocorticoid levels further inhibit the release of TSH with a concomitant reduction in T3 and T4 production and release (95). The animal's response may reflect past experience in coping with stress, so that it may lash out aggressively at any perceived stressor, become anxious or engage in displacement behavior. Humans with hypothyroidism have a reduction in reasoning ability, and in animals this may further limit their ability to behave appropriately.

Treatment

Once hypothyroidism has been diagnosed, treatment is 0.1 mg per 4.5–6.8 kg of body weight of L-thyroxine sodium PO q12 h. This dosage reduces activity to acceptable levels, and aggression is markedly reduced or extinguished within 3 weeks (96). While we have not experienced aggressive, hypothyroid dogs that have failed to respond to L-thyroxine, there are dogs in which other clinical signs either fail to resolve or are only partially ameliorated. This appears to be due to a failure to convert T4 into T3 in the liver. In these cases, supplementing the L-thyroxine with 2.2 μg/kg of liothyronine sodium (synthetic T3) PO q8–12 h has proven effective.

While aggression in hypothyroid dogs is generally responsive to thyroid supplementation in the majority of cases, we have found that some dogs do not respond either to this or to other behavioral or pharmacological intervention. In several of these cases there is evidence of serious cerebral dysfunction resulting from a history of disease or prolonged hypoxia. See Case Study 3.3 for an example of hypothyroid interdog aggression.

Case Study 3.3.   Hypothyroid interdog aggression

Signalment. A 62 lb, 7-year-old, spayed female German Shepherd dog, owned by a professional dog trainer.

Problem. Long-term fear-aggression directed toward people and especially other dogs.

Previous therapy. Clomipramine 25 mg PO q12 h, which had no appreciable effect.

Thyroid panel. TT3: 86 ng/dL (normal range 125–225 ng/dL)
TT4: 1.39 μg/dL (normal range 3–5 μg/dL)
FT3: 2.6 pg/mL (normal range 2–4 pg/dL)
FT4: 0.92 ng/dL (normal range 2–4 ng/dL)

Therapy. Clomipramine was reduced to 25 mg PO q24 h 10 days prior to thyroid testing, with no appreciable change in behavior. After the results of the thyroid panel were received, the dog was started on levothyroxine sodium (Soloxine) 0.4 mg PO q12 h.

Outcome. The owner took the dog to a nearby park 5 days after initiation of thyroxine supplementation, and, with some trepidation, let her off leash. The dog played happily with all other dogs present, played tug-of-war with a puppy with a stick, and showed no aggression whatsoever. In subsequent weeks, the bitch lost some excess weight and shed out her coat normally (which she had not done previously). Her behavior with people and other dogs moderated. She no longer behaved like a puppy, as she had initially, but as a somewhat arthritic matron. She displayed normal "aggression" only, reprimanding a puppy for unruly behavior, but never aggressively attacked other dogs or people.

STEROID HORMONES

Testosterone

To some extent the effect of testosterone on aggression is species dependent. In most species, elevation in testosterone levels during the mating season produces an increase in aggression toward males of the same species. For those species that live alone and aggressively guard territories against both male and female animals of the same species for the majority of the year, the seasonal elevation in testosterone generally produces a reduction in aggression directed toward females of the same species. Frequently, however, aggression toward females also rises, as the male bites and/or claws at the female during the act of mating. In animals living in mixed-sex groups, both aggression and plasma levels of testosterone are significantly higher in dominant versus subordinate animals. Dominant squirrel monkeys have plasma testosterone levels ten times greater than those of subordinate males in the same colony during the mating season (202.9 ± 13.4ng/mL vs. 28 ± 6.2ng/mL); and even in the nonmating season, dominant male testosterone levels are significantly higher than those of subordinates (55.2 ± 23.7ng/mL vs. 7.3 ± 1.7ng/mL) (97).

In the stallion, dominance displays are a normal testosterone-linked characteristic. However, this aggression may become excessive and may be directed either against mares or human handlers. Stallions that strike out at both humans and mares are a more difficult problem. Exogenous progestins reduce stallion aggression (e.g., megestrol acetate, 65–85mg per 500kg horse PO q24h; repositol progesterone, 100mg per 500kg horse IM every 4 days, or 200mg per 500kg horse IM every 7 days; altrenogest, 1mL of a 0.22% solution per 500kg horse PO q24h) (98); however, as they also reduce spermatogenesis, they can only be used as part of a retraining protocol.

Elevated testosterone levels have been reported to produce an increased aggression toward other horses in mares. These animals are dominant and show other stallion-like behaviors. The elevated testosterone levels are generally the result of an ovarian granulosa cell tumor but may be produced by adrenal or pituitary abnormalities (99).

Progestins have also been used with varying success to treat aggression in male dogs and cats. Medroxyprogesterone acetate has been used at a dose of 10mg/kg IM or SQ for dogs and 10–20mg/kg SQ for cats not to exceed three treatments per year (100,101). Alternatively, an initial dose of 100mg IM, subsequently reduced by one-third to one-half, given every 30 days has been used for male cats (102). Voith and Marder (97) also suggest a dose of megesterol acetate of 1.1–2.2mg/kg PO q24h for 2 weeks, then 0.5mg/kg PO q24h for 2 weeks in conjunction with a behavior modification program for the treatment of excessive aggression in male dogs.

Although it is clearly not an option for breeding animals, castration may also be performed to control aggression. While castration is generally more effective if it is performed before the aggression appears, clinical surveys have shown a 60% and 90% reduction in canine and feline intermale aggression, respectively, following castration of adult males. In approximately two-thirds of the dogs and one-half of the cats, this behavioral change occurred rapidly (103,104). As aggression appears to be at least partially inherited, castration is frequently recommended as part of the treatment for all aggressive male animals, as it prevents perpetuating this trait through future generations.

Estrogen

Estrogen increases interfemale aggression in some animals, and ovariectomy may reduce estrus-linked interfemale aggression. One study comparing the behavior of 150 bitches preoperatively with that 6 months postspaying showed a significant increase in dominance aggression toward family members postoperatively (105). However, the effect was most marked in puppies less than 1 year old that had already shown signs of aggression. Of these, 50% showed increased aggression, but in the other half the aggression diminished. This compared to 14% showing increased aggression and 86% with reduced aggression in the unspayed control group.

Other Steroids

Endogenous and exogenous corticosteroids are normally associated with feelings of euphoria but may produce aggression in some dogs. The use of anabolic steroids (e.g., stanozolol, boldenone undecylenate, mibolerone) to treat anorexia/cachexia and unthriftiness, to inhibit estrous in adult bitches, and to increase weight gain and muscle mass in cattle has also been associated with increased aggression.

As geldings age, some show stallion-like behavior, including aggression, herding of animals pastured with them, flehmen, excessive interest in fresh manure, and even mounting. Houpt (unpublished data 1996), who refers to this constellation of signs as "sexy gelding syndrome," has suggested that the behavior may result from an adenoma of the pars intermedia of the pituitary gland, with the associated elevation of circulating adrenocorticotropic hormone (ACTH) stimulating an increase in adrenal androgen release. These tumors are relatively common in older horses, although they are seen more often in mares, and are frequently an incidental finding at necropsy. The more commonly associated signs are polydipsia/polyuria; shaggy, brittle, curly hair coat; and a swaybacked, pot-bellied appearance. Polyphagia is common, but animals lose condition despite adequate caloric intake and often experience muscle weakness (106). Recommended therapy is with cyproheptadine HCl tablets to be administered in the morning; the dose starts at 8 mg orally and gradually increases over 30 days to a maximum dose of 88 mg. Cyproheptadine has been used as an antidepressant for treating human patients. It is a potent serotonin $5\text{-}HT_2$ receptor antagonist but does not appear to affect the $5\text{-}HT_{1A}$ receptor (107).

Trauma and Aggression

CRANIAL INJURY

Cranial injury can frequently lead to aggressive behavior as a result of damage to the cerebrum or limbic system. A recent study in humans has shown that buspirone is effective in reducing trauma-induced aggression as well as nonspecific organic aggression (108). Of the twenty patients in the study, aggression was reduced in eighteen (90%), and reduction was greater than 50% in twelve (60%) of the patients. In some cases, initiation of therapy was followed by an increase in aggression, which was in turn followed by subsequent substantial reductions, but the full effect of treatment was not achieved until 3 months into the study in some cases. Therapeutic levels required were somewhat higher than those used to treat psychiatric disorders, and this may indicate reduced receptor sensitivity. Side effects were not apparent at the higher doses used. In dogs and cats suffering posttraumatic aggression, an initial dose of 4 mg/kg PO q12h is recommended.

PAIN AND AGGRESSION

Aggression as a protective response to pain appears appropriate in order to prevent further injury. The only research on this subject, however, suggests that the response is not purely defensive. Pairs of male rats exposed to electric shock showed three stages of response. Initially they attempted to escape from the chamber; in the second stage, aggression was defensive; but in the third stage, the rats began to attack each other (109). It is possible that the attacking rat perceived the other rat as the cause of pain, or the aggression may have been simply redirected. Similarly, animals suffering traumatic injury may react aggressively to those trying to help them, even before there has been an attempt to touch the animal. However, because a violation of the animal's safety zone has already occurred with its injury, defensive aggression could be postulated.

Central pain perception and modulation involve the thalamus, hypothalamus, brain stem, reticular formation, limbic system, and parietal and frontal cortices. Animals experiencing pain respond with stimulation of the sympathetic autonomic nervous system. Elevated catecholamine levels reduce the aggressive threshold (110). Animals experiencing pain respond by releasing natural opioids and neurotransmitters which produce antinociception. Serotonin is a potent antinociceptive agent. Aberrant pain perception in human patients suffering from fibromyalgia has been shown to result from a deficiency of serotonin (111). The central analgesic tramadol produces its effect by increasing the level of serotonin in neurons of the frontal cortex (112). Tricyclic antidepressants, including amitryptiline and clomipramine, have also proved effective analgesics, acting on the endogenous opioid system and via serotonergic and noradrenergic pathways (113). The use of amitryptiline or clomipramine in animals exhibiting pain-related aggression would be very appropriate, as it would address both issues. Oral L-tryptophan, a serotonin precursor, is being used experimentally in human patients for the management of chronic pain and could prove useful for veterinary patients as well (114).

Genetic Causes of Aggression

In wild, pack-living canids, only the alpha pair normally reproduce. Within the litter, a dominance hierarchy quickly becomes apparent, as it does in litters of domestic dogs and cats. The litter as a whole may also be more or less dominant relative to others of the same breed or species. For group living animals that usually produce only single offspring, the status of the progeny frequently reflects that of its dam. It would appear that aggression is frequently a familial trait, particularly in dogs and horses. Dogs bred for guarding and fighting are those most likely to display unacceptable levels of aggression. Different breeds are associated with particular forms of aggression (dominant vs. fear-induced).

Genetic and metabolic studies of a large related human group in the Netherlands—in which many of the male members exhibited borderline mental retardation, impulsive aggression, arson, attempted rape, and exhibitionism—identified a rare point mutation of a gene (single cytosine/thymine base switch) on the X chromosome; the gene codes for the activity of monoamine oxidase A (MAOA), which metabolizes serotonin, dopamine, and noradrenaline. MAO inhibition increases shock-induced aggression in rats and reduces REM sleep, which has also been shown to increase aggression (115). MAOA activity varies widely in the general population, and it may be that MAOA does not have to be completely absent for aggression to increase. However, Breakefield (116) has pointed out that even within this family there were individuals with the mutation who did not show excessive aggression, suggesting that environment can override a genetic propensity for aggression, at least in some instances.

A strain of mice has been produced in which the gene for the serotonin 5-HT1B receptor has been knocked out. This receptor is found in several parts of the mouse brain, including the limbic system. The resulting mice have an explosive increase in aggression directed against male intruders. They also are less fearful than normal mice in stressful situations (117).

Progressive ataxia is a neurologic condition that occurs in Charolais calves 6 to 36 months of age and is believed to be caused by a recessive gene. The animals become aggressive and show musculoskeletal and proprioceptive deficits (118). The condition is progressive, and there is no treatment. The nature of this genetic defect has not been described. It is possible that this and other conditions relate to defects in the serotonergic pathways.

It should be noted that some of the conditions previously discussed are also inherited; these include seizures, alpha-mannosidosis, fucosidosis, lissencephaly, and hypothyroidism.

Conclusion

Aggression is the most prevalent behavior problem in the dog and horse, and the second most common in the cat. Aggression is a normal and sometimes acceptable behavioral trait; however, even normal aggression can at times be unacceptable in the domestic animal. Centuries of selective breeding have created many of the breeds with which we share our lives. Food animals have on the whole been bred for tractability. Some breeds of horses and dogs were created for warfare, fighting, or protection, and in these breeds aggression was desirable. Of course, this is frequently at odds with the companionship role we may now expect from them.

Apart from a genetic predisposition for aggression, thyroid abnormalities and partial seizure disorders, including feline hyperesthesia, are those most likely to present at the behavior specialty practice. For these, behavioral signs may be the most obvious and frequently are the only ones seen at presentation, whereas animals afflicted with the other conditions described here generally exhibit aggression as a secondary sign of disease.

Until we started testing dogs for hypothyroidism on a fairly regular basis, we did not diagnose the condition. Now we are finding that not only is aggression frequently related to autoimmune thyroiditis, but so are other "behavior" problems, including global fear, separation anxiety, obsessive-compulsive problems, hyperactivity, and seizures. While correcting the thyroid imbalance may not provide a complete resolution of the behavior problems, it is an extremely rare animal that shows no improvement, and certainly none shows a deterioration in behavior following treatment. In the future, it is possible that if we test for other endocrine and metabolic parameters, we will discover additional links between systemic conditions and behavior problems.

References

1. Vite CH. Neurology for the behaviorist. Presented at the American Veterinary Society of Animal Behavior Special Symposium on Animal Behavior, Orlando, FL, January 1995.
2. Centerwall BS. In: Jan Volovka, ed. Review of: Neurobiology of violence, Washington, DC: American Psychiatric Press, 1995. N Engl J Med 1995;333:1653.
3. Yeh S-R, Fricke RA, Edwards DH. The effect of social experience on serotonergic modulation of the escape circuit of crayfish. Science 1996;271:366–369.

4. Weiger WA, Bear DM. An approach to the neurology of aggression. J Psychiatr Res 1988;22:85–98.

5. Egger MD, Flynn JP. Further studies on amygdaloid stimulations and ablation on hypothalamically elicited attack behavior in cats. In: Adey WR, Tokizane T, eds. Progress in brain research: structure and function of the limbic system. Amsterdam and New York: Elsevier, 1967.

6. Darwin C. The Expression of emotions in man and the animals. London, 1873: Reprint. New York: Philosophical Library, 1955.

7. Kravitz EA. Hormonal control of behavior: amines and the biasing of behavioral output in lobsters. Science 1988;241:1775–1781.

8. Bard P. A diencephalic mechanism for the expression of rage with special reference to the sympathetic nervous system. Am J Physiol 1928;84:490–515.

9. Wasman M, Flynn JP. Directed attack elicited from the hypothalamus. Arch Neurol 1962;6:222–227.

10. Smith DE, King MD, Hoebel BG. Lateral hypothalamic control of killing: evidence for cholinoceptive mechanism. Science 1970;167:900–901.

11. Roberts WW. Escape learning without avoidance learning motivated by hypothalamic stimulation in cats. J Comp Physiol Psychol 1958;51:391–399.

12. Wheatley MD. The hypothalamus and affective behavior in cats: a study of experimental lesions with anatomic correlations. Arch Neurol Psychiatry 1944;52:296–316.

13. Reeves AG, Plum F. Hyperphagia, rage and dementia accompanying a ventromedial hypothalamic neoplasm. Arch Neurol 1969;20:616–624.

14. Haugh RM, Markesbery WR. Hypothalamic astrocytoma: syndrome of hyperphagia, obesity and disturbances of behavior and endocrine and autonomic function. Arch Neurol 1983;40:560–563.

15. Bear D. Neurological perspectives on aggressive behavior. J Neuropsychiatry 1991;3 (suppl):S3–S8.

16. Bear DM, Rosenbaum JF, Norman R. Aggression in cat and man precipitated by a cholinesterase inhibitor. Psychosomatics 1986;26:535–536.

17. Metcalf DR, Holmes JH. EEG, psychological and neurological alterations in humans and organophosphate exposure. Ann NY Acad Sci 1969;160:357–365.

18. Bowers MB, Goodman E, Sim VM. Some behavioral changes in man following anticholinesterase administration. J Nerv Ment Dis 1964;138:383–389.

19. Gershon S, Shaw FH. Psychiatric sequelae of chronic exposure to organophosphorus insecticides. Lancet 1961;1:1371–1374.

20. Egger MD, Flynn JP. Effects of electrical stimulation of the amygdala on hypothalamically elicited attack behavior in cats. J Neurophysiol 1963;26:705–720.

21. Kluver H, Bucy PC. Preliminary analysis of functions of the temporal lobes in monkeys. Arch Neurol Psychiatry 1939;42:979–1000.

22. Horel JA. Recovery from the behavioral effects of occipital temporal disconnection. Anat Rec 1971;169:342–343.

23. Keating EG. Somatosensory deficit produced by parieto-temporal disconnection. Anat Rec 1971;169:353–354.

24. Screiner L, Kling A. Behavioral changes following rhinencephalic injury in cat. J Neurophysiol 1953;16:643–659.

25. Rosvold HE, Mirsky AF, Pribram KH. Influence of amygdalectomy on social behavior in monkeys. J Comp Physiol Psychol 1954;47:173–178.

26. Minor R. Rabies in the dog. Vet Rec 1977;101:516–512

27. Owen R, Ap R. Rabies in the horse. Vet Rec 1978;191:69.

28. Papez J. A proposed mechanism of emotion. Arch Neurol Psychiatry 1937;38:725–743.

29. Marlowe WB, Mancall EL, Thomas JJ. Complete Kluver-Bucy syndrome in man. Cortex 1975;11:53–59.

30. Terzian H, Ore JD. Syndrome of Kluver and Bucy reproduced in man by bilateral removal of temporal lobe. Neurology 1955;5:373–380.

31. Allen BD, Cummings JF, deLahunta A. The effects of prefrontal lobotomy on aggressive behavior in dogs. Cornell Vet 1974;64:201–216.

32. Blumer D, Benson DF. Personality changes with frontal and temporal lobe lesions. In: Benson DF, Blumer D, eds. Psychiatric aspects of neurologic disease. New York: Grune & Stratton, 1975.

33. Devinsky O, Bear DM. Varieties of aggressive behavior in temporal lobe epilepsy. Am J Psychiatry 1984;141:651–656.

34. Kligman D, Goldberg DA. Temporal lobe epilepsy and aggression, problems in clinical research. J Nerv Ment Dis 1975;160:324–339.

35. Buhl EH, Otis TS, Mody I. Zinc-induced collapse of augmented inhibition by GABA in temporal lobe epilepsy model. Science 1996;271:369–373.

36. Breitschwerdt EB, Breazile JE, Broadhurst JJ. Clinical and electroencephalographic findings associated with ten cases of suspected limbic epilepsy in the dog. J Am Anim Hosp Assoc 1979;15:37–50.

37. Dodman NH, Miczek KA, Knowles K, et al. Phenobarbital-responsive episodic dyscontrol (rage) in dogs. J Am Vet Med Assoc 1992;201:1580–1583.

38. Dodman NH, Knowles KE, Shuster L, et al. Behavioral changes associated with suspected complex partial seizures in Bull Terriers. J Am Vet Med Assoc 1996;208:688–691.

39. Cromwell-Davis SL, Lappin M, Oliver JK. Stimulus-responsive psychomotor epilepsy in a Doberman Pinscher. J Am Anim Hosp Assoc 1989;25:57–60.

40. Moon-Fanelli AA, Dodman NH. (in press).

41. Falco MJ, Barker J, Wallace ME. The genetics of epilepsy in the British Alsatian. J Small Anim Pract 1974;15:685–692.

42. van der Velden NA. Fits in Tervueren Shepherd dogs: a presumed hereditary trait. J Small Anim Pract 1968;9:63–70.

43. Wallace ME, Keeshonds: a genetic study of epilepsy and EEG readings. J Small Anim Pract 1975;16:1–10.

44. Beaver BV. Mental lapse aggression syndrome. J Am Vet Med Assoc 1980;16:937–939.

45. Millichap G. Anticonvulsant drugs in the management of epilepsy. Mod Treat 1969; 6:1217–1232.

46. Podell MJ. The use of diazepam per rectum at home for the acute management of cluster seizures in dogs. J Vet Intern Med 1995; 8:68–74.

47. Sheard MH. Clinical pharmacology of aggressive behavior. Clin Neuropharmacol 1988;11:483–492.

48. Barratt ES, Kent TA, Bryant SG, Felthous AR. A controlled trial of phenytoin in impulsive aggression (letter). J Clin Psychopharmacol 1991;11:388–389.

49. Austin VH. The skin. In: Catcott EJ, ed. Feline medicine and surgery, 2nd ed. Santa Barbara CA: American Veterinary Publications, 1975:461–484.

50. Mosier JE. Common medical and behavioral problems in cats. Mod Vet Pract 1975:56:699–703.

51. Reister M. Good nutrition shines through. Cat Fancy 1995;38:10–14.

52. Moisier JE. Hyperesthesia syndrome and treatment with primadone (letter). Feline Pract 1977;7:5–6.

53. Dow C, McFerran JB. Aujeszky's disease in the dog and cat. Vet Rec 1963;75:1099–1102.

54. Dow C, McFerran JB. The pathology of Aujeszky's disease in cattle. J Comp Pathol 1962;72:337–347.

55. Crandell RA. Selected animal herpesviruses: new concepts and technologies. Adv Vet Sci Comp Med 1985;29:281–327.

56. Pederson NC, Ho EW, Brown ML, Yamamoto JK. Isolation of a T-lymphotropic virus from domestic cats with an immunodeficiency-like syndrome. Science 1987;235:790–793.

57. Dow SW, Dreitz MJ, Hoover EA. Exploring the link between feline immunodeficiency virus infection and neurologic disease in cats. Vet Med 1992;87:1181–1184.
58. Plowright W, Herniman AJ, Jessett DM, et al. Immunization of cattle against the herpesvirus of malignant catarrhal fever: failure of inactivated culture vaccines with adjuvant. Res Vet Sci 1975;19:159–166.
59. Lansbury PT, Caughey B. The chemistry of scrapie infection: implications of the "Ice 9" metaphor. Chem Biol 1995;2:1–5.
60. Gibbs CJ, Gajdusek DC. Transmission of scrapie to the cynomolgus monkey (Macaca fascicularis). Nature 1972;236:73–74.
61. Bachmann PA, ter Meulen V, Jentsch G, et al. Sporadic bovine meningo-encephalitis—isolation of a paramyxovirus. Arch Virol 1975; 48:107–120.
62. Allen JR, Barbec DD, Boulton CR. Brain abscesses in a horse: diagnosis by computerized axial tomography and successful surgical treatment. Equine Vet J 1987;19:552–555.
63. Kuttler KL, Craig TM. Isolation of bovine *Theileria*. Am J Vet Res 1975;36:323–325.
64. Dill SG. Polioencephalomalacia in ruminants. In: Howard JL, ed. Current veterinary therapy: food animal practice 2. Philadelphia: Saunders, 1986:868–869.
65. Phillips RW. Water soluble vitamins. In: Booth NH, McDonald LE, eds. Veterinary pharmacology and therapeutics, 6th ed. Ames, IA: Iowa State University Press, 1988:698–702.
66. Dodman NH, Reisner I, Shuster L, et al. Effect of dietary protein content on behavior in dogs. J Am Vet Med Assoc 1996;208:376–379.
67. Schwarte LH, Biester HE, Murray C. A disease of horses caused by feeding moldy corn. J Am Vet Med Assoc 1937;90:76–85.
68. Biester HE, Schwarte LH, Reddy CH. Further studies on moldy corn poisoning (leukoencephalomalacia) in horses. Vet Med 1940;35:636–639.
69. Needleman HL, Riess JA, Tobin MJ, et al. Bone lead levels and delinquent behavior. JAMA 1996;275:363–369.
70. Louis-Ferdinand RT, Brown DR, Fiddler SF, et al. Morphometric and enzymatic effects of neonatal lead exposure in the rat brain. Toxicol Appl Pharmacol 1978;43:351–360.
71. Hatch RC. Poisons causing nervous stimulation or depression. In: Booth NH, McDonald LE, eds. Veterinary pharmacology and therapeutics, 6th ed. Ames, IA: Iowa State University Press, 1988:1088–1089.
72. Ramsey DT, Castel SW, Faggella AM, et al. Use of orally administered succimer (*meso*-2,3-dimercaptosuccinic acid) for treatment of lead poisoning in dogs. J Am Vet Med Assoc 1996;208:371–375.
73. Alroy J, Orgad U, Ucci AA, Gavris VE. Swainsonine toxicosis mimics lectin histochemistry of mannosidosis. Vet Pathol 1985;22:311–316.
74. Smith MO, Wenger DA, Hill SL, Matthews J. Fucosidosis in a family of American-bred English Springer Spaniels. J Am Vet Med Assoc 1996;209:2088–2090.
75. Mullen KD, Szauter KM, Kaminsky K, et al. Detection and characterization of endogenous benzodiazepine activity in both animal models and humans with encephalopathy. In: Butterworth RF, Layrargues GP, eds. Hepatic encephalopathy, pathophysiology and treatment. Clifton, NJ: Humana, 1989:287–294.
76. van der Rijt CC, Schalm SW, Meulstee J, Stijnen T. Flumazenil therapy for hepatic encephalopathy: a double blind cross-over study. Gastroenterol Clin Biol 1995;19:572–580.
77. de Lahunta A. Feline ischemic encephalopathy—a cerebral infarction syndrome, In: Kirk RW, ed. Current veterinary therapy, Vol. 1. Small animal practice. Philadelphia: Saunders, 1977:906–908.
78. Bernstein NM, Fiske RA. Feline ischemic encephalopathy in a cat. J Am Anim Hosp Assoc 1986;22:205–206.

79. Barr WG, Merchut MP. Systemic lupus erythematosus with central nervous system involvement. Psychiatr Clin North Am 1992;15:439–454.

80. van Dam AP. Diagnosis and pathogenesis of CNS lupus. Rheumatol Int 1991;11:1–11.

81. Jones DRE, Hopkinson ND, Powell RJ. Autoantibodies in pet dogs owned by patients with systemic lupus erythematosus. Lancet 1992:339:1378–1380.

82. Greene CE, Vandevelde M, Braund K. Lissencephaly in two Lhasa Apso dogs. J Am Vet Med Assoc 1976;169:405–410.

83. Dodman NH, Bronson R, Gliatto J. Tail chasing in a bull terrier. J Am Vet Med Assoc 1993;202:758–760.

84. Broussard JD, Peterson ME. Changes in the clinical and laboratory findings in hyperthyroid cats from 1988–1992. J Vet Intern Med 1993;7:112. Abstract.

85. Joseph RJ, Peterson ME. Review and comparison of neuromuscular and central nervous system manifestations of hyperthyroidism in cats and humans. Prog Vet Neurol 1992; 3:114–119.

86. Atterwill CK, Bunn SJ, Atkinson DJ, et al. Effects of thyroid status on presynaptic alpha-2-adrenoreceptor function and beta-adrenoreceptor binding in the rat brain. J Neural Transm 1984;59:43–55.

87. Savard P, Merand Y, Di Paolo T, Dupont A. Effects of thyroid state on serotonin, 5-hydroxyindoleacetic acid and substance P contents in discrete brain nuclei of adult rats. Neuroscience 1983;10:1399–1404.

88. Peterson ME, Becker DV. Radioiodine treatment of 524 cats with hyperthyroidism. J Am Vet Med Assoc 1995;207:1422–1428.

89. Meric SM. Diagnosis and management of feline hyperthyroidism. Comp Cont Educ 1989; 11:1053–1062.

90. Peterson ME, Kintzer PP, Hurvitz AI. Methimazole treatment of 262 cats with hyperthyroidism. J Vet Intern Med 1988;2:150–157.

91. Trepanier LA, Peterson ME, Aucoin DA. Methimazole pharmokinetics in the normal cat. ACVIM 1989,50:1037. Abstract.

92. Aronson LP, Dodman NH, DeNapoli JS, Dodds WJ. The behavioral implications of canine hypothyroidism (in press).

93. Henley WN, Chen X, Klettner C, et al. Hypothyroidism increases serotonin turnover and sympathetic activity in the adult rat. Can J Physiol Pharmacol 1991;69:205–210.

94. Cameron DL, Crocker AD. The hypothyroid rat as a model of increased sensitivity to dopamine receptor agonists. Pharm Biochem Behav 1990;37:627–632.

95. Whybrow PC. Behavioral and psychiatric manifestations of hypothyroidism. In Braverman LE, Utiger RD (eds). Werner and Ingbar's The Thyroid; a fundamental and clinical text (7th edition). Philadelphia. Lippincott-Raven 1996:886–870.

96. Dodman NH, Mertens PA, Aronson LP. Aggression in two hypothyroid dogs; behavior case of the month. J Am Vet Med Assoc 1995;207:1168–1171.

97. Winslow JT, Miczek KA. Androgen dependency of alcohol effects on aggressive behavior: a seasonal rhythm in high-ranking squirrel monkeys. Psychopharmacol 1988; 95:92–98.

98. Beaver BV. Aggressive behavior problems. Vet Clin North Am Equine Pract 1986;2:635–644.

99. Beaver BV, Amoss MS. Aggressive behavior associated with naturally elevated serum testosterone in mares. Appl Anim Ethol 1982;8:425–428.

100. Voith VL, Marder AR. Canine behavioral disorders. In: Morgan RV, ed. Handbook of small animal practice. New York: Churchill-Livingstone, 1988:1033–1043.

101. Voith VL, Marder AR. Feline behavior disorders. In: Morgan RV, ed. Handbook of small animal practice. New York: Churchill-Livingstone, 1988:1045–1051.

102. Beaver BV. Disorders of behavior. In: Sherding RG, ed. The cat: diseases and clinical managment. New York: Churchill-Livingstone 1989:163–184.

103. Hopkins SG, Schubert TA, Hart BL. Castration of adult male dogs: effects on roaming, aggression, urine marking and mounting. J Am Vet Med Assoc 1976;168:1108–1110.

104. Hart BL, Barrett RE. Effects of castration on fighting, roaming, and urine spraying in adult male cats. J Am Vet Med Assoc 1973;163:290–292.

105. O'Farrell V, Peachey E. The behavioral effects of ovariohysterectomy on bitches. J Small Anim Pract 1990;31:595–598.

106. Beech J. Tumors of the pituitary gland (pars intermedia). In: Robinson NE, ed. Current equine therapy, vol. II. New York: Saunders, 1987:182–185.

107. Greenway SE, Pack AT, Greenway FL. Treatment of depression with cyproheptadine. Pharmacotherapy 1995;15:357–360.

108. Stanislav SW, Fabre T, Crismon ML, Childs A. Buspirone efficacy in organic-induced aggression. J Clin Psychopharmol 1994;14:126–130.

109. Rylov AL, Dolgov ON, Anaskin AN. Deistvitel'no li agressiia, vyzvannaia bol'iu, iavliaetsia oboronitel'noi formoi dannogo (Is pain-induced aggression actually a defensive form of that behavior?). Zh Vyssh Nerv Deiat 1986;36:892–897.

110. Higley JD, Mehlman PT, Taub DM, et al. Cerebrospinal fluid monoamine and adrenal correlates of aggression in free-ranging Rhesus monkeys. Arch Gen Psychiatry 1992;49: 436–441.

111. Russell IJ, Michalek JE, Vipraio GA, et al. Platelet 3H-imipramine uptake receptor density and serotonin levels in patients with fibromylagia/fibrositis syndrome. J Rheumatol 1992; 19:104–109.

112. Driessen B, Reimann W. Interaction of the central analgesic, tramadol, with the uptake and release of 5-hydroxytryptamine in the rat brain in vitro. Br J Pharmacol 1992;105:147–151.

113. Valverde O, Mico JA, et al. Participation of opioid and monoaminergic mechanisms on the antinociceptive effect induced by tricyclic antidepressants in two behavioral pain tests in mice. Prog Neuropsychopharmacol Biol Psychiatry 1994;18:1073–1092.

114. Haze JJ. Toward the understanding of the rationale for the use of dietary supplementation for chronic pain management: the serotonin model. Cranio 1991;9:33–43.

115. Brunner HG, Nelen M, Breakefield XO, et al. Abnormal behavior associated with a point mutation in the structural gene for monoamine oxidase A. Science 1993;262:578–580.

116. Breakefield XO, quoted in Mann CC. Behavioral genetics in transition. Science 1994;264:1686–1689.

117. Hen R. Mean genes. Neuron 1996;16:17–21.

118. Montgomery DL, Mayer JC. Progressive ataxia in Charolais cattle. Southwestern Vet 1986;37:247–250.

II FEAR AND ANXIETY

Fear and Anxiety: Mechanisms, Models, and Molecules

Berend Olivier

Klaus A. Miczek

A major human illness such as anxiety cannot be reproduced fully in animals, but it does have an evolutionary precursor in species other than humans. Anxiety or fear are hypothetical mental states that all healthy persons will experience occasionally in everyday life, for example, in situations of physical danger or in social interactions. However, when anxiety becomes too extreme, chronic, or disproportionate to external stimuli, clinical anxiety disorders may emerge that usually lead an individual to seek professional help; this occurs in 2 to 4% of the human population (1). By extrapolation, anxiety-like responses are identified in animals, particularly in mammals, and increasingly in veterinary medicine concerned owners are seeking help for animals that have clinical anxiety-related disorders.

Using the diagnostic criteria of the American Psychiatric Association (*Diagnostic and Statistical Manual of Mental Disorders*, Fourth Edition [DSM-IV], 1994), anxiety disorders can be divided into generalized anxiety disorder, panic disorder, obsessive-compulsive disorder, posttraumatic stress disorder, and phobias. A similar classification could be employed for veterinary patients. Whether these categories are directly relevant to veterinary concerns remains to be established. Table 4.1 shows a plausible comparison.

Generalized anxiety disorder is characterized by a continuous increased level of ("free-floating") anxiety, whereas the anxiety in panic disorder comes in spells of intense fear. These so-called panic attacks include an intense fear of dying, insanity, or uncontrollability, and are generally accompanied by severe autonomic symptoms, such as tachycardia, trembling, sweating, dizziness, choking, or fainting. Cognitive factors are important in the etiology and maintenance of panic disorder, as stimuli associated with prior panic attacks may become potent triggers for future attacks. Obsessive-compulsive disorder can be described by the occurrence of obsessive acts

Table 4.1.   Relationship of human anxiety disorders to anxiety-related veterinary behavioral conditions

DSM IV Disorder	Putative Veterinary Behavioral Equivalent
Generalized Anxiety Disorder* (GAD)	Excessive chronic generalized anxiety with multiple fears (animate, inanimate, and situational)
Panic Disorder* (PD)	Separation anxiety, fear of car travel, fear of veterinarian office
Post-traumatic stress disorder** (PTSD)	Enhanced/Exaggerated fearfulness appearing as GAD or PD which develops following acute trauma/stress, e.g., following gunshot
Phobias	Noise phobia (e.g., thunderstorm phobia) and other animate and inanimate phobias
Obsessive-compulsive Disorder (OCD)***	Stereotypy/compulsive disorder

* Discussed in next chapter by Mertens and Dodman.
** Discussed in chapter by Thompson.
*** Discussed in section on Compulsive Disorders (Section III).

(compulsions), such as hand washing, or obsessive thoughts (obsessions), like counting. Both obsessions and compulsions are thought to reduce anxiety levels. Posttraumatic stress disorder may arise after severe traumas such as war experiences. Phobic disorders can be divided into agoraphobia, social phobia, and simple phobias, like arachnophobia (fear of spiders). Anxiety disorders not falling in these categories form a residual group of "atypical anxiety disorders." This human psychiatric framework has guided veterinary behavioral pharmacology.

Barbiturates represented the first generation of pharmacologic treatment for anxiety disorders in the first half of the twentieth century. Meprobamate in the 1950s was followed by the benzodiazepines (BZDs) in the 1960s. The BZDs are very effective and safe anxiolytics and are still widely prescribed. These drugs were found to enhance gamma-aminobutyric acid (GABA)-ergic neurotransmission in a modulatory fashion by acting at the BZD site of the $GABA_A$-BZD receptor complex. Other compounds with less selective anxiolytic actions, like the barbiturates and alcohol, have their own specific binding sites at this receptor complex (2).

Aside from their potent anxiolytic activity, BZDs exert other physiologic and behavioral effects that may be regarded as unwanted or unnecessary side effects in the treatment of anxiety disorders: for example, their sedative, anticonvulsive, muscle-relaxant, hypnotic, and amnestic effects. In addition, under some conditions they may produce tolerance to the anxiolytic action, as well as physiologic and psychological dependence, and may induce severe withdrawal symptoms in some individuals (3). These problems have led—and in fact still lead—to the search for new anxiolytic compounds with fewer side effects and maximal anxiolytic activity. As a result, novel anxiolytic drugs emerged acting at the serotonin (5-HT) system, such as 5-HT_{1A} receptor agonists (4) and 5-HT uptake inhibitors (5).

According to present psychiatric knowledge, generalized anxiety disorder is effectively treated with BZDs, like diazepam or chlordiazepoxide, and with the partial 5-HT_{1A} receptor agonist buspirone (4). Panic disorder and obsessive-compulsive disorder, on the other hand, respond better to 5-HT uptake inhibitors, like clomipramine, fluoxetine, or fluvoxamine (5). BZDs in general (6), as well as partial 5-HT_{1A} receptor agonists (7), are not very effective treatments for panic disorder and obsessive-compulsive disorder. Panic disorder, however, is effectively suppressed by the triazolobenzodiazepine alprazolam (8), a BZD-ligand from a different class of molecular structures, unrelated to the "classic" BZDs. The other groups of anxiety disorders do not have such a clear pharmacotherapeutic profile and are probably less frequently treated with drugs.

There is very limited research regarding the role of psychoactive drugs in anxiety disorders in veterinary patients. In general, BZDs are used on a pragmatic basis—not supported by appropriate placebo-controlled studies—although the available data suggest that the drugs used are as effective in veterinary patients as in laboratory rodents or humans.

This chapter begins with a description of frequently used preclinical experimental procedures to detect anxiolytic drug effects. The effects of BZDs, 5-HT_{1A} receptor agonists, and selective serotonin reuptake inhibitors (SSRIs) in these procedures are discussed. The chapter ends with a short outline of new developments in the field of putative anxiolytics, especially those in the serotonergic field.

Animal Models of Anxiety

One model is implemented by experimental procedures that suppress or inhibit behavior; a drug is considered to have potentially anxiolytic activity when it attenuates or reverses the behavioral suppression or inhibition. A second model relies on procedures, usually involving aversive events, that engender a distinctive behavior; a drug with anxiolytic potential attenuates or blocks this induced or elicited behavior (9). These procedures can be based on conditioned behavior and involve responses controlled by operant or classic conditioning procedures. Other procedures involve unconditioned behavior that do not require specific training. Often the latter models rely on species-specific responses (e.g., social interaction, ultrasonic vocalization) and are sometimes referred to as "ethologically-based" models. Table 4.2 summarizes the models currently used to study the anxiolytic effects of drugs.

Table 4.2. Preclinical experimental procedures frequently used in the study of anxiolytic drug effects

(1) Conditioned	(2) Unconditioned
A. Behavioral Suppression or Inhibition due to Punishing Consequences	
Conflict procedures:	Suppressed exploration in rodents:
(a) food reinforced lever pressing	(a) Elevated Plus Maze
(b) water reinforced licking	(b) Light Dark Exploration
(c) food reinforced key pecking	(c) Open Field Test
	(d) Suppressed Social Interactions
B. Aversively Stimulated Behavior	
Fear-potentiated Startle	
Separation Distress Vocalization in Pups	
Vocalizations in Response to Pain, Startle, Attack, and Drug Withdrawal	
Defensive Burying	
Stress-induced Hyperthermia	
Stretched Approach Posture	

BEHAVIORAL SUPPRESSION OR INHIBITION DUE TO PUNISHING CONSEQUENCES

Conflict Procedures

In conflict procedures, ongoing behavior is suppressed by the presentation of aversive consequences for the behavior. The experimental protocols involving the suppression of behavior are summarized in Table 4.3. Punishing consequences suppress either lever-pressing that is reinforced by food in hungry rats (10), key-pecking reinforced by food intake in hungry pigeons (11), or water-licking in thirsty rats (12). Signaled or unsignaled delivery of electric shock pulses may be used as an aversive consequence. The release of suppressed behavior without affecting the levels of unpunished responding following pharmacologic intervention predicts an "anxiolytic" effect. In rodents, pigeons, and primates BZDs are consistently found to be effective in these models. The activity of putative anxiolytics like the SSRIs is difficult to detect using such conflict procedures.

In rat conflict models, non-BZD anxiolytics such as buspirone have little or no anxiolytic effect (13). Increases in punished responding in rats after 5-HT_{1A} receptor agonists are more likely seen when water licking (Vogel-type procedure) is used than when food-reinforced lever pressing (Geller conflict procedure) is studied (13). In contrast, anxiolytic activity of 5-HT_{1A} receptor agonists in pigeons has been extended to mixed 5-HT1 receptor agonists and 5-H_{T2} receptor antagonists, although to a lesser extent (13).

A related and simple test is the four-plate test, introduced by Boissier et al (14). In this procedure, mice are placed into a novel test cage; the floor is

Table 4.3. Overview of anxiety models and their sensitivity to pharmacological treatments

Release of suppressed behavior

Model	Description of anxiolytic effect	Pharmacological class		
		BZD	5-HT$_{1A}$	5-HTupt.
Conditioned Responses				
Geller-Seifter conflict test	increase of punished response	+	0	0
Vogel conflict test	increase of punished drinking	+	+/0	0
Conflict in pigeon	increase of punished food reinforced pecking	+	+	nt
Conditioned emotional response	increase of suppressed responding	+/0	+	nt
Unconditioned Responses				
Four-Plate Test	increase of punished crossings (exploration)	+	+/0	+/0
Open Field test	increase of exploration in center of a large illuminated circular arena	+	nt	nt
Elevated Plus Maze	increase of open arm exploration	+	0/−	0/−
Light Dark Box	increase of exploration in bright light	+	+/0	0
Social Interaction test	increase of social interaction in lit unfamiliar cage	+	+/0	0

Legend: BZD = benzodiazepines; 5-HT$_{1A}$ = 5-HT$_{1A}$ receptor agonists; 5-HTupt. = 5-HT uptake inhibitors; + indicates anxiolytic effect; 0 indicates inactive; − indicates anxiogenic effect; nt = not tested.

divided into four metal plates. Crossing from one plate to the other is punished by electric shock. BZD-receptor ligands like classic BZDs (15), but also certain beta-carbolines, are effective in this test as indicated by the increased number of crossings (16). However, the specificity of this test has been questioned (15). Moreover, 5-HT$_{1A}$ receptor agonists and SSRIs are not active in this procedure (17).

Elevated Plus-Maze

The elevated plus-maze, based on Montgomery's maze (18), is a procedure that relies on the exploratory behavior of rats placed in an elevated maze, which consists of two opposite open alleys and two walled alleys (in a plus configuration). Rats and mice will explore the different alleys, as tallied by their total number of entries. Typically, rats enter the open arms less than the walled ones, presumably due to the aversive nature of open spaces. Anxiolytic drugs reduce the inhibition of open alley exploration, presumably by causing less fear. The ratio of open-arm entries to the total of arm entries is interpreted as an index of the anxiolytic-like effect of a drug, and this measure is not very sensitive for general effects on exploration.

In this model, the anxiolytic activity of BZDs can be reliably demonstrated by the increase in percentage of open-arm entries and time spent in the open arms. Drugs stimulating the 5-HT_{1A} receptor, such as 8-hydroxy-dipropylaminotetralin (8-OH-DPAT), buspirone, and ipsapirone, have either been reported to be ineffective or to show an opposite effect (i.e., decreasing the percentage of entries or time spent in the open arms) (19). This latter effect may be due to some anxiogenic effects of these drugs, but it may also represent a false-negative in this test. SSRIs are either inactive or anxiogenic in the elevated plus-maze. While this model requires no conditioning, inexperienced animals are necessary for each test, since habituation to novelty is relatively rapid.

Open Field Test

In one of the simplest procedures for studying anxiety-like responses in animals, rats or mice are placed in a novel and relatively large arena. This arena is often divided into outer and inner circles or into squares; sometimes the center is brightly lit and the walled edge is dimly lit. Drug effects are assessed on exploratory behavior such as walking across lines as an index of locomotion, sniffing, grooming, and on autonomic activity such as urination and bolus counts. BZD anxiolytics reduce these behavioral and autonomic "anxiety" parameters in this model. However, the procedure also yields false-positives with psychostimulants and anticholinergics, and it does not reliably detect 5-HT_{1A} receptor agonists and SSRIs.

Light-Dark Exploration

This procedure is based in principle on the aversion of mice and rats for brightly lit places. In a two-compartment box, one dark and the other brightly lit, the total activity, the time spent in the light compartment, and the number of crossings between the light and dark compartments provide information about the preference of the animal for the dark compartment. As anxiolytics should reduce the impact of aversive consequences, the essential feature of this model is that anxiolytic drugs increase the number of crossings and/or the time spent in the light compartment. The latter parameter is generally considered to be the most relevant. BZDs are reliably detected in this model (20). Also, the 5-HT$_{1A}$ receptor agonists have been reported to show an anxiolytic profile in this model (21).

Social Interaction Test

When rats or mice are unfamiliar with each other and are placed in a novel test arena, they interact for a short time. File (22) systematically varied the test conditions and found the most suppression of social interactions when the arena was brightly lit and unfamiliar to both animals. Typically, the time spent by the animals in social interaction is measured in addition to locomotor activity. BZDs increase the time spent in social interaction. A similar effect has been reported for the 5-HT$_{1A}$ receptor agonists buspirone and ipsapirone (23), though not always (24). For other putative anxiolytics ambivalent data have been reported, and the test does not appear to detect potential anti-panic, anti-phobic, or anti-OCD effects of drugs (25).

AVERSIVELY STIMULATED BEHAVIOR (TABLES 4.4 AND 4.5)

Fear-Potentiated Startle Response

The experimental procedures for stimulating animals aversively and studying anxiolytics and SSRIs on the resulting behavioral responses are summarized in

Table 4.4. Overview of anxiety models and their sensitivity to pharmacological treatments. Inhibition of stress-evoked behavior: Conditioned responses.

Model	Description of anxiolytic effect	Pharmacological class		
		BZD	5HT$_{1A}$	5HTupt.
Startle response	startle amplitude	+	+	0
Pentylenetetrazol discrimination	decrease in choice for PTZ-cue	+	0	nt
Shock-induced USV	decrease in USV	+	+	0
Startle-induced USV	decrease in USV	+	+	nt
Conditioned social defeat	decrease in USV and physiological stress reactions	0	+	nt
Conditioned USV	decrease in USV	+	+	+

Legend: BZD = benzodiazepines; 5-HT$_{1A}$ = 5-HT$_{1A}$ receptor agonists; 5-HTupt. = 5-HT uptake inhibitors; + indicates active; 0 indicates inactive; nt = tested.

Table 4.5. Overview of anxiety models and their sensitivity to pharmacological treatments. Inhibition of stress-evoked behavior: Unconditioned responses.

Model	Description of anxiolytic effect	Pharmacological class		
		BZD	5HT$_{1A}$	5HTupt.
Defensive Burying	decrease in shock prod burying	+	+	0/−
Stretched Approach Posture (SAP)	decrease in SAP	+	+	+
Stress-induced Hyperthermia	decrease in hyperthermia in anticipation of handling + injection	+	+	0
Rat pup isolation USV	decrease in USV	+	+	+
Guinea pig pup isolation calls	decrease in vocalizations	+	+	+
BZD Withdrawal	decrease in USV	+	+	nt

Legend: BZD = benzodiazepines; 5-HT$_{1A}$ = 5-HT$_{1A}$ receptor agonists; 5-HTupt. = 5-HT uptake inhibitors; + indicates active; 0 indicates inactive; − indicates anxiogenic-like response; nt = not tested.

Tables 4.4 and 4.5. The fear-potentiated startle response consists of both classically conditioned and unconditioned behavior (26). The startle response of a rat to a loud tone can be augmented by prior Pavlovian fear conditioning. During the fear conditioning phase, a light stimulus (serving as the conditioned stimulus) signals the imminent delivery of a shock (unconditioned stimulus). During the startle response measurement, presentation of the shock-associated light will only augment the startle amplitude. Both the anxiolytic effect of BZDs and the anxiogenic effect of yohimbine and DMCM can be detected in this model (26–28). The partial 5-HT$_{1A}$ receptor agonists buspirone and gepirone (29), and the full 5-HT$_{1A}$ receptor agonist flesinoxan (28), are also effective in this model. However, other 5-HT$_{1A}$ receptor agonists such as the full agonist 8-OH-DPAT and the partial agonist ipsapirone are not effective, and the effect of buspirone could not be antagonized by 5-HT receptor antagonists or by lesioning of the 5-HT system (29,30). The latter findings suggest that 5-HT$_{1A}$ receptor stimulation is not involved in the anxiolytic profile of buspirone in this model. SSRIs, notably fluvoxamine (27,28), are ineffective in this procedure.

Pentylenetetrazol Discrimination

In typical drug discrimination methodology, the injection with a specific drug dose or its control vehicle (placebo) signals to the animal which of two response options will be reinforced. After approximately 30 daily training trials with alternating pentylenetetrazol (PTZ) and vehicle conditioning, rats will respond on the PTZ-appropriate lever more than 80 to 90% of the time after being injected with PTZ (31). Human subjects report that PTZ induces feelings of anxiety, and it is assumed that the PTZ cue engenders a similar anxious state in animals (32).

Drugs that antagonize PTZ as a signal for PTZ-appropriate responding may be considered anxiolytics. Accordingly, BZD agonists block the PTZ cue, whereas anticonvulsants do not. This latter observation is significant because PTZ is a convulsant at higher doses. The lack of antagonism by anticonvulsants therefore suggests that the cue is not based on the convulsant or preconvulsant effect of PTZ, but rather on the anxiety-like activity.

Drugs such as inverse BZD agonists generalize to the PTZ cue, supporting the interpretation of this drug state as anxiogenic (33). There is no evidence that 5-HT$_{1A}$ receptor agonists are able to antagonize the PTZ cue (3), whereas SSRIs have not yet been studied systematically with this procedure.

Vocalizations in Aversive Social Situations

Adult male rats emit ultrasonic vocalizations (USV) (approximately in the 20–28 kHz range) of distress under various aversive conditions such as, for example, in the presence of a predator (14) or an aggressive male opponent (34), or after exposure to a painful shock (35) or a loud acoustic (36,37) or tactile startle stimulus (38). Interestingly, rats can also produce USVs in association with a prior aversive event without the actual physical presence of threat. This latter feature may have face validity with regard to situational panic attacks, where environmental stimuli may acquire aversive properties and become triggers for panic attacks (35). USVs in adult rats may represent affective expressions by rats exposed to threatening, startling, or painful stimuli (9).

Socially experienced rats emit USVs at a higher rate after being withdrawn from chronic treatment with opioid drugs in a time- and dose-dependent manner (39). Similarly, when rats are startled 24 hours after the last of ten diazepam injections, they emit high rates of USVs (37). These USVs during withdrawal from diazepam can be attenuated with 5-HT$_{1A}$ partial agonist gepirone or with diazepam (39). Withdrawal from cocaine, which was administered long-term either in the drinking fluid or by intravenous self-administration in "binges," produces large increases in USVs in rats, mimicking the clinically observed "crash" phase (38).

Anxiolytics targeting to 5-HT$_{1A}$ and GABA$_A$-BZD receptors decrease these ultrasounds (20–30 kHz) when rats are exposed to acoustic startle stimuli (36) or to footshock—but not when exposed to tail shock (40–42)—and also when they are anticipating a confrontation with an aggressive opponent (43).

Under a conditioning procedure, when rats were exposed to the environment where they had received electric footshock previously, they emitted fewer USVs after treatment with 5-HT$_{1A}$ receptor agonists, but not with BZDs, except for alprazolam (35). This pattern of results suggests that this experimental procedure may serve as model for detecting antipanic activity.

Ultrasonic Vocalization in Mouse and Rat Pups   In rodents, removal of the pup from its nest, mother, and littermates engenders ultrasonic calling (Table 4.5). These types of ultrasounds are in the frequency range of 30 to 50 kHz. The primary function of calling is probably to alert the mother and to stimulate her to search and retrieve the pup (44). In rats, ultrasonic calling shows a characteristic developmental pattern. USVs increase gradually to peak levels at about 9 to 11 days (45). Thereafter, they gradually decrease and disappear at 16 to 18 days of age.

Ultrasonic calling is sensitive to treatment with clinically proven anxiolytics as well as with putative anxiolytic compounds (46). BZDs reduce ultrasounds in rats and mice (47,48). Conversely, BZD inverse agonists can increase ultrasounds (48), suggestive of anxiogenic drug effects. Also, 5-HT$_{1A}$ anxiolytics, like the full agonists 8-OH-DPAT and flesinoxan; the partial agonists buspirone, gepirone, and ipsapirone; and the 5-HT reuptake inhibitors, such as fluvoxamine, zimelidine, and clomipramine, reduce pup ultrasounds (9,46,49,50). Despite the immature nervous system and the limited physiologic thermoregulation and behavioral repertoire, the BZDs and 5-HT$_{1A}$ anxiolytics that have been tested to date consistently reduce separation-induced ultrasounds.

Distress Vocalizations in Guinea Pig Pups   Guinea pig pups emit distress vocalizations when separated from their mother and littermates (51). These calls are mainly in the audible range for humans (52). Previously, morphine and the antidepressants imipramine and fluvoxamine were found to reduce isolation distress calls in guinea pigs (51,53,54). In recent systematic studies, BZDs (diazepam, alprazolam), alcohol, the full 5-HT$_{1A}$ agonists (8-OH-DPAT, flesinoxan), but *not* the partial 5-HT$_{1A}$ agonist buspirone, reduced calling in guinea pig pups (55). Furthermore, antidepressants with different mechanisms of action (SSRIs, monoamine oxidase inhibitors [MAOIs], noradrenergic uptake inhibitors) also decreased calling. Neuroleptic and psychostimulant drugs were inactive and can be considered "correct rejections." The effectiveness of both anxiolytics and antidepressants on vocal responses in separation-distress in guinea pigs complement the findings in rodents and establish the utility of this experimental preparation.

Stress-Induced Hyperthermia

Recently, stress-induced hyperthermia (SIH) was described in group-housed mice (56). When removed one by one from their housing cage, the mice removed last always had higher rectal temperatures than those removed first. This phenomenon has been interpreted as being caused by anticipatory fear or the stress of an aversive event (e.g., handling, disturbance in the cage). Similarly, the body temperature of group-housed rats also increases when they are handled and recorded sequentially (57). Such findings have been considered as a conditioned response in anticipation to handling and/or insertion of the rectal probe (58). Temperature rises can be conditioned to stimuli occurring in anticipation of events such as forced exercise (59), or drug injections and rotarod measurements (60).

Interactions between body temperature and emotional states also occur in humans (61,62), and it is customary to include changes in autonomic functioning (like temperature) in the diagnosis of generalized anxiety disorders and panic disorder (e.g., in DSM-IV). Moreover, the stress-induced increase in rectal temperature could be prevented by administration of BZDs and 5-HT$_{1A}$ receptor agonists, but not by antidepressants or neuroleptics (56,63,64), supporting the view that SIH may be considered to be an animal model representing some form of anticipatory anxiety.

Defensive Burying

Defensive burying has been demonstrated in a number of rodents (rats (65), mice (31), gerbils (66), and ground squirrels (67)). Defensive burying is operationally defined by pushing and spraying of bedding material, with alternating thrusting movements of forepaws and shoveling movements of the snout, directed toward a discrete source of unfamiliar, aversive, or noxious stimuli. The behavior is interpreted as an unconditioned, species-specific response toward certain olfactory (68), tactile (31), and visual stimuli (69), which will prompt avoidance behavior under appropriate conditions. Together with flight, freezing, and certain forms of agonistic behavior, it constitutes the defensive behavioral repertoire in these species.

Defensive burying is also easily evoked as a conditioned response toward originally neutral stimuli having acquired aversive properties (e.g., by a one-trial association with an electric shock presentation through a wire-wrapped dowel (65)). Defensive burying, both as a conditioned and an unconditioned response, has been proposed as a useful experimental procedure for the screening of novel anxiolytic drugs (70).

Anxiolytics belonging to two different pharmacologic classes (i.e., BZDs, 5-HT$_{1A}$ receptor agonists) have been found to suppress defensive burying both in rats (71) and mice (72), though the behavioral selectivity of the effects of 5-HT$_{1A}$ receptor agonists has been questioned in mice (73). A number of 5-HT uptake-blocking drugs selectively reduced defensive burying (74).

Stretched Approach Posture

Ambivalent behavior is a universal response of humans and animals in conflict situations. It is the result of at least two incompatible tendencies that are engendered by an object or a subject, such as the fight-flight conflict in confrontations with an aggressive opponent, or an approach-avoidance conflict in interactions with a sexual partner (75).

Ambivalent behavior can also occur in a nonsocial context such as an approach-avoidance conflict toward an aversive object. These incompatible tendencies are combined into one behavioral pattern that displays elements of both underlying motivational states (75). In rats and mice, approach-avoidance ambivalence can be observed toward an aversive object that elicits fear and curiosity, which results in a behavioral pattern, described as stretched approach posture (SAP) (76). SAP can be observed in various situations as, for example, in passive avoidance situations, on the elevated plus-maze (77), or after a mild startle reaction due to physical contact with an electrified probe (78).

Suppression of SAP seems to provide a very attractive and ethologically valid model for the study of anxiolytic drugs. SAP is reduced by BZD full agonists, 5-HT_{1A} receptor agonists, and SSRIs (76,78,79).

Future Developments in Anxiolytic Drugs

An ideal anxiolytic drug should have the following properties (80): 1) rapid onset, without initial exacerbations; 2) full efficacy, i.e., working on all anxiety disorders; 3) no tolerance development; 4) no rebound upon discontinuation; 5) no interactions with sedative drugs such as alcohol; 6) no impairment of cognitive processes such as memory or performance; and 7) no euphoric actions that could lead to abuse. In fact, this is a description of the advantages of a potent BZD agonist, without its side effects.

Notwithstanding considerable efforts to improve ligands for the $GABA_A$-BZD receptor, including subtype selective ligands, partial agonists, or neurosteroids (cf. 81), up to now no real breakthroughs in this area have occurred (cf. 9; 82).

For short-term veterinary applications, BZDs may be the first choice for general use. In the near future, the potential of BZD partial agonists as anxiolytic agents devoid of sedation and muscle-relaxant properties will be investigated. It is suggested that this class of compounds could lead to less tolerance and withdrawal.

Compounds, exerting anxiolytic effects via non-BZD mechanisms may fulfill an important role in the future treatment of anxiety. One such approach is represented by 5-HT_{1A} receptor agonists. 5-HT_{1A} receptors are one type of 5-HT receptors, of which at least fourteen others are known ($5\text{-HT}_{1A, 1B, 1D, 1E, 1F}$; $5\text{-HT}_{2A, 2B, 2C}$; 5-HT_3; 5-HT_4; $5\text{-HT}_{5A, 5B}$; 5-HT_6; and 5-HT_7 receptors). Although a role for various 5-HT receptors in anxiety has been suggested (e.g., $5\text{-}HT_{1D}$, $5\text{-}HT_{2C}$, $5\text{-}HT_3$), only the $5\text{-}HT_{1A}$ receptor has been shown to exert a modulatory role in various anxiety processes. However, the exact role of full (e.g., flesinoxan) or partial (e.g., buspirone, gepirone, ipsapirone) $5\text{-}HT_{1A}$ receptor agonists, certainly in veterinary applications, has yet to be established.

The role of SSRIs (fluoxetine, fluvoxamine) in anxiety disorders is surprisingly large. SSRIs enhance serotonergic neurotransmission and exert therapeutic efficacy only after weeks of administration. SSRIs are particularly active in obsessive-compulsive disorder and in panic disorder. It is unclear which 5-HT receptor is particularly influenced by SSRIs, and future studies with selective 5-HT ligands should shed light on this problem. There is considerable evidence that SSRIs are also active in various obsessive-compulsive disorder–like behaviors and pathologies in veterinary practice (82a,83).

Various additional neurophysiologic mechanisms of action, other than the ones discussed here, are also involved in anxiety. For example, corticotropin-releasing hormone (CRH) and cholecystokinin (CCK) are activated. The evidence that both CRH receptors (stress) and CCK receptors are involved in anxiety processes is strong, although until now, no effective ligands for these receptors have been developed.

References

1. Green S, Hodges H. Animal models of anxiety. In: Willner P, ed. Behavioral models in psychopharmacology. Oxford: Oxford University Press, 1991:21–49.
2. Richards G, Schoch P, Jenck F. Benzodiazepine receptors and their ligands. In: Rodgers RJ, Cooper SJ, eds. $5\text{-}HT_{1A}$ agonists, $5\text{-}HT_3$ antagonists and benzodiazepines: their comparative behavioral pharmacology. Chichester, England: John Wiley & Sons, 1991:1–30.
3. Stephens DN, Andrews JS. Screening for anxiolytic drugs. In: Willner P, ed. Behavioral models in psychopharmacology. Oxford: Oxford University Press, 1991:50–75.
4. Goa KL, Ward A. Buspirone: a preliminary review of its pharmacological properties and therapeutic efficacy as an anxiolytic. Drugs 1986;32:114–129.
5. Den Boer JA, Westenberg HGM, Kamerbeek WDJ, et al. Effect of serotonin uptake inhibitors in anxiety disorders: a double-blind comparison of clomipramine and fluvoxamine. Int Clin Psychopharmacol 1987;2:21–32.
6. McNair DM, Kahn RJ. Imipramine compared with a benzodiazepine for agoraphobia. In: Klein DF, Rabkin J, eds. Anxiety: new research and changing concepts. New York: Raven, 1981:69–80.
7. Robinson DS, Shrotriya RC, Alms DR, et al. Treatment of panic disorder: nonbenzodiazepine anxiolytics including buspirone. Psychopharmacol Bull 1989;25:21–26.
8. Boissier JR, Simon P, Aron C. A new method for rapid screening of minor tranquilizers in mice. Eur J Pharmacol 1968;4:145–151.
8. Chouinard G, Annable L, Fontaine R, Solyon L. Alprazolam in the treatment of generalized anxiety and panic disorders: a double-blind, placebo-controlled study. Psychopharmacology 1982;77:229–233.
9. Miczek KA, Weerts EM, Vivian JA, Barros HM. Aggression, anxiety and vocalizations in animals: $GABA_A$ and 5-HT anxiolytics. Psychopharmacology 1995;121:38–56.

10. Geller I, Seifter J. The effects of meprobamate, barbiturates, d-amphetamine and promazine on experimentally induced conflict in the rat. Psychopharmacology 1960;9:482–492.

11. Barrett JE, Witkin JM, Mansbach RS, et al. Behavioral studies with anxiolytic drugs. III. Antipunishment actions of buspirone in the pigeon do not involve benzodiazepine receptor mechanisms. J Pharmacol Exp Ther 1986;238:1009–1013.

12. Vogel JR, Beer B, Clody DE. A simple and reliable conflict procedure for testing anti-anxiety agents. Psychopharmacology 1971;1:1–7.

13. Barrett JE, Gleeson S. Anxiolytic effects of 5-HT$_{1A}$ agonists, 5-HT$_3$ antagonists and benzodiazepines: conflict and drug discrimination studies. In: Rodgers RJ, Cooper SJ, eds. 5-HT$_{1A}$ agonists, 5-HT$_3$ antagonists and benzodiazepines; their comparative behavioral pharmacology. Chichester, England: John Wiley & Sons, 1991:59–105.

14. Blanchard RJ, Blanchard DC, Agullana R, Weiss SM. Twenty-two kHz alarm cries to presentation of a predator, by laboratory rats living in visible burrow systems. Physiol Behav 1991;50:967–972.

15. Aron C, Simon P, Boissier JR. Evaluation of a rapid technique for detecting minor tranquillizers. Neuropharmacologia 1971;10:459–469.

16. Stephens DN, Kehr W. β-carbolines can enhance or antagonize the effects of punishment in mice. Psychopharmacology 1985;85:143–147.

17. Molewijk HE, Van der Heyden JAM. Psychopharmacological profile of fluvoxamine. In: Olivier B, Mos J, eds. Depression, anxiety and aggression: preclinical and clinical interfaces. Houten: Medidact, 1988:31–42.

18. Montgomery KC. The relation between fear induced by novel stimulation and exploratory behavior. J Comp Physiol Psychol 1955;48:254–260.

19. Pellow S, Johnston AL, File SE. Selective agonists and antagonists for 5-hydroxytryptamine receptor subtypes, and interactions with yohimbine and FG7142 using the elevated plus-maze test in the rat. J Pharm Pharmacol 1987;39:917–928.

20. Crawley JN. Neuropharmacologic specificity of a simple animal model for the behavioral actions of benzodiazepines. Pharmacol Biochem Behav 1981;15:695–699.

21. Kilfoil T, Michel A, Montgomery D, Whiting RL. Effects of anxiolytic and anxiogenic drugs on exploratory activity in a simple model of anxiety in mice. Neuropharmacology 1989;28:901–905.

22. File SE. The use of social interaction as a method for detecting anxiolytic activity of chlordiazepoxide-like drugs. J Neurosci Methods 1980;2:219–238.

23. Schuurman T, Spencer DG, Traber J. Behavioral effects of the 5-HT$_{1A}$-receptor ligand ipsapirone (TVX Q7821): A comparison with 8-OH-DPAT and diazepam. Psychopharmacology 1987;89(suppl):S54.

24. File SE. Animal models for predicting clinical efficacy of anxiolytic drugs. Neuropsychobiology 1985;13:55–62.

25. Barrett JE. Animal behavioral models in the analysis and understanding of anxiolytic drugs at serotonin receptors. In: Olivier B, Mos J, Slangen JL, eds. Animal models in psychopharmacology. Basel: Birkhäuser Verlag, 1991:37–52.

26. Davis M. Pharmacological and anatomical analysis of fear conditioning using the fear-potentiated startle paradigm. Behav Neurosci 1986;100:814–824.

27. Hijzen TH, Houtzager SWJ, Joordens RJE, et al. Predictive validity of the potentiated startle response as a behavioral model for anxiolytic drugs. Psychopharmacology 1995;118:150–154.

28. Joordens RJE, Hijzen TH, Peeters BWMM, Olivier B. Fear-potentiated startle response is remarkably similar in two laboratories. Psychopharmacology 1996;26:104–109.

29. Kehne JH, Cassella JV, Davis M. Anxiolytic effects of buspirone and gepirone in the fear-potentiated startle paradigm. Psychopharmacology 1988;4:8–13.

30. Mansbach RS, Geyer MA. Blockade of potentiated startle responding in rats by 5-HT$_{1A}$ receptor ligands. Eur J Pharmacol 1988;56:375–383.
31. Broekkamp CL, Rijk HW, Joly-Gelouin D, Lloyd KL. Major tranquillizers can be distinguished from minor tranquillizers on the basis of effects on marble-burying and swim-induced grooming in mice. Eur J Pharmacol 1986;126:223–229.
32. Shearman GT, Lal H. Generalization and antagonism studies with convulsants, GABA-ergic and anticonvulsant drugs in rats trained to discriminate pentylenetetrazole from saline. Neuropharmacology 1980;19:473–479.
33. Lal H, Emmett-Oglesby MW. Behavioral analogues of anxiety. Neuropharmacology 1983;2:1423–1441.
34. Vivian JA, Miczek KA. Diazepam and gepirone selectively attenuate either 20–32 kHz or 32–64 kHz ultrasonic vocalizations during aggressive encounters. Psychopharmacology 1993;112:66–73.
35. Molewijk HE, Van der Poel AM, Mos J, et al. Conditioned ultrasonic distress vocalisations in adult male rats as a behavioral paradigm for screening anti-panic drugs. Psychopharmacology 1995;117:32–40.
36. Kaltwasser MT. Acoustic startle-induced ultrasonic vocalizations in the rat: a novel animal model of anxiety? Behav Brain Res 1991;3:133–137.
37. Miczek KA, Vivian JA. Automatic quantification of withdrawal from 5-day diazepam in rats: ultrasonic distress vocalizations and hyperreflexia to acoustic startle stimuli. Psychopharmacology 1993;110:379–382.
38. Barros HMT, Miczek KA. Withdrawal from oral cocaine in rats: ultrasonic vocalizations and tactile startle. Psychopharmacology 1996;125:379–384.
39. Vivian JA, Miczek KA. Ultrasounds during morphine withdrawal in rats. Psychopharmacology 1991;104:187–193.
40. Cuomo V, Ciagiano R, Salvia MA, et al. Ultrasonic vocalization in response to unavoidable aversive stimuli in rats: effects of benzodiazepines. Life Sci 1988;43:485–491.
41. De Vry J, Benz U, Schreiber R, Traber J. Shock-induced ultrasonic vocalization in young adult rats: a model for testing putative anti-anxiety drugs. Eur J Pharmacol 1993;249:331–339.
42. Sanchez C. Effect of serotonergic drugs on footshock-induced ultrasonic vocalization in adult male rats. Behav Pharmacol 1993;4:269–277.
43. Tornatzky W, Miczek KA. Alcohol, anxiolytics and social stress in rats. Psychopharmacology 1995;121:135–144.
44. Allin JT, Banks EM. Effect of temperature on ultrasound production by infant albino rats. Dev Psychobiol 1971;4:49–156.
45. Hård E, Engel J, Musi B. The ontogeny of defensive reactions in the rat: influence of the monoamine transmission systems. Scand J Psychol Suppl 1982;1:90–96.
46. Winslow JT, Insel TR. Infant rat separation is a sensitive test for novel anxiolytics. Progr Neuropsychopharmacol Biol Psychiatry 1991;5:745–757.
47. Gardner CR, Budhram P. Effects of agents which interact with central benzodiazepine binding sites on stress-induced ultrasounds in rat pups. Eur J Pharmacol 1987;134:275–283.
48. Nastiti K, Benton D, Brain PF. The effects of compounds acting at the benzodiazepine receptor complex on the ultrasonic calling of mouse pups. Behav Pharmacol 1991;2:121–128.
49. Winslow JT, Insel TR. Serotonergic modulation of rat pup ultrasonic isolation call: studies with 5-HT$_1$ and 5-HT$_2$ subtype-selective agonists and antagonists. Psychopharmacology 1991;105:513–520.
50. Mos J, Olivier B. Ultrasonic vocalizations by rat pups as animal models for anxiolytic activity: effect of serotonergic drugs. In: Archer T, Bevan P, Cools, eds. The behavioral pharmacology of 5-HT. New York: Lawrence Erlbaum Inc., 1989:361–366.

51. Herman BH, Panksepp J. Effects of morphine and naloxone on social attachment in infant guinea pigs. Pharmacol Biochem Behav 1978;9:213–219.

52. Berryman JC. A study of guinea pig vocalizations: with particular reference to mother-infant interactions. Thesis, University of Leicester, 1974:1–299.

53. Olivier B, Mos J, Bradford LD. Serotonergic and opiate involvement in an animal model of affiliative behaviour: distress vocalizations in guinea pigs. In: Olivier B, Mos J, eds. Depression, anxiety and aggression: preclinical and clinical interfaces. Houten: Medidact, 1988;71–84.

54. Pettijohn TF. Effects of imipramine on infant pig distress vocalizations. Psychol Rep 1979;44:918.

55. Molewijk HE, Hartog K, Van der Poel AM, et al. Reduction of guinea pig pup isolation calls by anxiolytic and antidepressant drugs. Psychopharmacology 1996;128:31–28.

56. Borsini F, Lecci A, Volterra G, Meli A. A model to measure anticipatory anxiety in mice? Psychopharmacology 1989;98:207–211.

57. Eikelboom R, Stuart J. Conditioned temperature effects using morphine as the unconditioned stimulus. Psychopharmacology 1979;61:31–38.

58. Eikelboom R. Learned anticipatory rise in body temperature due to handling. Physiol Behav 1986;37:649–653.

59. Gollnick PD, Ianuzzo CD. Colonic temperature response of rats during exercise. J Appl Physiol 1968;24:747–750.

60. York JL, Regan SC. Conditioned and unconditioned influences on body temperature and ethanol hyperthermia in laboratory rats. Pharmacol Biochem Behav 1982;7:119–124.

61. Reeves DL, Levinson DM, Justesen DR, Lubin B. Endogenous hyperthermia in normal human subjects: experimental study of emotional states (II). Int J Psychosom 1985;32: 18–23.

62. Yoshiue S, Yoshizawa H, Ito H, et al. Analysis of body temperature at different sites in patients having slight fever caused by psychogenic stress. In: Lomax P, and Schonbaum S, eds. Thermoregulation: research and clinical applications. Basel: Karger, 1989:169–172.

63. Zethoff TJJ, Heyden van der JAM, Tolboom JTBM, Olivier B. Stress-induced hyperthermia in mice: a methodological study. Physiol Behav 1994;55:109.

64. Zethof TJJ, Van der Heyden JAM, Olivier B. Stress-induced hyperthermia as putative anxiety model. Eur J Pharmacol 1995;294:125–135.

65. Pinel JPJ, Treit D. Burying as a defensive response in the rat. J Comp Physiol Psychol 1978;92:708–712.

66. Davis SF, Moore SA, Cowen CL, et al. Defensive burying in the Mongolian gerbil (Meriones unguiculatus) as a function of size and shape of the test chamber. Anim Learn Behav 1982;10:516–520.

67. Heynen AJ, Sainsbury RS, Montoya CP. Cross-species responses in the defensive burying paradigm: a comparison between Long-Evans rats (Rattus norvegicus), Richardson's ground squirrels (Spermophilus richardsonii), and thirteen-lined ground squirrels (Catellus tridecemlineatus). J Comp Psychol 1989;103:184–190.

68. Jackson RL, Garbin CP, Hollingsworth EM. Defensive burying of aversive fluids in rats: the possible role of odor. Learn Motiv 1984;5:85–105.

69. Pinel JPJ, Treit D, Wilkie DM. Stimulus control of defensive burying in the rat. Learn Motiv 1980;11:150–163.

70. Treit D. Anxiolytic effects of benzodiazepines and 5-HT$_{1A}$ agonists: animal models. In: Rodgers RJ, Cooper SJ, eds. 5-HT$_{1A}$ agonists, 5-HT$_3$ antagonists and benzodiazepines: their comparative behavioral pharmacology. Chichester, England: John Wiley & Sons, 1991:107–131.

71. Groenink L, Van der Gugten J, Verdouw PM, et al. The anxiolytic effects of flesinoxan, a 5-HT1A receptor agonist, are not related to its neuroendocrine effects. Eur J Pharmacol 1995;280:185–193.

72. De Boer SF, Van der Gugten J, Slangen JL. Behavioral and hormonal indices of anxiolytic and anxiogenic drug action in the shock prod defensive burying/avoidance paradigm. In: Olivier B, Mos J, Slangen JL, eds. Animal models in psychopharmacology. Basel: Birkhäuser Verlag, 1991:81–96.

73. Broekkamp CLE, Berendsen HHG, Jenck F, Van Delft AML. Animal models for anxiety and response to serotonergic drugs. Psychopathology 1989;22(suppl 1):2–12.

74. Njung'e K, Handley SL. Effects of 5-HT uptake inhibitors, agonists and antagonists on the burying of harmless objects by mice: a putative test for anxiolytic agents. Br J Pharmacol 1991;104:105–112.

75. Hinde RA. Behaviour in conflict situations. In: Hinde RA, ed. Animal behaviour: a synthesis of ethology and comparative psychology. New York: McGraw Hill, 1970:270–290.

76. Kaesermann HP. Stretched attend posture, a non-social form of ambivalence, is sensitive to a conflict-reducing drug action. Psychopharmacology 1986;9:31–37.

77. Cole JC, Rodgers RJ. An ethological analysis of the effects of chlordiazepoxide and bretazenil (Ro 16-6028) in the murine elevated plus-maze. Behav Pharmacol 1990;4:573–580.

78. Molewijk HE, Van der Poel AM, Olivier B. The ambivalent behaviour 'stretched approach posture' in the rat as a paradigm to characterize anxiolytic drugs. Psychopharmacology 1995;121:81–90.

79. Pollard GT, Howard JC. Effects of chlordiazepoxide, pentobarbital, buspirone, chlorpromazine and morphine in the stretched attend posture (SAP) test. Psychopharmacology 1988;94:433–434.

80. Nutt DJ. Anxiety and its therapy: today and tomorrow. In: Briley M, File SE, eds. New concepts in anxiety. New York: Macmillan, 1991:1–12.

81. Rabow LE, Russek SJ, Farb DH. From ion currents to genetic analysis: recent advances in $GABA_A$ receptor research. Synapse 1995;21:189–274.

82. Doble A, Martin IL. The $GABA_A$/Benzodiazepine receptor as a target for psychoactive drugs. New York: Chapman and Hall, 1996:1–274.

82a. Dodman NH, Olivier B. In search of animal models for obsessive-compulsive disorder. CNS Spectrums 1996;1:10–15.

83. Insel TR, Mos J, Olivier B. Animal models of obsessive compulsive disorder: a review. In: Olivier E, Zohar J, Marazzati, Olivier B, eds. Current insights in obsessive compulsive disorder. Chichester, England: John Wiley & Sons, 1994:17–35.

Pharmacologic Treatment of Fear and Anxiety in Animals

Petra A. Mertens

Nicholas H. Dodman

Fear is a conscious, rational, and emotional response to stimuli in the face of danger. An adaptive fear reaction protects the threatened individual and consists of species-specific behaviors including fight, flight, or immobility (1,2). Fear responses may become exaggerated, even maladaptive, in animals that have suffered adverse experiences. Anxiety is a diffuse, often longer lasting state of fear that exists without an obvious distinct cause or threat. In animals, anxiety manifests as hyperactivity, restlessness, apparent insecurity, hypervigilance, enhanced reactivity, inappetence, and frequent elimination (3). The development of anxiety depends on several factors including heredity and experience. Phobias (see Chap. 6) are fear reactions that are out of proportion, inducing extreme and irrational avoidance reactions (4).

About one third of all patients admitted to behavior clinics in veterinary teaching hospitals present with fear-related problems (1,5). Some animals become frightened of people or other animals of the same or different species, whereas others fear inanimate cues such as loud noises. Fears can also be situationally motivated, as exemplified by separation anxiety. Many animals have multiple fear-related conditions, perhaps due to some genetic or acquired predisposition. In some dogs, excessive anxiety or fearfulness appears to be an underlying trait from which specific fears develop.

Etiology

INHERITANCE AND ANXIETY

Intensive breeding of dogs for different purposes has led to unexpected medical and behavioral problems (6). Most animal behaviorists acknowledge that there are breed predilections for temperament and, consequently, behavior problems (7). Spaniels and terriers frequently display dominance aggression (5,8) and

German Shepherds and other herding dogs seem predisposed to anxiety-based conditions. Breed differences in temperament were confirmed by the work of Fuller (9) who showed that beagles, when isolated, showed reduced activity, whereas terriers became more active. The influence of inheritance on anxiety and fearfulness is illustrated by a genetically nervous strain of pointers maintained at the National Institutes of Health (10). Affected dogs display excessive timidity, hyperstartle, rigidity in the presence of humans, and marked inhibition of environmental exploration (11). Recently, increased anxiety and fearfulness has been found to be associated with subclinical hypothyroidism in some dogs (Dodman NH, Aronson L, Dodds J, unpublished data, 1997). For further information on this subject, see Chapter 3, Systemic Causes of Aggression and Their Treatment.

LEARNING AND ANXIETY

Negative early experiences, especially those occurring during sensitive periods of development, may have profound and long-lasting effects on an animal's behavior. If the same portentous situation is encountered repeatedly, anxiety and apprehension may develop from anticipation of the noxious stimulus, thereby making the experience progressively more distressing for the animal in the future (i.e., sensitization) (2,12). To some extent, this compounding of the response is dependent on stimulus intensity and frequency. Mild stressors (e.g., painless restraint) occurring frequently may have an opposite effect and result in desensitization to the stressor (13). This is the basis of systematic desensitization, the primary behavior modification strategy in the treatment of fears. However, individual factors do play a role in determining which animals will have enhancement or reduction of the adrenocortical response pattern when exposed to chronic stress (13).

Physiologic Response

CENTRAL MECHANISMS

The central nucleus of the amygdala is a key area involved in the generation of the signs and symptoms of fear and anxiety (14,15). In the process of mediating fear responses, this nucleus makes connections with many other areas, such as the hypothalamus, dorsal motor nucleus of the vagus, parabrachial nucleus, locus coeruleus, and paraventricular nucleus. Four neurotransmitter systems, acting in concert, are instrumental in the development of fear and anxiety (16,17).

Noradrenergic System
The central noradrenergic system, and in particular noradrenergic neurons projecting from the locus coeruleus, mediates a broad range of behaviors and

physiologic responses associated with anxiety and fear (18). Increases in tha-lamic transmission accompanying activation of the locus coeruleus may lead to increased vigilance and superior signal detection in a state of fear and, via trigeminal and motor nuclei, facial expressions of fear (14). The "fight-flight" reaction that typifies fear is coordinated by activation of the sympathetic nervous system, including the adrenal release of epinephrine and norepineph-rine (12,19). Activation of the beta-adrenergic system in situations of emo-tional arousal affects long-term memory of negative events through plastic changes in central adrenergic mechanisms (20). This enhancement of memory is adaptive for the animal concerned. The amygdala appears to be the primary site of the memory-enhancing effects of catecholamines (21).

Dopaminergic System

Certain populations of dopamine neurons are selectively activated in stress, a response that is attenuated by anxiolytics (22). Dopamine release occurs mainly in the meso-prefrontal cortex, but other areas, such as the meso-amygdaloid area, are also involved. The limbic system, in which the amygdal-oid area is situated, is a phylogenetically ancient part of the brain that governs a variety of emotional and viscerosomatic functions (23).

Serotonergic System

Serotonin (5-HT) is involved in the mediation of anxiety, though its role is not clearly defined. The 5-HT system, particularly that located in the dorsal raphe nuclei, inhibits adaptive and social attachment behavior (24–27). Stress and anxiety increase 5-HT release (28), and adequate serotonin release is instru-mental in some fear responses (29). However, no strict relationship exists between the release of 5-HT and the performance of anxiety-driven behavior (30). The anxiety-related increase in hippocampal 5-HT release exhibited by rats is not exhibited by peers raised in isolation, suggesting that the responsive-ness of the 5-HT system may be, in part, determined by prior experience. (30).

GABA-ergic System

Gamma-aminobutyric acid (GABA)-mediated neurotransmission is known to be affected by stress (31). GABA is an important inhibitory neurotransmitter that influences tone in serotonergic and noradrenergic networks, the former being instrumental in its anxiolytic effects (see Chap. 4, Fear and Anxiety: Mechanisms, Models, and Molecules). As a corollary, $GABA_A$ blockade pro-duces anxiogenic-like effects in rats and cardiovascular and respiratory activa-tion (32).

PERIPHERAL MECHANISMS

Fear and anxiety in animals produce physiologic responses similar to those that occur in humans, including trembling, tachycardia, tachypnea, and gastrointestinal disturbances (33). These symptoms result from increased activity of the sympathetic nervous system as the fight-flight response is activated. Other signs of sympathetic activation include dilation of the pupils, peripheral vasoconstriction, increased arousal/alertness, piloerection, and the secretion of thick viscid saliva from the submandibular salivary glands. Animals that are fearful also exhibit increased startle potential, increased grooming, and may adopt freezing postures (34).

Discharge of the anal glands is a manifestation of fear in dogs, cats, and some other species. Anal gland secretions may contain a fear pheromone that signals the site of the fear-inducing event.

Clinical Manifestations of Fear and Anxiety

Fears can be thought of as comprising either: 1) fear of living things (animate fears); 2) fear of inanimate cues; or 3) fear of situations. The interrelationship of these components of fear responses is illustrated in Figure 5.1.

CANINE ANIMATE FEARS

Dogs that are fearful of animate cues will display signs of fear when confronted with the fear-inducing stimulus by changes in affect, posture, and purposeful or

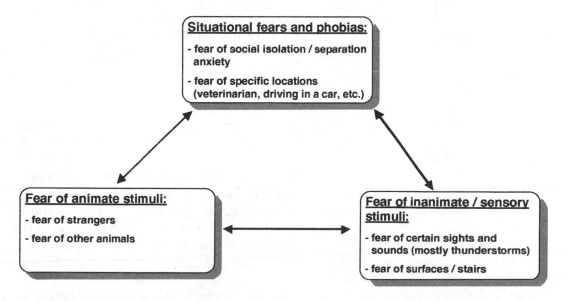

Figure 5.1.
Common fears and phobias in animals. A subdivision of fear-related problems into three categories simplifies the discussion of problems and their treatment. One has to keep in mind that this subdivision is artificial. The individual patient is often suffering from multiple fear-related problems that require treatment.

apparently purposeless operant behavior. Operant responses include fight, flight, freezing, and displacement behaviors, such as pacing or circling. Signs of autonomic arousal are apparent. As dogs with fears of this nature mature and gain confidence, some of the more dominant ones employ aggression as a defensive strategy, capitalizing on early successes and escalating their approach. Systematic desensitization is the basis for treatment of animate fears and other fear-induced behavioral conditions; however, fear-alleviating medication can be an invaluable adjunct to behavior modification therapy.

CANINE INANIMATE FEARS

Auditory, visual, tactile, or olfactory cues can precipitate fear in susceptible animals. Fears of this type are usually conditioned through pairing with a fear-inducing event. One common inanimate fear is fear of thunderstorms, which can present at various levels of intensity ranging from mild apprehension during storms to a full-blown phobia (see Chap. 6, Pharmacology of Acquired Fears and Phobias).

CANINE SITUATIONAL FEARS

Separation anxiety is a common situational fear that affects approximately 4% of the nation's 55 million dogs. Between 2% and 34% of all dogs presented to veterinary behaviorists are diagnosed with separation anxiety (35–37). Dogs are highly social animals and require social interaction to maintain individual security (5). Puppies normally react with increased activity and vocalization if they are separated from their dams; the function of this behavior is to bring about an early reunion. The strong emotional attachment of dogs to their owners supplants this intraspecific social bonding. Following adoption, normal pups learn to tolerate separation from their owners for extended periods of time, but social deprivation during a sensitive period of development (3–12 weeks of age) may have profound and long-lasting effects on their confidence.

Typically, dogs with separation anxiety have experienced suboptimal bonding experiences. Some dogs have had multiple owners and some have developed separation anxiety after spending time in a pet store or animal shelter while young (37). Separation anxiety may intensify when the owner's schedule changes or the dog is brought into a new environment. Separation anxiety is common in young dogs that have not yet adjusted to their new environment, but it is also the most common behavior problem in dogs older than 10 years (38). The latter finding may be attributable to comorbid medical problems (39). Clinical signs of separation anxiety include following the owner around the house, becoming anxious as the owner prepares to leave, vocalization shortly after the owner's departure, panic leading to frantic attempts to escape ("barrier frustration"), damage to property (often around doors and windows), salivation, inactivity (perhaps related to learned helplessness/depression), psychogenic anorexia, inappropriate elimination, and exuberant greeting behavior on the owner's return. Not all signs are present in all affected animals, but if five or more signs are present a diagnosis of separation anxiety probably applies if differential diagnoses (medical and behavioral) have been excluded.

FELINE ANIMATE FEARS

Fear of strangers is a common feline behavioral complaint. Inadequate socialization and adverse early experiences are usually at the root of the problem. Feral cats' mistrust of humans serves as an extreme example of the importance of early socialization. Fear of other cats is another common problem that may result in conflict. Fear of other housecats, from whom there is no escape, may lead to a variety of neurotic conditions, such as inappropriate elimination and psychogenic alopecia.

In cats, signs of animate fears are analogous to those in dogs and include pupillary dilation, piloerection, and rotation of the pinnae. Behavioral responses include fight, flight, the adoption of postures designed to intimidate an adversary, and displacement grooming.

FELINE INANIMATE FEARS

Like dogs, cats can become fearful of inanimate cues they have previously associated with an unpleasant event or novel stimulus portending danger. Many such fears go unnoticed by cat owners, possibly because frightened cats usually flee and hide. Thunderstorm phobia is rarely if ever reported in cats.

FELINE SITUATIONAL FEARS

Cats frequently develop separation anxiety, fear of visits to the veterinarian's office, and fear of car travel. The latter two conditions present as an unwillingness to enter the cat carrier. Signs of separation anxiety in cats are not as blatant as those in dogs. Cats do not exhibit obvious barrier frustration but may disturb neighbors by excessive vocalization. Overattachment to the owner and inappropriate urination are more likely presenting signs of separation anxiety in cats. Many cases of feline separation anxiety probably are undiagnosed.

EQUINE ANIMATE FEARS

Horses frequently develop fear of people or other horses. Other animate fears, such as fear of flying insects, are also encountered. Undersocialization and harsh treatment are sometimes to blame for the development of fear of humans, especially if adverse experiences occur in a sensitive period of development. Fear aggression possibly develops when dominance fuels a proactive approach toward dealing with the animate fear. Fear aggression toward people is extremely dangerous for the persons concerned, and treatment should be undertaken with this in mind.

EQUINE INANIMATE FEARS

Horses are normally suspicious of anything unfamiliar and will react by shying or bolting. A plethora of inanimate fears is found in all but the most well-trained horses. Many horses exhibit fear of shadows, strange objects, unusual surfaces, and so on. Fear of storms can result if a horse is exposed to some aversive experience during a storm.

EQUINE SITUATIONAL FEARS

Trailering is one of the most common situational fears encountered in horses. Trailer shyness arises partly because horses have a natural fear of small spaces and are sometimes not allowed sufficient time to overcome this fear when they are first introduced to loading. The experience is thus remembered as an unpleasant one that the horse will subsequently attempt to avoid. Adverse experiences during a journey can also create loading problems in horses.

Separation anxiety is a common equine situational fear. Under some circumstances, horses develop close relationships with one another and separation of a bonded pair can result in much whinnying and, sometimes, disastrous physical attempts by one horse to be reunited with its mate.

Treatment of Fear-based Conditions

Nonpharmacologic treatment of situational fears and other fear-related problems in animals involves applying specific behavior modification techniques, such as desensitization, counterconditioning, and flooding, which are described in detail elsewhere (40,41). Success rates of nonpharmacologic behavior modification therapy vary because most of these techniques require a high level of owner compliance and commitment to the program. One of the most daunting aspects of behavior modification therapy for owners is the time that it takes to effect noticeable change. Also sticking points are often encountered during the desensitization programs in which progress is barely discernible or nonexistent. Adjunctive pharmacologic therapy often expedites recovery by circumventing these sticking points and encouraging owner compliance with the program. Pharmacologic therapy alone will sometimes permit spontaneous desensitization to a previously feared stimulus/situation, although this is not usually the optimum approach.

Before any treatment program is instituted, it is important to conduct a detailed behavioral interview with the client and to examine the patient to confirm the nature of the problem, establish a behavioral diagnosis, and rule out the possibility that a medical condition may be contributing to the problem. In some cases, laboratory tests or other diagnostic procedures, such as radiography or electroencephalography, are required to fully evaluate a patient. A complete blood count (CBC), chemistry profile, thyroid panel, and urinalysis provide useful background information when medical conditions are thought to be involved.

Pharmacotherapy

The majority of drugs used to alleviate fear and anxiety (Table 5.1) have not been approved as safe or effective for use in animals by the Food and Drug Administration's Center for Veterinary Medicine. However, their legitimate use in nonfood animals has recently been approved in the Animal Medicinal Drug Use Clarification Act (1994).

In the past, veterinarians prescribed two main classes of drugs for behavioral therapy of fear-based conditions: phenothiazines and benzodiazepines (42,43). More recently other drugs, including the tricyclic antidepressants and azapirones, have been used with increasing frequency. The interaction of some commonly used pharmacologic agents with various neurotransmitters is depicted in Figure 5.2.

BENZODIAZEPINES

Benzodiazepines have been the most frequently prescribed antianxiety drugs for humans as well as for animals. For years drugs like diazepam and clorazepate have been employed for the treatment of various fear-related conditions in pets, including animate fears, sound phobia, and separation anxiety (43,44).

The mechanism of action of benzodiazepines is based on a drug-receptor interaction throughout the CNS. Different types of benzodiazepine receptors have been identified in the limbic system, brain-stem arousal centers, cerebellum, hippocampus, cortex, and spinal cord (45). When benzodiazepines bind to benzodiazepine receptors, there is increased chloride influx into the cell and consequent hyperpolarization. The net effect is inhibition of neurotransmission involving the noradrenergic, dopaminergic, and serotonergic systems (46). This mechanism is responsible for alleviation of anxiety as well as effects such as sedation, ataxia, muscle relaxation, impaired learning and memory, and elevation of the seizure threshold.

A rare, but lethal hepatopathy in cats treated with low doses of diazepam, for even a short period of time, has recently been reported (47). It is not known whether other benzodiazepines might also cause this effect in cats, but for the time being, it may be prudent to employ alprazolam in this

Table 5.1. Drugs used to alleviate fear and anxiety

Drug class	Commonly used drug	Indication	Suggested canine dosage	Suggested feline dosage	Potential side effects	Contraindications	Onset of drug action
Azapirone	Buspirone (Buspar)	Situational fears, especially cases of generalized fear	2.5–10.0 mg PO bid *per dog*	2.5–5.0 mg PO bid or tid *per cat*	Sedation, arousal	Potentiates diazepam	2–4 wks
Benzodiazepine	Diazepam (Valium)	Short-term sedation for fear of infrequently encountered situations	0.55–2.20 mg/kg PO prn	1–2 mg PO bid *per cat*	Sedation; increased seizure threshold; ataxia, muscle relaxation	Chronic fears and phobias; treatment requiring learning	Rapid
Beta-blocker	Propranolol (Inderal)	Mild manifestations of situational fears, or in combination with other anxiolytics, like buspirone	Propranolol, 5–40 mg PO tid *per dog* (depending on weight)	2.5–5.0 mg PO bid or tid *per cat*	Urinary incontinence	Medical problems involving heart and circulation	Generally within 60 min after medication

Phenothiazine	Acepromazine maleate (Acepromazine)	Short-term sedation for fear of infrequently encountered situations	0.55–1.1 mg/kg PO; 0.055–0.110 mg/kg IM, SQ, IV	1.1–2.2 mg/kg PO; 0.11–0.22 mg/kg IM, SQ, IV	Sedation, agitation, reduced social and exploratory behavior	Chronic anxiety; animals showing paradoxical effects	Rapid (1–2 hrs)
Serotonin reuptake inhibitor	Fluoxetine (Prozac)	Chronic situational fears; conditions occurring in combination with other problems	1 mg/kg PO sid	None	Decreased appetite, vomiting, restlessness		Approximately 4–6 wk
Tricyclic antidepressant	Amitriptyline (Elavil) Clomipramine (Anafranil)	Separation anxiety, chronic situational fears conditions occurring in combination with other problems	2.2–4.4 mg/kg PO bid 1–3 mg/kg PO sid	5–10 mg PO sid per cat; 1 mg/kg PO sid	Sedation, dry mouth, constipation, urinary retention, cardiac conduction	Animals suffering from cardiac conditions or problems involving the urinary tract (especially infections)	After 4 wk

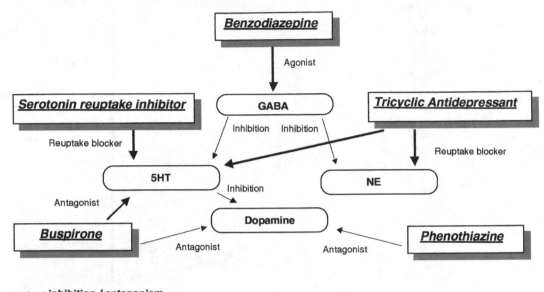

Figure. 5.2.
Drug-neurotransmitter interaction. (GABA = gamma-aminobutyric acid; 5-HT = 5-hydroxytryptamine [serotonin]; NE = norepinephrine [noradrenaline]).

species. Alprazolam is structurally different from other benzodiazepines and has different metabolites. In addition, alprazolam produces fewer side effects than the classic 1,4-benzodiazepines (48–50) and has analgesic effects (51).

One of the main disadvantages of benzodiazepines in any species is that they are dependence-producing, and abrupt discontinuation can precipitate withdrawal. This has been suggested as one of the main reasons for the high recidivism rate (90%) following diazepam treatment of anxiety-related inappropriate elimination behavior in cats (52). Optimally, benzodiazepines should be tapered off gradually, over 1 or 2 months following treatment, depending on the patient's response to the tapering schedule (53).

Benzodiazepines often cause troublesome side effects, such as sedation, ataxia, hyperphagia, and weight gain. Although tolerance to some of these side effects occurs fairly rapidly, their occurrence is nonetheless a drawback of benzodiazepine use. We reserve benzodiazepines for short-term therapy of patients in acute situations in which sedation and ataxia are less important than the overall effect of controlling the animal's emotional reaction to a stimulus or situation. For longer term treatment, more specific anxiolytic drugs, such as buspirone, often produce similar effects with fewer or no side effects and with no risk of inducing pharmacologic dependence.

NEUROLEPTICS

Neuroleptic drugs exert their therapeutic and extrapyramidal effects by blocking dopamine receptors in the brain. Phenothiazines, such as acepromazine, promazine, and chlorpromazine, are the most frequently prescribed agents in this group and have been the mainstays of pharmacologic behavior modification in the past. They have proved effective in the suppression of symptoms associated with a variety of anxious or fearful behaviors, including fear aggression, excess timidity, sound phobia, separation anxiety, and other situational fears; however, their effects are anything but selective, being inseparable from associated CNS depression. Sedation, a primary feature of the action of phenothiazines, may be desirable when phenothiazines are employed for chemical restraint, but it is a disadvantage during long-term behavior modification therapy. Within the three decades during which neuroleptics have been used in veterinary medicine, idiosyncratic reactions of severe aggression have been reported a few times related to the use of acepromazine and chlorpromazine in dogs (53a). Although these episodes are reported rarely, one should be aware of this potential side effect when using phenothiazines for treatment of behavior problems related to fear and anxiety.

Physiologic consequences of the administration of phenothiazines include hypotension (as a result of alpha-adrenergic blockade), hypothermia, smooth muscle relaxation, antiemesis, reduction of the seizure threshold, and an increase in prolactin secretion. High-potency neuroleptics, such as butyrophenones, haloperidol, and droperidol, produce less sedation but are more likely to induce extrapyramidal side effects than low-potency neuroleptics. Though less sedating, butyrophenones are more effective than phenothiazines in inhibiting spontaneous and conditioned learning behavior. Butyrophenones have weaker antiadrenergic properties than phenothiazines, are potent antiemetics, and increase prolactin secretion.

Neither high- nor low-potency neuroleptics are ideal for use in behavior modification therapy, but newer neuroleptics might eventually play a valuable role in pharmacologic behavior modification therapy. Two such drugs are clozapine and risperidone. Clozapine is a dibenzazepine derivative with antagonistic action at multiple dopamine receptors and significant anticholinergic effects. Site specificity has been suggested as an explanation for the low incidence of extrapyramidal effects with this drug (54). Clozapine also has high affinity for $5\text{-}HT_2$ receptors where it acts as an antagonist. Clozapine causes salivation and other minor side effects in dogs and can trigger seizures, but it does not cause agranulocytosis in this species (54; Sandoz Pharmaceutical, unpublished data, 1997). Risperidone is a novel antipsychotic with potent D2 and $5\text{-}HT_2$ antagonistic properties. The D2 blocking effects, in particular, may help prevent agitation and facilitate socialization (55). Although promising, clozapine and risperidone (and other novel antipsychotics) remain unproven in veterinary behavioral pharmacology, but the way things are going it is only a matter of time.

BETA-BLOCKERS

Beta-blockers have been reported to be effective antianxiety drugs for the treatment of situational fears in humans. For example, propranolol decreases cardiovascular complaints and tremor associated with anxiety in humans (56,57,58). Beta-blockers have also been shown to have beneficial effects in animal models of anxiety (59). We have used beta-blockers with some success to treat animate fears, sound phobias, and separation anxiety in dogs. The mechanism of action of beta-blockers may be more complex than simply attenuating the fight-flight response. It appears that they may reduce apprehension by resetting muscle spindles (60), thus attenuating proprioceptive impulses to the reticular activating system (RAS). As proprioceptive afferents' bombardment of the RAS maintains alertness, the net effect is to decrease vigilance and reactivity. In addition, beta-blockers that cross the blood-brain barrier block 5-HT1 receptors, thereby increasing serotonin release. This secondary action may contribute to the behavioral and mood stabilizing effects of beta-blockers.

Beta-blockers cause bradycardia and hypotension and are contraindicated in some cardiac conditions; beyond this, however, they produce few, if any, problematic side effects and have no potential for producing dependence. Given orally, they take effect in about 1 to 2 hours and their effect appears to last a few hours depending on the compound used. They may either be administered empirically, usually on a three times daily basis or given as needed, depending on the frequency of the fear-inducing event. Alternatively, long-acting preparations can be employed on a once or twice daily schedule.

BUSPIRONE

Buspirone is a member of a new class of anxiolytic drugs (azaspirodecanedione derivatives) that are chemically unrelated to other anxiolytics. It is highly specific in its action and does not produce the unwanted side effects of sedation, ataxia, or drug dependence (61,62). The term "anxioselective" has been coined to describe buspirone's action and to distinguish it from less specific agents. In a laboratory model of separation distress in rat pups, buspirone's anxiolytic properties mimicked those of benzodiazepines (63). Clinical studies comparing buspirone and diazepam confirm the anxiolytic effectiveness of both drugs in humans (64–68), though information about buspirone's anxiolytic use in domestic animals is only at the clinical report stage. In humans, buspirone appears more effective in patients that have not been previously treated with benzodiazepines (69).

Buspirone's effects involve multiple neurotransmitter systems, though 5-HT1A receptors located in the dorsal raphe, hippocampus, and frontal cortex are the primary sites of its anxiolytic action. Buspirone also acts as a weak dopamine antagonist (70–72). Although therapeutic blood levels of buspirone are attained quite rapidly after an oral dose, the anxiolytic effects build up progressively, with maximum efficacy being achieved only after 3 or 4 weeks of treatment (72). The half-life of buspirone ranges from 1 to 11 hours in humans but is probably less in domestic small animals (73). For this reason, multiple daily dosing (bid or tid) is recommended.

We have found buspirone effective in the treatment of various small animal fears, including canine separation anxiety, noise phobia, and fear of strangers. Its effect is palliative rather than fully therapeutic, so adjunctive behavior modification therapy is usually required. In humans, potential adverse reactions to treatment with buspirone include nausea, sedation, headaches, and dizziness. These symptoms occur in a much lower percentage of patients treated with buspirone than with diazepam or clorazepate (74,75). A veterinary study in cats reports side effects of buspirone as increased affection to owners, occasional spats of intraspecific aggression, and transient agitation shortly after dosing (52).

TRICYCLIC ANTIDEPRESSANTS

Tricyclic antidepressants, especially tertiary amines, including amitriptyline, imipramine, and clomipramine, are effective treatments for panic attacks and agoraphobia in humans (76), and chronic treatment with desipramine is effective in preventing anxiety-related behavior in rats subjected to conflict situations (33). The neurotransmitter effects of tricyclic antidepressants include anticholinergic, antihistaminic, serotonergic, adrenergic, and noradrenergic effects (68), and tricyclics may be classified according to their potency in inhibiting or recapturing these neurotransmitters. Most antidepressants, including tricyclic antidepressants and serotonin reuptake inhibitors, increase 5-HT neurotransmission (77). Clomipramine is more selective than imipramine or amitriptyline in this respect (78). Tricyclic antidepressants may work by modifying receptor site sensitivity rather than by a direct action at the receptor site, as the anxiolytic effects are only seen after several weeks of treatment (77,79).

As serotonin is known to influence social attachment behaviors, it is logical that tricyclic antidepressants should effect separation distress during isolation of animals from groupmates. Imipramine has been found to reduce signs of separation anxiety in isolated young rhesus monkeys (80), and amitriptyline has been successfully used in cases of severe separation anxiety in dogs (37,44). In dogs with separation anxiety treated with behavior modification therapy and amitriptyline, beneficial effects were first noticed after approximately 4 weeks of treatment, though the effect continued to build to a peak within 6 months of therapy (37). If the condition is stabilized at a satisfactory level for 1 to 2 months, the medication can then be gradually withdrawn over several weeks, at a rate determined by the patient's response. If there is a relapse, the dose can be adjusted to a previously effective level for a further or indefinite period. Clomipramine has been used successfully to treat separation anxiety in dogs. Results from a multicenter, blinded, placebo controlled, clinical trial (n = 77) show that clomipramine leads to significant improvements in dogs treated for separation anxiety when used at a dosage of 2 mg/kg bid PO in conjunction with behavior modification techniques. These effects were more pronounced at this dose than in a group treated with clomipramine at a lower dose (1 mg/kg bid PO) and a placebo group. Improvements are reached faster using the higher dose, which is also clearly improving owner compliance. The only side effect that was attributed to the use of clomipramine during an observation period of 84 days was temporary vomiting, observed in 12.5% of the dogs treated at the higher and in 11.1% of the cases at the lower dose (80a).

In humans, side effects observed during therapy with tricyclic antidepressants include dry mouth, arrhythmias, and tachycardia. Gastrointestinal side effects are also common. In addition, patients treated with antidepressants may experience excessive sleepiness and dizziness. Similar observations have been made by the owners of dogs treated with amitriptyline. Side effects in dogs include polydipsia (presumably caused by dryness of the mouth), vomiting, and urinary retention (37). Similar side effects may be seen in cats treated with clomipramine though, in addition, we have noticed a paradoxical syndrome of social withdrawal in this species. Many of the side effects of antidepressants result from blockade of muscarinic and H1-histaminic receptors.

SELECTIVE SEROTONIN REUPTAKE INHIBITORS

Third-generation antidepressants show great promise in veterinary medicine. Fluoxetine, a dicyclic antidepressant, is the best known member of this group and is effective for treatment of a variety of different problems, including aggression, obsessive-compulsive disorder, and fear-related problems (81–83). Although selective serotonin reuptake inhibitors (SSRIs) are marketed for the treatment of depression, they are also effective treatments for fear and anxiety-related conditions. Animal experiments measuring anxiolytic drug effects by reduction of cries of rat pups during separation distress show that SSRIs like fluoxetine have strong anxiolytic potencies (84).

Inhibition of serotonin reuptake at the presynaptic neuronal site induces enhanced serotonergic transmission, which in turn is thought to lead to downregulation of postsynaptic receptors (85). Enhanced 5-HT levels initially lead to activation of 5-HT$_{1A}$ somatodentric receptors, reducing 5-HT release (86). Tolerance to this latter effect develops, subsequently reversing the effect and possibly causing augmentation of synaptic concentrations of serotonin.

Advantages of SSRIs over tricyclic antidepressants include less sedation, fewer anticholinergic side effects, and minimal effects on cardiac conduction. Known side effects of fluoxetine are mostly related to the gastro-intestinal tract, but inappetence, weight loss, and restlessness also sometimes occur.

Conclusion

Psychotropic drugs may be helpful adjuncts in treating fear-related problems in veterinary medicine. The advantages and disadvantages of the different drugs previously discussed should be evaluated in light of the behavioral application and individual patient requirements. Understanding the biochemical interactions, side effects, contraindications, and design of treatment protocols is essential for safe and effective pharmacologic treatment of all behavior problems in animals, including those that are fear based. Constant monitoring and modification of treatment programs, including adjustments of the type and dose of the medications, is key to the success of treatment and is necessary for the safety of the patient.

References

1. Shull-Selcer E, Stagg W. Advances in the understanding and treatment of noise phobias. Vet Clin North Am 1991;21:353–367.
2. Webster J. Animal welfare: a cool eye towards Eden. Oxford: Blackwell Science, 1995.
3. Rowan AN. Animal anxiety and animal suffering. Appl Anim Behav Sci 1988;20:135–142.
4. Marks I. Fears, phobias, and rituals. panic, anxiety, and their rituals. New York: Oxford University Press, 1987.
5. Mertens PA, Dodman NH. The diagnosis of behavior problems in dogs, cats, birds, and horses: characteristics of 323 cases (July 1994–June 1995). Kleintierpraxis 1996;41:197–206.
6. Scott JP, Fuller JL. Genetics and social behavior of the dog. Chicago: University of Chicago Press, 1965.
7. Hart BL, Hart LA. Behavioral aspects of selecting and raising dogs and cats. In: Canine and feline behavioral therapy. Philadelphia: Lea & Febiger, 1985:185–206.
8. Sherman CK, Reisner IR, Taliaferro LA, Houpt KA. Characteristics, treatment, and outcome of 99 cases of aggression between dogs. Appl Anim Behav Sci 1996;47:91–108.
9. Fuller JL. Experimental deprivation and later behavior. Science 1967;158:1645–1652.
10. Lucas LA, DeLuca DC, Newton JEO, Angel CA. Animal models for human psychopathology: the nervous pointer dog. In: Gershon ES, Matthysse S, Breakefield XO, Ciaranello RD, eds. Genetic research strategies for psychobiology and psychiatry. Pacific Grove: Boxwood Press, 1981.
11. Tancer ME, Stein MB, Bessette BB, Uhde TW. Behavioral effects of chronic imipramine treatment in genetically nervous pointer dogs. Physiol Behav 1990;48:179–181.
12. Broom DM, Johnson KG. Stress and animal welfare. London: Chapman and Hall, 1993.
13. Ladewig J, De Passillé AM, Rushen J, et al. Stress and the physiological correlates of stereotypic behavior. In: Lawrence AB, Rushen J, eds. Stereotypic animal behavior: fundamentals and applications to welfare. CAB International, 1993.
14. Davis M. The role of the amygdala in fear-potentiated startle: implications for animal models of anxiety. TIPS 1992;13:35–41.

15. Barinaga M. Watching the brain remake itself. Science 1994;266:1475–1476.

16. Trimble MR. The neurological basis of anxiety. Br J Clin Pract 1985;39:10–13.

17. Dubovsky SL. Generalized anxiety disorder: new concepts and psychopharmacologic therapies. J Clin Psychiatry 1990;51:3–10.

18. Charney DS, Woods SW, Nagy LM, et al. Noradrenergic function in panic disorder. J Clin Psychiatry 1990;51:5–11.

19. Cannon WB. Stresses and strains of homeostasis. Am J Med Sci 1935;189:1–14.

20. Cahill L, Prins B, Weber M, McGaugh JL. β-adrenergic activation and memory for emotional events. Nature 1994;371:702–704.

21. McGaugh JL. Affect, neuromodulatory systems, and memory storage. In: Christianson S, ed. The handbook of emotion and memory research and theory. Hillsdale: Lawrence Erlbaum Assoc, 1992:245–268.

22. Coco ML, Kuhn CM, Ely TD, Kilts CD. Selective activation of mesolimbic dopamine neurons by conditioned stress: attenuation by diazepam. Brain Res 1992;590:39–47.

23. Kelly D. Physiological changes during operations on the limbic system in man. Conditional Reflex 1972;7:127–138.

24. Charney DS, Woods SW, Goodman WK, Heininger GR. Serotonin function in anxiety. II. Effects of the serotonin agonist MCPP in panic disorder patients and healthy subjects. Psychopharmacology 1987;92:12–24.

25. Molliver ME. Serotonergic neuronal systems: what their anatomic organization tells us about function. J Clin Psychopharmacol 1987;7:3–23.

26. Mench JA, Shea-Moore MM. Moods, minds and molecules: the neurochemistry of social behavior. Appl Anim Behav Sci 1995;44:99–118.

27. Paul SM. Anxiety and depression: a common neurobiological substrate? J Clin Psychiatry 1988;49:13–16.

28. Yoshioka M, Matsumoto M, Togashi H, Saito H. Effects of conditioned fear stress on 5-HT release in the rat prefrontal cortex. Pharmacol Biochem Behav 1995;51:515–519.

29. Chen C, Rainnie DG, Greene RW, Tonegawa S. Normal fear response and aggressive behavior in mutant mice deficient for α-calcium-calmodulin kinase II. Science 1994; 266:291–294.

30. Wright IK, Upton N, Marsden CA. Resocialization of isolation-reared rats does not alter their anxiogenic profile on the elevated X-maze model of anxiety. Physiol Behav 1991;50:1129–1132.

31. Hamon M. Neuropharmacology of anxiety. TIPS 1994;15:36–39.

32. Shekhar A. Effects of treatment with imipramine and clonazepam on an animal model of panic disorder. Biol Psychiatry 1994;36:748–758.

33. Bass C. Physical symptoms of anxiety. Br J Clin Pract 1985;39:343–380.

34. Davis M. Animal models of anxiety based on classical conditioning: the conditioned emotional response (CER) and the fear-potentiated startle effect. Pharmacol Ther 1990;47:147–165.

35. Wright JC, Fillingin R, Nesselrobe M. Classification of behavioral problems in dogs: influence of age, breed, sex and reproductive status. Presented at the Meeting of the Animal Behavior Society, Raleigh NC, 1985.

36. Beaver BV. Owner complaints about canine behavior. J Am Vet Med Assoc 1994;12:1953–1955.

37. Mertens PA, Dodman NH, Unshelm J. Separation anxiety—pharmacological treatment of a yuppie-puppy syndrome. Presented at the Meeting of the International Association for Anthrozoology, Cambridge, United Kingdom, July 1996.

38. Chapman RB, Voith VL. Behavioral problems in old dogs: 26 cases (1984–1987). J Am Vet Med Assoc 1990;196:1070–1072.

39. Dodman NH. Will you still need me, will you still feed me? In: The dog who loved too much. New York: Bantam, 1996.

40. Borchelt PL, Voith VL. Treatment and diagnosis of separation anxiety problems. Vet Clin North Am Advan Compan Anim Behav 1982:12:625–636.

41. Tuber DS, Hothersall D, Peters MF. Treatment of fears and phobias in dogs. Vet Clin North Am 1982:12:607–624.

42. Voith VL. Pharmacological approaches to treating behavioral problems. In: Anderson RS, ed. Nutrition and behavior in dogs and cats. Oxford: Pergamon, 1984:227–234.

43. Hart BL. Behavioral indications for phenothiazine and benzodiazepine tranquilizers in dogs. J Am Vet Med Assoc 1985;163:1192–1194.

44. Marder AR. Psychotropic drugs and behavioral therapy. In: Marder AR, Voith VL, eds. Vet Clin North Am Advan Compan Anim Behav 1991;21:329–342.

45. Doble A, Martin IL. Multiple benzodiazepine receptors: no reason for anxiety. TIPS 1992;13:76–81.

46. Hindmarch I. Anxiety, performance and anti-anxiety drugs. Br J Clin Pract 1985;39:53–57.

47. Center SA, Elston TH, Rowland RH, et al. Fulminant hepatic failure associated with oral administration of diazepam in 11 cats. J Am Vet Med Assoc 1996;209:618–625.

48. Fabre LF, McLendon FM. A double-blind study comparing the efficacy and safety of alprazolam with diazepam and placebo in anxious outpatients. Curr Ther Res 1979;26:519–526.

49. Cohn JB. Multicenter double-blind efficacy and safety study comparing alprazolam, diazepam, and placebo in clinically anxious patients. J Clin Psychiatry 1982;42:347–351.

50. Rickels K, Csanalosi I, Greisman P, et al. A controlled clinical trial of alprazolam for the treatment of anxiety. Am J Psychiatry 1983;140:82–85.

51. Forman LJ, Estilow-Isabell S, Harwell M, et al. Possible opiate action in the anxiolytic and antinociceptive actions of alprazolam. Res Commun Chem Pathol Pharmacol 1991;71: 259–271.

52. Hart BL, Eckstein RA, Powell KL, Dodman NH. Effectiveness of buspirone on urine spraying and inappropriate urination in cats. J Am Vet Med Assoc 1993;203:254–258.

53. Burrows GD. Managing long-term therapy for panic disorder. J Clin Psychiatry 1990;51: 9–12.

53a. Meyer EK. Rare, idiosyncratic reactions to acepromazine in dogs. J Am Vet Med Assoc 1997,210:1114–1115.

54. Michals ML, Crismon ML, Roberts S, Childs A. Clozapine response and adverse effects in nine brain injured patients. J Clin Psychopharmacol 1993;13:198–203.

55. Leysen JE, Janssen PMF, Gommeran W, et al. In vitro and in vivo receptor binding and effects on monoamine turnover in rat brain regions of the novel antipsychotics risperidone and ocaperidone. Mol Pharmacol 1991;41:494–509.

56. Grainviller-Grossmann KL, Turner P. Effect of propranolol on anxiety. Lancet 1996;1:788–790.

57. Tyrer P, Lader M. Physiological respiration with propranolol and diazepam in chronic anxiety. Pharmacology 1974;1:387–390.

58. Hallstromm C, Tresaden I, Edwards JG. Diazepam, propranolol and diazepam in chronic anxiety. Br J Psychiatry 1981;139:417–421.

59. Durel LA, Krantz DS, Barrett JE. The antianxiety effect of beta-blockers on punished responding. Pharm Biochem Behav 1991;11:398–399.

60. Ratey JJ, Morrill R, Oxenkrug G. Use of propranolol for provoked and unprovoked episodes of rage. Am J Psychiatry 1983;140:1356–1357.

61. Goldberg HL. Buspirone hydrochloride: a unique new anxiolytic agent. Pharmacotherapy 1984;4:315–324

62. Goa KL, Ward A. Buspirone: a preliminary review of its pharmacological properties and therapeutic efficacy as an anxiolytic. Drugs 1986;32:114–129.

63. Winslow JT, Insel TR. The infant rat separation paradigm: a novel test for novel anxiolytics. TIPS 1991;12:402–404.

64. Goldberg H, Finnerty RJ. Comparative efficacy of buspirone in two different studies. Am J Psychiatry 1982;43:87–91.
65. Rickels K, Weisman K, Norstad N. Buspirone and diazepam in anxiety: a controlled study. J Clin Psychiatry 1982;43:81–86.
66. Bond A. The psychological effects of buspirone. Br J Clin Pract 1985;39:83–89.
67. Tyrer P, Murphy S, Owen RT. The risk of pharmacological dependence with buspirone. Br J Clin Pract 1985;39:91–93.
68. Petracca A, Nistia C, McNir D, et al. Treatment of generalized anxiety disorder: preliminary clinical experience with buspirone. J Clin Psychiatry 1990;51:31–39.
69. Olajide D, Lader M. A comparison of buspirone, diazepam, and placebo in patients with chronic anxiety states. J Clin Psychopharmacol 1987;7:148–152.
70. Eison MS, Van der Maeleu CP, Matheson GK, et al. Interactions of the anxioselective agent buspirone with central serotonin systems. Soc Neurosci Abstr 1983;9:436.
71. Leonard BE. Neuropharmacological profile of buspirone: a nonbenzodiazepine anxiolytic with specific mid-brain modulating properties. Br J Clin Pract 1985;38:74–81.
72. Peroutka SJ. Selective interaction of novel anxiolytics with 5-hydroxytryptamine 1A receptors. Biol Psychiatry 1985;20:971–979.
73. Gammans RE, Mayol RF, Labudde JA. Metabolism and disposition of buspirone. Am J Med 1986;80:41–51.
74. Newton RE, Casten GP, Alms DR, et al. The side effects profile of buspirone in comparison to active controls and placebo. J Clin Psychiatry 1982;43:102–107.
75. Knapp JE. Clinical profile of buspirone. Br J Clin Pract 1985;38:95–99.
76. Liebowitz MR, Fyer AJ, Gorman JM, et al. Tricyclic therapy of the DSM-III anxiety disorders: a review with implications for further research. J Psychiatry Res 1988;22:7–33.
77. Blier P, de Montigny C, Chaput Y. Modifications of the serotonin system by antidepressant treatments: implications for the treatment response in major depression. J Clin Psychopharmacol 1987;7:24–35.
78. Balant-Gorgia AE, Gex-Fabry M, Balant LP. Clinical pharmacokinetics of clomipramine. Clin Pharmacokinet 1991;20:447–462.
79. de Montigny C, Agajanian GK. Tricyclic antidepressants: long term treatment increases responsivity of rat forebrain neurons to serotonin. Science 1978;202:1303–1306.
80. Suomi SJ, Seaman SF, Lewis JK, et al. Effects of imipramine treatment of separation-induced social disorders in rhesus monkeys. Arch Gen Psychiatry 1978;35:321–325.
80a. Simpson B. Treatment of separation-related anxiety in dogs with clomipramine. Results from a multicentre, blinded, placebo controlled clinical trial. Proceedings of the First International Conference on Veterinary Behavioural Medicine. Birmingham, UK 1.-2. April 1997:143–154.
81. Dodman NH, Donnelly RD, Shuster L, et al. Use of fluoxetine to treat dominance aggression in dogs. J Am Vet Med Assoc 1996;209:1585–1587.
82. Dodman NH, Moon-Fanelli AA, Mertens PA, Stein DJ. Animal models for obsessive compulsive disorder. In: Hollander E, Stein DJ, eds. Obsessive compulsive disorder. New York: Marcel Dekker, 1997 (in press).
83. Dodman NH. Has fluoxetine (Prozac) been found to be truly effective for behavior modification? Vet Med 1997 (in press).
84. McKinney WT. Separation and depression: biological markers. In: Reite M, Field T, eds. The psychobiology of attachment and separation, vol. 6. Orlando: Academic Press, 1985:201–222.
85. Olivier B, Tulp M, Mos J. Serotonergic receptors in anxiety and aggression: evidence from animals pharmacology. Hum Psychopharmacol 1991;6:73–78.
86. Rickels K, Schweizer E. Clinical overview of serotonin receptors: effector systems, physiological roles and regulation. Psychopharmacology 1987;92:267–277.

Pharmacologic Treatment of Phobias

Steven B. Thompson

Fear-related behaviors in companion animals are well recognized. These include fear of loud noises, separation, strange environments, strangers, and novel objects (1–5), although reactivity can be associated with stimuli that are no longer novel (6). This chapter focuses on the diagnosis, development, and treatment of excessive fears, termed *phobias*.

Diagnostic Criteria, Classification, and Neurobiology

Veterinarians are a pet owner's initial contact for medical, nutritional, management, and behavioral advice (7). Pet owners often present the companion animal to a practitioner with a diagnosis based on their own interpretation of the pet's behavior and their recognition of the situational stressor. However, pets may also be presented for behavior problems like destruction or excess vocalization that have their origins in a fear or phobia the owners have yet to recognize.

A thorough behavioral history and appropriate medical workup are essential to fully elucidate factors involved in the propagation and maintenance of behavior problems. Numerous articles have extolled the virtues of incorporating a behavioral history form into practice protocols and of having access to a behavior consultant (8–11). Additional time is required to administer and interpret a behavioral history form, and it is critical that fee structures reflect this, just as fee structures should reflect extended consultations on medical case discussions for patients with diabetes mellitus or hyperadrenocorticism (12). The information gathered through an appropriate history allows the practitioner to rule in or out various behavioral disorders as a cause for the presenting condition. Practitioners must resist the quick-fix diagnosis of "behavior disorder" or "stress" and should proceed through a logical thought process, just as if evaluating a medical symptom, such as polyuria.

Although progress has been made in the classification of anxiety disorders in animals, this field is still in its infancy. As is the case with anxiety-based conditions in the field of child and adolescent psychiatry (13), much work remains to be done on basic issues such as diagnostic reliability, diagnostic validity, natural course, outcome, and treatment. Understanding and being able to diagnose normal and abnormal fear responses is critical before implementing any therapeutic plan, whether it includes owner education regarding species-typical behaviors, behavior modification therapy, or the use of pharmacotherapy.

THE FEAR RESPONSE

When a threat is recognized, an animal manifests a self-protective response. Typical stimuli that naturally evoke fear responses include: 1) direct predator stimuli (e.g., proximity, specific and sudden movements, visual features, olfactory and auditory cues); 2) situations or events associated with the threat of predation; 3) environmental or physical dangers such as heights, noise, or temperature extremes; 4) perceived danger in the form of novel or unfamiliar objects or locations; and 5) behaviors of conspecifics, including threats, intrusion into territorial or personal space, and initial interactions with strangers (2,14). The fear response is a complex integration of three components: behavioral, physiological, and emotional (1).

Fearful dogs and cats, like most mammals, have three major defensive behavior strategies known as the three Fs: *flight*—from the threat; *fight*—defensive aggression involving actual attack or threat of attack in self-defense; and *freezing*—immobility, lying still to avoid attracting attention (15). With regard to the latter, for years veterinarians have used lift-tables and slick surfaces to capitalize on fear-induced immobility in order to accomplish a thorough physical examination on a previously fractious pet. The few minutes of immobility provided often allows sufficient time for an organized individual with technical assistance to perform the physical examination, obtain needed laboratory samples, and administer necessary treatments. When captured, prey species often will show a tonic immobility that may facilitate release by a predator. Unlike the immobility seen when prey species are hiding and their exploratory behavior gradually returns, captured animals are prepared to escape immediately following this tonic immobility state (15).

Dogs and other group species, including humans, demonstrate a fourth type of reaction to fear-inducing stimuli, *fiddling*. This takes the form of deflection or appeasement in an effort to convince the threatener that it is not worth the bother or risk of attack (16). In companion animals, the presence of a human, such as the owner, can be a determining factor in the behavior demonstrated (1).

The physiologic component of the fear response includes activation of the autonomic and neuroendocrine systems. This activation has been ascribed to the brain's response to differences between set values and actual values for any homeostatic variable monitored and controlled by the CNS (17). This physiologic response shows extreme variance and reflects individual variability, the intensity and duration of the fear response, and situational requirements (1,18).

The two main sources of variance are genetic variance and variance due to storage of information (learning or memory) dependent on the CNS (17). Ursin (17) has proposed two stages in emotional behaviors that relate to fear responses in particular. Initially, there is an *affective phase*, with high activation, that gradually transfers to an *instrumental phase*, with lower activation. When a behavior pattern (e.g., cat runs to hide under the bed) achieves a desired instrumental effect (e.g., visitors are less threatening), there is a reducing effect on the activation response and the somatic state of the animal. Within this context, *coping* is defined as the particular effect of instrumental behavior (17). The behavioral and physiologic responses of two individuals responding to one stimulus may therefore be quite different (2,17).

The emotional component of the fear response is the subjective awareness of fear. Humans can describe feelings of fear and rank its intensity. Presumably, companion animals also "feel afraid," but an owner or clinician is only able to interpret a pet's "emotional behavior." *Emotional behavior* is characterized by the activation processes, and the experience of these processes is an important component of emotions (17).

The three components of the integrated fear response do not necessarily correlate well; physiologic responses to a stimulus may not correlate well either (1). Investigations into the characterization and correlation of these responses in humans with anxiety disorders, including panic attacks and phobias, have increased in frequency in the psychiatry literature from 3% of the total number of articles in 1980 to 16% in 1990 (19). While literature on animals includes information on responses to stress, pain, and experimentally conditioned fears, information on naturally occurring fear disorders in companion animals is quite limited. This information is critical to understanding mechanisms behind fear-related disorders and should help improve treatment options (1).

FUNCTIONAL CLASSIFICATION SCHEMES

Traditionally, companion animal behavior problems have been categorized using a functional classification system that attempts to identify the relationship between the animal, its behavior, and the environment (including the owner) (20). However, genetic predispositions, developmental factors, stimulus-response relationships, physiologic states, and disease also have an effect. Usually, fears and phobias are clustered together and considered distinct diagnoses from other fear-related conditions, such as fear aggression and separation anxiety, although a fearful animal may present to a practitioner with more than one or all of the above-mentioned problems (20). A three-category system has been used that is dependent on the contexts in which the behaviors occurred (6). Based on interpretations of development and exploratory behavior mechanisms (21), the *stimulus-reactivity* category is used to characterize behaviors that demonstrate excessive approach or avoidance in reaction to a stimulus. The other two categories are *aggression* (i.e., agonistic behaviors) and *separation-related disorders*. Phobic reactions are included in the stimulus-reactivity category. Animals may display heightened arousal or reactivity during an event or submissive postures and trembling associated with withdrawal from the stimulus (6).

The American Psychiatric Association's *Diagnostic and Statistical Manual of Mental Disorders*, Fourth Edition (DSM-IV; 22) is the standard reference for discussing mental disorders in the medical community. Most phobias recognized in companion animals would best fall within the diagnostic criteria used for anxiety disorders in human psychiatry. Diagnostic criteria are readily applicable to animal patients in most categories. Overall (23) has modified criteria from DSM-IV to establish "necessary and sufficient conditions" for behavioral diagnoses in companion animals, while stressing that diagnoses are not diseases and correlation is not causality (see Chapter 9). The necessary and sufficient conditions for noise phobia include: sudden and profound, nongraded, extreme response to noise, manifest as intense, active avoidance, escape, or anxiety behaviors associated with the activities of the sympathetic branch of the autonomic nervous system; behaviors can include catatonia and mania concomitant with decreased sensitivity to pain or social stimuli; repeated exposure results in invariant patterns of response (23).

SPECIFIC PHOBIA (PHOBIAS OF OBJECTS)

The DSM-IV now uses the term *specific phobia* (formerly *simple phobia*) to describe a phobic response (22). According to DSM-IV (22), the seven diagnostic criteria for a specific phobia include:

A. Marked and persistent fear that is excessive or unreasonable, cued by the presence or persistence of a specific object or situation.

B. Exposure to the phobic stimulus almost invariably provides an immediate anxiety response, which may take the form of a situationally bound or situationally predisposed panic attack. *Note*: In children, the anxiety may be expressed by crying, tantrums, freezing, or clinging.

C. Patient recognition of excessive fear. *Note*: This feature may be absent in children.

D. The phobic situation is avoided or else is endured with intense anxiety or distress.

E. The avoidance, anxious anticipation, or distress in the feared situations interferes significantly with their normal routine, functioning, or social relationships.

F. In individuals less than 18 years, the duration is at least 6 months.

G. The anxiety, panic attacks, or phobic avoidance associated with the specific object or situation is not better accounted for by another mental disorder such as posttraumatic stress disorder, separation anxiety disorder, social phobia, or panic disorder with agoraphobia, or obsessive-compulsive disorder.

With extrapolation and if the social maturation date is changed from a human time frame to a species typical time frame, these criteria can be utilized by the veterinary practitioner to define a specific phobia in companion animals. For example, "less than 18 years old" in humans would be equivalent to less than 1.5 to 3 years of age in dogs and cats. In animals, fear-related aggression may be the equivalent of tantrums in children. The DSM-IV also has a list of subtypes that are used to better classify the specific phobias (22).

- The *animal type*, which generally begins in childhood in humans, would include phobias to other species including insects. For pets, examples of common animal-type phobias might include snakes, children, or individuals of another race.
- The *natural environment type*, which also begins in childhood in humans, accounts for phobias to storms, heights, and water.
- The *blood-injection-injury type* is recognized as a unique subtype in humans, is cued by injury, injections, or other invasive medical procedures, and is known to be highly familial and characterized by a strong vasovagal response. Whether some veterinary hospital phobias after vaccine visits or diagnostic workups fit this phobia subtype has yet to be examined in companion animals. There is considerable support that this subtype may deserve a separate classification from the other phobic disorders. True syncopal episodes on exposure to the stimulus are not uncommon in patients with this phobia, and this is not a characteristic of other anxiety disorders (24).
- The *situational type* is designated if the fear is cued by specific situations like elevators, flying, driving, or enclosed places. Most veterinary visit phobias would likely be categorized this way, as would show ring phobias. This subtype in humans has a bimodal age distribution during childhood and then early adulthood (mid 20s), which is similar to that seen with panic disorder and agoraphobia.
- The "*other*" category includes miscellaneous stimuli not covered already. Common specific phobias in humans that fall into this category include "space" phobias such as fear of being out in an open area and childhood fears of loud noises and costumed individuals (22). The remaining companion animal noise phobias due to gunshots, fireworks, appliances, vacuums, or lawn mowers would be classified as "other," as would fear of objects like storm sewers, bikes, or farm machinery.

POSTTRAUMATIC STRESS DISORDER

Posttraumatic stress disorder (PTSD) is by definition the only psychiatric disorder requiring that a particular stressor should precede its appearance (25).

PTSD is generally recognized as a neurobiologic disturbance produced by severe, unexpected, and/or uncontrollable stress. Traumatic events in humans are primarily combat related, but include sexual abuse, burn injury, criminal victimization, and hurricanes (25). PTSD is characterized by avoidance of stimuli associated with the severe stressor. It has been reported that some people with diagnosed combat-related PTSD exhibit an exaggerated startle response to loud noises (26,27).

Several situations in companion animals may correlate with the diagnostic criteria for PTSD: 1) development of fear of vehicles in animals hit by a car or when passengers during a car accident; 2) excessive, irrational fear of particular strangers following known abuse by unscrupulous individuals; 3) panic manifested by an animal that has previously been stung by an insect whenever it hears an insect buzzing; and 4) generalized noise phobia in animals that have observed an explosion or have been in close contact with a lightning strike. Each of these is a potential example of PTSD that still requires confirmation.

In contrast to patients with panic disorder, PTSD patients characteristically exhibit hyperarousal and have difficulties sleeping (25). PTSD has been explained and characterized primarily as representing phasic sympathetic hyperarousal, and there appears to be dysfunction in the hypothalamic-pituitary-adrenal axis; this contrasts with panic disorder, in which such changes have not been clearly identified (25). Sleep history may therefore be a valuable adjunct to behavioral histories on companion animal pets and should assist with their classification using appropriate diagnostic criteria. Studies are just now beginning to look at startle responses in normal and phobic dogs (28) and behavioral responses to stimuli during sleeping and waking in dogs (29).

SOCIAL PHOBIA (PHOBIAS OF FUNCTION)

Social phobia is the most common human anxiety disorder in the United States, with a lifetime prevalence of 11.3% (30). Social phobias often coexist with other psychiatric disorders, the most common being simple or specific phobia (59% of patients with social phobia), and panic attacks may occur in social phobia on exposure to the feared situation (30). Diagnostic criteria for social phobia or social anxiety disorder require evidence of the capacity for age-appropriate social relationships with familiar people, and the anxiety must occur in peer settings (22). Several difficulties arise in determining whether animals exhibit social phobias as they are currently defined in psychiatry, because the criteria necessitate social interaction with similar species. This may exclude cats, ferrets, and other "asocial" species from the classification scheme. Interaction with other species is better classified as a specific phobia, *animal subtype*. However, dogs, horses, and hand-raised psittacines may readily relate to people as fellow pack, herd, or flock members. A second criterion, still more difficult to extrapolate, is the need for awareness of humiliation or embarrassment. Neither race or performance horses nor show dogs commonly show humility, disappointment, frustration, or regret after not winning or after placing last in an event. Based on our current understanding of their emotional and communication capacities, this type of phobia does not readily apply to companion animals.

PANIC DISORDER

Panic disorders (PD) are considered a common illness in humans. Between 4 and 8% of the adult population will meet the criteria for PD within any year (31), and approximately 10% of adults will qualify for the diagnosis at some time (32). Anxious and phobic animals seem to demonstrate characteristics similar to those recognized in human panic attacks and can reasonably be interpreted as having PD (2,16,33,34).

The DSM-IV definition of a panic attack requires a discrete period of intense fear or discomfort in which four or more of the following symptoms develop abruptly and reach a peak within 10 minutes (22). These could include: 1) some palpitations, pounding heart, or accelerated heart rate; 2) sweating; 3) trembling or shaking; 4) sensations of shortness of breath or smothering; 5) feelings of choking; 6) chest pain or discomfort; 7) nausea or abdominal distress; 8) feeling dizzy, unsteady, lightheaded, or faint; 9) feelings of unreality or being detached from oneself; 10) fear of losing control or going crazy; and 11) fear of dying. These can contribute to a sense of terror, escape attempts, or a desire to flee (22). A panic attack usually lasts for several minutes, but rarely for more than 1 hour, during which symptoms can be very intense. Descriptions of phobic pets have included presenting symptoms and client complaints of varying intensity. Mild, low-intensity reactions might include pacing, trembling, cowering, or dependence on being in the presence of or in contact with the owner. More severe, higher intensity reactions can include whining, panting, salivating, eliminating, running, and frantic escape behavior, which might include scratching or chewing at barriers and jumping through windows or screens.

In humans, PD is familial, with evidence suggesting a genetic predisposition (22,25). In some patients, situational events appear to facilitate onset and maintenance of the disorder. PD usually begins in the third decade of life and runs a chronic course, with waxing and waning of symptoms. The onset is as late at the sixth decade in some patients (35). The genetic components of PD in companion animals await further study.

AGORAPHOBIA (PHOBIAS OF SITUATIONS)

Agoraphobia is commonly linked with PD, although PD can occur spontaneously without agoraphobia, and agoraphobia without a history of PD is an entity in human psychiatry. In DSM-IV (22), agoraphobia has been defined by the following criteria:

A. Anxiety about being in places or situations from which escape might be difficult (or embarrassing) or in which help might not be available in the event of having an unexpected or situationally predisposed panic attack or panic-like symptoms. Agoraphobic fears typically involve characteristic clusters of situations that include being outside the home alone, being in a crowd, standing in a line, being on a bridge, or traveling in a bus, train, or automobile. *Note*: Consider the diagnosis of specific phobia if the avoidance is limited to one or only a few specific situations, or social phobia if the avoidance is limited to social situations.

B. The situations are avoided or else are endured with marked distress or with anxiety about having a panic attack or panic-like symptoms, or require the presence of a companion.

C. The anxiety or phobic avoidance is not better accounted for by another mental disorder, such as social phobia, specific phobia, obsessive-compulsive disorder, PTSD, or separation anxiety.

Most show ring, veterinary hospital, and performance phobias in dogs and horses are better classified as specific phobias, *situational type*, as defined earlier. The more difficult distinction is in the timid dog that responds poorly in most novel, social, or outdoor environments and who often requires owner presence when outside, interacting with people, or in unfamiliar surroundings. Most agoraphobic individuals feel more comfortable when accompanied by a friend or relative (24). Antisocial or "unfriendly" cats that do not tolerate forced interactions with visitors or veterinarians may also fit the criteria for agoraphobia. Some of these dogs and cats cope by displaying fear aggression, while others have panic attacks and "go crazy" such that the owner lacks the ability to control the animal. Whether PD with agoraphobia is an accurate diagnosis in these companion animals awaits further investigation.

Fear aggression, separation anxiety, and situational phobias are covered elsewhere in this text so this chapter deals primarily with acquired fears and phobias that include specific phobias and panic attacks.

Development of Fears and Phobias

The normal fear response is adaptive because it increases the chances of survival. Fear is abnormal or maladaptive (i.e., a phobia) when it is not justified by the stimulus that provokes it (i.e., out of context of danger) or when the intensity of the fear is in excess of the response requirements of the real situation (1,24). Using these criteria, one phobic scenario might involve a pet demonstrating physiologic changes and actions in response to a non-threatening stimulus, as in the case of a dog afraid of a bike or a child when there have been no prior negative experiences associated with either. This type of reaction may be explained by neophobia, lack of early socialization, or the expression of appropriate coping mechanisms. In humans, these spontaneous phobias, if they persist, are the most "irrational" ones. For example, ailurophobic individuals may state that they know they should not be afraid of cats but may still respond physiologically to and acknowledge terror in the presence of cats.

The more common scenario for phobias in companion animals focuses on the disruptive, disorganized, maladaptive fears and anxieties to potentially dangerous or threatening situations, as is the case for thunderstorm and other noise phobias in dogs. In contrast to the expectation that pets should adapt to loud noises and threats that do not materialize via habituation, noise-phobic animals have been described as having the following characteristics: 1) the vast majority of noise phobias in dogs are to a limited set of sound stimuli; 2) the fear is enhanced rather than extinguished by repeated natural exposure to the sound stimulus; and 3) in many cases in which a precipitating event is known, a high-intensity phobia is established after only one exposure. These findings support a more primitive biological/evolutionary basis for fear disorders (1,18). Caution has been urged when extrapolating data from laboratory-conditioned fear reactions reported in the experimental literature to naturally occurring phobias, because acquisition of phobias in companion animals does not seem to fit the classic conditioning model of learning that has been traditionally proposed (1,3).

Rachman's model of phobia acquisition (36) suggests three possible etiologic components in the development of phobias: direct conditioning, indirect conditioning (involving vicarious acquisition), and informational and/or instructional acquisition. While this model proposes that conditioned fears have a more severe intensity phobia than indirectly acquired fears, a study examining human fear of dogs (37) indicates that conditioning does not make severity worse and that conditioning actually corresponded to less severe anxiety during a stimulus exposure. Despite dividing the conditioning events into those involving pain and those that were frightening (without bites or scratches), conditioning events were equally likely to have occurred in the fearful group and in the nonfearful control group (37). If conditioning events do contribute to human fear of dogs, other factors must determine whether a phobia develops. An expectation of fear or panic was characteristic of fear of dogs (37) and phobias of small animals (38), of which snake phobias accounted for almost half of the animal phobias described. None of the patients with small animal phobias had experienced a painful conditioning event, whereas 50% of those fearful of dogs had been harmed during a previous dog interaction.

An expectation of harm appears to play a significant role in human-dog fears. In one study, 100% of humans who were fearful of dogs expected dogs to harm them (37), whereas only 41% of individuals who were fearful of small animals believed that they would be harmed physically (38). Fearful individuals who were previously frightened or injured by a dog tended to be less anxious and more likely to touch a dog during a behavior approach test than fearful individuals who lacked such a conditioning event (37). Physiologic arousal in the form of elevated heart rate was demonstrated in all individuals, dog-fearful and nonfearful, who had a prior conditioning event and was highest in those dog-fearful individuals who had not reported a conditioning event (indirect conditioning); this arousal was not sufficient to cause a phobia to develop (39). Further studies are needed to examine the applicability of these observations to companion animals that have experienced injections or other painful procedures in the veterinarian's office, the boisterous play of a child, or the fear of a sudden loud noise.

EPIDEMIOLOGY

PD in humans has a strong likelihood of heritability, as was indicated in a recent literature review (25). Specific phobias, like *blood-injection-injury* and *situational subtypes*, have also been shown to have a genetic basis (22). Anxiety disorders in general, including PD, have been reported to be more common in women, and women develop specific phobias about twice as frequently as men (24).

A familial transmission of fear of loud noises and other fears has been demonstrated in a strain of German Shorthaired Pointers inbred for timidity (40). A German study (33) conducted at a behavior consultant's practice indicated 9 (60%) of 15 German Shepherds and crosses had evidence of familial transmission of fear disorders. In this report, separation anxiety was grouped with phobias, and it indicated a 2:1 ratio of male-female anxiety incidence (33).

Males also presented more frequently than females in a Georgia behavior consultant practice, although in this study phobias were clustered in a diagnostic classification system defined as stimulus reactivity (6). This category included both approach and avoidance reactivity, which unfortunately makes these results difficult to compare with other classification schemes. Interestingly, when reproductive status was taken into account, intact males and neutered females were shown to be the most likely to be referred for stimulus-reactivity problems (6). Separation-related problems were also classified and did not show a statistical difference in sex or reproductive status (6). Several other reports indicate no apparent sex predilection exists for fears and phobias in dogs (1,2).

Phobias can occur in any breed, though German Shepherds, Golden Retrievers, and Chow Chows were overrepresented in one incidence study (41), accounting for almost 30% of the phobic patients presented to three behavior referral practices; however, the number of dogs in this study was quite low (n = 27). The German study previously mentioned (33) indicated that one-third of its fearful dogs were German Shepherds and crosses, although it did not compare this population with the breed distribution of the pet population sampled. The only study that has surveyed the population incidence of anxiety in dogs reported an overall incidence of 2.1% in 658 dogs presented to a veterinary hospital (42). This study classified separation anxiety with phobias and other fear-related behaviors, excluding aggression. When only problem dogs were considered, fear and anxiety disorders accounted for 5.5% (42). This is a much lower incidence than the 26% incidence of fear and anxiety disorders reported in the German study (33), approximating more closely the incidence of fear-based conditions and phobias presented to North American behavior consultant practices, 6% (41) and 9.8% (43), respectively.

The German study reporting the higher incidence may lend support to the presumed hereditary basis for some canine anxiety disorders, as German Shepherds, a known anxious breed, were probably overrepresented in the population sampled. Tuber et al (3) have reviewed the dynamics within unique canine populations, and this report also lends support to a hereditary basis for fear. Nineteen percent of guide dogs, including German Shepherds, Labradors, and Golden Retrievers, were frightened by loud noises, 15% by cars or farm machinery, 12% by other animals, 4% by bikes, and 18% were fearful of unspecified miscellaneous situations. (It was not stated how much any one dog contributed to each of these percentages.) In another special group of German Shepherds, 11% showed an oversensitivity to tactile stimuli, and 11% an oversensitivity to auditory stimuli (3). Environmental and geographical variation cannot be ruled out as contributing to the higher incidence in these studies, however, and more research is needed to clarify these issues.

In humans, phobic disorders usually begin in the late teens or early adulthood and are generally sudden in onset, with the cause of symptoms usually not immediately apparent (24). Fears and phobias in dogs can develop at any age (1–3,6), though noise phobias appear to develop more frequently prior to age 6, with 78% occurring when dogs are between 1 and 5 years old (1). One study examining geriatric dogs with behavior problems reported that 26% presented for fears, restlessness, or startle (44). Early on, aggressive dogs, which are the majority of dogs presenting to behaviorists, may lose the opportunity to develop or contribute to these geriatric incidence numbers if they fail to remain welcome pets in their household.

NEUROBIOLOGY

Increased biologic understanding of the anxiety disorders, paired with phenomenologic, demographic, natural history, and treatment-response variables, will likely lead to more specific and effective pharmacologic treatments (24). Review articles evaluating animal and human studies of anxiety have postulated important roles for numerous cortical, limbic, and brain-stem structures. Chapters 4 and 5 have discussed the neuroanatomic importance of the locus coeruleus (LC), median raphe nucleus, nucleus reticularis paragigantocellularis, hypothalamus, amygdala, hippocampus, limbic system, and prefrontal cortex, and the central role of the noradrenergic system in the development and expression of anxiety and fear. Dysregulation of this system appears to lead to panic attacks and phobias, although no neuropathologic condition has been identified as a direct and exclusive cause of pathologic anxiety states (1,23).

Instead, these are likely multifactorial disorders, and neuroanatomic models and neurophysiologic challenges have provided differing results based on moderate anxiety, phobic anxiety, and panic attack (23,25). A wide array of panicogens is recognized, and neurochemical theories proposed for panic disorder include substances or systems related to adenosine, cholecystokinin (CCK), gamma-aminobutyric acid (GABA)-benzodiazepine, isoproterenol (beta-adrenergic), lactate, norepinephrine (NE), respiratory/carbon-dioxide, and serotonin (5-HT) (25). (See previous chapters as well as recent reviews of the literature (25,45,46) for more discussion of this subject).

One group of investigators (47) offers a three-part neuroanatomic model to explain differences in anxiety, panic, and phobia. This model suggests that panic attacks are initiated in the brain stem, that the limbic system modulates anticipatory anxiety, and that phobic anxiety is modulated by centers in the prefrontal cortex. Pathologic panic would therefore be caused by an oversensitivity of the brain-stem centers, usually by an inappropriate signal received at the LC, which then activates the panic circuit. This model leaves open the possibility that limbic dysfunction could initiate a pathologic panic attack (47). Positron-emission tomography (PET) scans that have revealed parahippocampal asymmetry (48,49) in patients with PD suggest that both structural and neurochemical imbalances resulting in panic attacks, and support a model that includes limbic dysfunction. Epileptiform discharges in this region have also been recognized in patients presenting with panic attacks (50).

Diagnostic criteria for phobic disorders that may represent distinct biologic subgroups (45) should be established. Animal models may provide valuable information in this process, as anticipatory anxiety and cognitive variables during experimental trials may be less in animals than in human subjects. SPECT and PET scans on patients with specific phobias have resulted in apparently contradictory findings, which have been explained by differences in experimental technique and variability depending on the nature of the phobic exposure (45). Brain activity, as measured by whole brain and regional blood flow, has been shown to demonstrate subtle differences based on the context of the anxiety condition and likely reflects variables due to input from imaginal, visual, tactile, or auditory pathways (45). These studies have supported the role of the thalamus as a relay station for emotionally relevant sensory information during anxiety states. Future studies are needed to clarify the roles of the basal ganglia, limbic structures, and midbrain structures in specific phobias.

The rate of carbon-dioxide–induced panic attacks in patients with specific phobias, while greater than in nonanxious controls, is less than in patients with PD and similar to that of patients with social phobia and general anxiety disorder (51). When specific phobias were separated into *situational* and *animal subtypes*, however, only the situational phobics were associated with abnormal sensitivity, and the animal subtypes were essentially identical to controls (52). Unfortunately *natural environmental* or *noise phobias* were not examined, and carbon-dioxide challenge studies have not been performed in companion animals with naturally occurring phobias.

Panic and Phobias: Treatment Options

BEHAVIOR MODIFICATION THERAPY

Since the publication of a ground-breaking article by Tuber et al (53), behavior modification therapy has been the mainstay of long-term successful management of phobias in companion animals. Applications of standard principles derived from the concepts of learning theory are well reported and have provided successful treatment outcomes in small animals (1–3,5,54) and horses (55,56). It is vital that, when attempting to manage companion animal phobias successfully, the practitioner understand the terminology associated with behavior modification and tailor its use to each individual patient or work closely with a behavior consultant. This is especially important when dealing with phobias because, as a general rule, specific phobias do not appear to respond to pharmacologic intervention (24), and in humans, behavior therapy is considered the treatment of choice for phobias. A successful long-term outcome therefore depends on incorporating behavior modification techniques.

The use of *cognitive behavior therapy* (i.e., seeking to modify a person's perspectives on potential anxiety-provoking stimuli), is showing great promise in managing specific fears, social anxiety, and social phobia. Behavioral methods do not fare as well with severe phobias, including panic attacks, although improvement sufficient enough to allow some patients to lead reasonably active lives has been reported (24). *Supportive therapy*, on an emotional level, is as important when treating a mental disorder as when treating any illness. Therefore, owners, behaviorists, and practitioners must attempt to set animals up for success if they are to overcome the phobic situation. This requires progressing at a rate that all involved can accept, as well as periodic reassessment to maintain a realistic expectation of outcomes.

Behavior therapy can be difficult to administer for a number of reasons. A defined stimulus is necessary to begin exposure techniques; however, achieving realism (e.g., in the replication of a thunderstorm) is sometimes the first major difficulty encountered when desensitization and counterconditioning are planned. Locally made recordings (57), high-fidelity commercial recordings, and a musical instrument amplifier have been recommended to replicate the sounds of a thunderstorm (1). On occasion, strobe lights for lightning and a hose or sprinkler aimed at a window may also be required to replicate a storm "realistically" (1–3). Second, few techniques are cost-effective or easy for the average practitioner to administer; exposure sessions with a behaviorist can be both time-consuming and expensive. Third, some owners may refuse to place their pet in a confrontational situation as part of the therapy. Fourth, panic attacks may persist when exposure to the real stimuli cannot be avoided outside a behavior therapy session. This is a common problem with thunderstorm phobias, although they usually have a seasonal course, providing ample time after the thunderstorm season for behavior therapy. Pharmacotherapy is often required to diminish the panic attacks during the season and to prevent escalation of panic attacks and the development of anticipatory anxiety (1).

PHARMACOTHERAPY

Because behavior therapy has limitations, consideration of adjunctive pharmacotherapy is often warranted (58). Combination therapy, using behavioral or management procedures with psychotropic drugs, is particularly helpful in two instances (59): 1) when conventional behavioral or management procedures are unlikely to resolve the problem alone or have failed; and 2) when a drug facilitates behavioral procedures that otherwise may not be an option for a client with limited time or resources. The importance of combining behavioral measures with drug therapy and gradual dose reduction over a span of 1 to 2 months or more has been stressed (59,60).

In recent controlled, double-blinded clinical trials, pharmacotherapy has been reported successful in controlling PDs, with and without agoraphobia, and to a lesser extent social phobias in humans (61). However, specific phobias in humans are reported to be unresponsive to drug therapy (62,63). Anecdotal case reports of successful treatment of phobias in companion animal species have not been followed up with randomized, controlled clinical trials. Therefore, caution must be exercised when evaluating case reports, case surveys, and prospective clinical trials (64). When choosing pharmacotherapy as an adjunct to therapy for any pet, the needs of the client and pet must be weighed against the benefits and limitations of these therapeutic trials, almost all of which involve extra-label use of drugs. Many factors must be considered when trying to select an appropriate therapeutic regimen for companion animals demonstrating phobias and panic attacks.

PETS AS CHILDREN?

Several correlations between the treatment programs for anxiety disorders in pets and in children and adolescents (13) are worth considering, especially because many owners believe that their pet is "like a child." It is especially important to maintain a good doctor-patient-client relationship throughout an extra-label drug trial. The clinician's role in the triad cannot be minimized, especially when medications are used. A great deal of time may be required in many cases, even when working with a qualified behaviorist. The general strategy in managing any anxiety disorder is to use medication to ameliorate the pet's subjective anxiety, while working with the owner and pet to modify the pet's avoidant behavior (13). Children and pets who are worried or fearful often become extremely demanding. It is common for parents and owners to react with a combination of guilt, fear, sorrow, puzzlement, helplessness, anger, or resentment. Therefore, clinicians should not only treat a pet with medication, they should also assist the owners to cope more effectively with their pet's behavior.

Treatment Plan

The psychopharmacologic treatment of an anxious pet must take place in the context of a comprehensive treatment plan. Simple prescription of medications with occasional monitoring is unacceptable. Following appropriate diagnosis, specific symptoms should be accurately documented, including symptom type, severity, frequency, and persistence. A side effect profile checklist should be completed prior to prescribing any medication in order to monitor possible emerging side effects or to identify currently existing somatic complaints that may be incorrectly attributed to medication side effects at a later date.

Assessment

Guidelines for children recommend that the assessment phase include medical history, physical examination, thyroid, metabolic, and electrolyte determinations and an ECG (13). A thorough medical history, physical exam, neurologic and cardiac assessment is necessary initially in companion animals. Metabolic assessment of veterinary patients should include routine hematology, chemistries, and urinalysis. Thyroid and adrenal function assessment is usually indicated as well, especially in older pets. A baseline ECG and tonometry are indicated prior to beginning medications that affect these systems.

Client Education

Following diagnosis and symptom assessments, owners should be educated about the phobic disorder and the pharmacologic treatment planned. Client informational handouts are available, and the author routinely distributes reading materials provided by Gaines Foods, including *Fear of Thunder and Other Loud Noises*, *The Fearful Dog . . . Easing Its Fright*, and *Strangers and the Family Dog* (65–67). An expected outcome should be qualified with a caveat: Medications will not solve all problems. A realistic view of what symptoms the medications are expected to relieve should be identified. An expected time course for treatment should be outlined as well as a rationale for multiple daily doses and proposed dosage increments, if necessary. The owner should be reminded that drugs alone seldom cure a condition, and that symptoms may return when the medication is discontinued (59). Education as to the expectation, potential severity, and duration of side effects can often mean the difference between compliance and noncompliance. Assessment of owner attitudes toward medications and expected outcome should also be addressed, and potential drug-drug interactions should be identified clearly.

Reassessment and Monitoring

A reassessment is usually planned for about 2 to 3 months after the initiation of treatment. Once medication is begun, however, patient monitoring should be done at appropriate intervals, ideally within the first 2 to 3 days after the initial drug dose. Weekly monitoring is then reasonable—with outcome and side effect scales completed—until the patient is stabilized at an acceptable dosage and symptoms are coming under control. During this maintenance phase, biweekly monitoring is acceptable, although a standardized monitoring procedure should be conducted at each appointment. The reassessment visit should critically review the patient's clinical course. Failure to achieve symptomatic control should lead to diagnostic reassessment, medical reevaluation, ancillary therapy assessment, compliance determination, possible dose adjustment, or a change to an alternate therapeutic agent. Continued treatment failures should lead to more intensive reassessments or referral (13).

Clinical Outlook

The current state of veterinary behavior management provides quite a bit less than the ideals previously described for managing children on psychoactive medications. This disparity will likely account for different overall success rates in animals when compared to human studies. Moreover, the economic realities of present-day veterinary medicine will likely delay acquisition of clinical information on the pharmacologic treatment of naturally occurring phobias. These economic realities, however, do not excuse clinicians from blame for haphazard drug trials or liabilities associated with pharmacotherapy.

It is the clinician's implicit responsibility to educate the client about the pet's illness, allay anxiety about the treatment, and establish a supportive relationship (57). Clearly, this cannot be accomplished in a standard office exam. Time needs to be set aside for proper discussion and consultation with a client, just as might be done for any chronic disease process. One important issue to address is sedation, which tends to be dose-related and usually subsides with continued drug use. Especially during dose adjustments, clients should be counseled to contact their veterinarian regarding questions or concerns. Remember that various antianxiety drugs are available, and finding one that works may require several attempts.

Pharmacotherapy for Phobias

CHOOSING A DRUG

Pharmacologic management of phobias essentially breaks down into acute management of panic attacks and chronic control during desensitization and counterconditioning. The amnesic effects of certain classes of drugs (i.e., benzodiazepines and barbiturates) make them less suitable for chronic use when behavior modification is also being attempted (1,60,68,69).

The seasonal nature of the most common noise phobias—thunderstorms, fireworks, and gunshots—may also require control of panic attacks during a specified time. Desensitization and counterconditioning can then be accomplished without medication during a subsequent "quiet" time of the year, typically late winter/early spring. For thunderstorm phobia, this winter/ early spring scheduling corresponds to a typically slower period in the veterinary community and is an opportune time to work with owners and pets who are otherwise cooped up due to shorter daylight hours or colder weather.

Key considerations in the choice of an anxiolytic medication include the following:

1. *Establish a tentative diagnosis.* A thorough history and physical exam, coupled with satisfying appropriate diagnostic criteria, are necessary to properly document a phobia and rule out other possible causes for the pet's symptoms. Workups may be required to rule out contributing cardiac, neurologic, endocrine, or other medical disorders.
2. *Select a drug with sufficient duration of action.* A duration of 8–10 hours is typically the minimum length for working households. Missed medications or low blood levels of a short-acting drug can result in relapsing panic attacks and are unacceptable, especially when behavior therapy is ongoing.
3. *Sufficiently rapid onset of action.* Not as critical as duration, but many times the severity of the panic attack requires almost immediate results to prevent psychological trauma to the patient, to stabilize the family's emotions, and to terminate any large economic losses associated with escape behaviors, destruction, elimination, or ptyalism. Most clients are open to a 1- to 3-week trial if necessary, and they should be made aware of potential outcomes.
4. *Acceptable side effects.* Any medication has potential side effects. Owner education, knowledge of pharmacology, and a thorough physical exam are the keys here. Factors including age, breed, results of metabolic screening, and concomitant medical disorders or other drug interactions must be accounted for when establishing a chemotherapeutic plan.

5. *Wide safety margins*. Medications with wide safety margins are preferred because many are given long-term, dose adjustments are commonplace, and effective dosages have not been established by clinical trials.

6. *Establish a client-patient-doctor relationship*. Communication will be necessary long-term, is critical to ensure compliance, and is necessary to allay personal concerns when extra-label drugs are prescribed, including some controlled drugs with abuse potential.

7. *Economic assessment*. The costs of the drugs themselves have rarely been a concern. More expensive drugs that work or that are more convenient and assist compliance are more cost-efficient than inexpensive drugs that do not work, although expensive does not necessarily mean better. Diagnostic workup and follow-up are typically much more of an expense. The economic cost of constant repairs or medical needs also usually outweigh drug costs.

Several reviews of pharmacologic agents used in companion animals are available in the literature and are a helpful beginning (1,60,67–73). However, for almost all medications, the dosages reflect extrapolations from human dosing, experimental toxicity studies, or therapeutic trials in individual cases. The reviews are an excellent place to start to understand possible mechanisms of action and side effects, but veterinary behavior pharmacotherapy is sorely lacking in peer-reviewed, randomized, controlled clinical trials on naturally occurring acquired fears and phobias.

A brief summary of the available veterinary literature follows, not all of which was peer-reviewed, with some comments on randomized, double-blind, placebo-controlled studies in the psychiatric literature as well. The use of *Physician's Desk Reference* in addition to the newer veterinary formularies (74) is prerequisite, so at the very least a practitioner is aware of a drug's therapeutic and toxic profiles in nonsimian primates (humans).

Benzodiazepines

Mechanism of Action

Benzodiazepines (BZDs) have been used in human psychiatry and veterinary medicine as mild tranquilizers (in addition to their uses for taming aggressive animals, especially zoo animals), as sedatives prior to anesthesia, as muscle relaxants, and for their anticonvulsant activities (75,76). BZDs modulate the coupling mechanism between GABA receptors and their associated chloride channels, which leads to an increased frequency in the opening of the chloride channels. GABA is the main inhibitory neurotransmitter in the CNS (77), and BZDs appear to depress the subcortical level of the CNS, primarily the limbic, thalamic, and hypothalamic regions. The major pharmacologic effects of BZDs are produced due to their binding to $GABA_A$ receptors in the CNS. BZDs have also been shown to decrease turnover of the neurotransmitters serotonin and norepinephrine, and this may be partially responsible for their clinical effects (77).

BZD-specific receptors have been located in the mammalian heart, kidney, liver, lung, and brain, although no receptors are present in the white matter (78). The peripheral-type BZD receptors are different from the GABA-BZD receptors and have a different affinity for certain BZDs. These peripheral-type receptors are found in the brain, where they are localized in mitochondria rather than at synaptic terminals. Additional investigation is needed to determine how GABA-BZD and peripheral-type BZD receptors are related, and to explain the physiologic and behavioral actions of BZDs (77,79).

Pharmacokinetics

Almost all BZDs have similar pharmacologic profiles, with individual differences being related to individual pharmacokinetics (77). Differences have been recognized among the 1,4 BZDs, which include the majority of the BZDs used clinically, and the 1,5 BZDs, which include newer drugs like clobazam (80). The pharmacologic properties of BZDs in animals are very species specific, particularly the reaction of the animal and the drug's duration of action (75). BZDs are well absorbed from the digestive tract.

In humans, peak serum concentrations are reached at 0.5 to 8 hours after oral administration. The BZDs are highly lipophilic and distribute readily to the CNS and tissues. BZD activity can be prolonged in extremely overweight or geriatric patients, who often have a higher ratio of fat to lean tissue (77). Most BZDs undergo extensive phase I oxidative metabolism with formation of active metabolites. Lorazepam, oxazepam, and temazepam are metabolized only through glucuronide conjugation. These three drugs are preferred in elderly patients at reduced dosages. BZDs are excreted almost entirely by the kidneys and elimination half-lives in humans range from 5 to 100 hours (81). Therapeutic drug monitoring does not seem to be helpful in BZD therapy (82), partly because the multiple metabolites can contribute to the clinical effect.

Side Effects and Limitations

Side effects of the BZDs have included sedation, muscle relaxation, increased appetite (especially in cats), and paradoxical excitation in 10 to 20% of animals (70). The paradoxical excitement can sometimes be alleviated by increasing the dose (68). Limitations to their use include their amnesic effects, dependence-producing properties, and potential for abuse (60,69).

While generally safer and less sedating than barbiturates, BZD side effects in elderly patients include paradoxical excitement, drowsiness, lethargy, slurred speech, ataxia, physical and psychologic dependence or compulsive use, general CNS depression, hypotension, dry mouth, headache, constipation, and urinary retention. Since there is decreased hepatic biotransformation in elderly patients, leading to higher doses of active drugs, lower doses of the BZDs should be used in these patients (83).

Interactions with other medications is a common concern with BZD use in humans. Cimetidine, erythromycin, isoniazid, disulfiram, and oral contraceptives including estrogen cause increased toxicity due to inhibition of BZD metabolism. Antacids and anticholinergics delay absorption. BZDs cause higher digoxin levels in patients on digoxin. Increased sedation can result when BZDs are administered along with neuroleptics, narcotics, antihistamines, sedative hypnotics, heterocyclic antidepressants, and alcohol (84). Patients receiving diazepam may show false-negative urine glucose results if using Diastix or Clinstix tests (78).

BZDs should be avoided in breeding animals because of reported teratogenic properties, causing cleft palate in mice and humans (85). Cautions include avoiding BZD use in fear-aggressive dogs, as aggressive behavior may be disinhibited (68–70). Gradual withdrawal is necessary to avoid the discontinuation syndrome (see below), and BZDs may interfere with the learning of conditioned responses (68,70). Chronically administered BZDs should be gradually withdrawn to prevent the potentiation of seizures (1).

BZD discontinuation syndrome comprises several overlapping phenomena (77). These include withdrawal, with its associated psychosensory symptoms, relapse, and rebound. *Withdrawal* is explained by the reverse of physiologic changes such as enhanced GABA activity and neuronal inhibition. *Relapse* is the return of the original symptoms; this is the typical situation in veterinary medicine, as seen in the 91% relapse rate for urine-marking cats after diazepam discontinuation (86). *Rebound* is the appearance of more severe symptoms than were initially present (77). Controlled studies related to BZD treatment of PDs have indicated that neither propranolol, clonidine, nor carbamazepine assist in minimizing BZD withdrawal and that buspirone may actually exacerbate it (87). Maintenance of high-dose therapy during a therapeutic trial has not been fully explored. Whether the typical clinician's desire to maintain lower doses over time during a therapeutic trial contributes to the high relapse rate is unknown (88).

A primary concern in prescribing BZDs is the potential for abuse by owners or other family members (35,60,69). Caution is urged when prescribing BZDs in households with teenagers, especially when they share responsibility for a pet's care. Veterinarians may need to be even more vigilant, since a pet's care may transiently be the responsibility of extended family, neighbors, groomers, trainers, or other pet care service providers (72). An up-to-date medical record, including all communications with doctors and staff, is critical, especially in multi-doctor practices and when working with a behaviorist or veterinary referral center. Therapeutic drug monitoring allows for assessment of client compliance and ensures that patients receive their medication. This is not commonly done for BZDs but is routine with phenobarbital, another potentially abusable medication. Warning signs that suggest the possibility of abuse include:

1. *Claims of lost or stolen prescriptions.* Even the first time this occurs should raise some questions. Give only 2 to 4 weeks of medication with limited or no refills initially.
2. *The need to have prescriptions filled ahead of time.* Conscientious owners do not want to risk future panic attacks in their pets; urgent requests for more medication made several weeks in advance should be noted.
3. *Escalating doses.* Owner requests for escalating doses of medication should prompt concerns.
4. *Evidence that the owner has sought medication from another practitioner.* Keep the medical record current with any client communications, including communications with all doctors in the practice and referral communications from behaviorists or specialty veterinary referral centers.
5. *Signs of intoxication.* Whether drug- or alcohol-related, any signs of owner intoxication should be a contraindication to use of any medication with abuse potential, especially BZDs.
6. *Information from a relative or friend suggesting abuse.* While family members may participate in some of the follow-up assessments, there is more potential for comment to general practitioners here. Listen to staff members who might share individual or community concerns about an owner.

Clinical Use

While amnesia may impair long-term behavior modification, this may be a beneficial component of as-needed therapy for single, well-defined, phobic situations. BZDs are well referenced for their taming effects on wild animals, notably ungulates and felidae, transported into captivity (75,85,89). BZDs are useful when excessive anxious behavior or PDs in a companion animal follow the death of a housemate or owner (89) and are this author's drug of choice for both dogs and cats in this situation. This author routinely uses BZDs in place of phenothiazines or phenobarbital for anticipatable noise phobias (e.g., fireworks) because the sedative effects of BZDs are of shorter duration than with the other drugs, and the patients seem calmer to their owners.

BZDs have long been considered the treatment of choice in human patients with panic and acute anxiety disorders due to their far more rapid onset compared to other classes of anxiolytics. Still, a sufficient response to control panic with BZDs often takes 1 to 2 weeks, with further gains being noted at 4 to 6 weeks (90).

BZDs have been successfully used for the treatment of thunderstorm and noise phobias in dogs. They must be administered 3 to 4 hours prior to the onset of the fearful event so that the drug level is sufficient to counteract the CNS and physiologic effects surrounding the stimuli (1,2,68,69). For thunderstorm phobias, BZDs should be administered no later than the earliest barometric pressure drop (69). Working owners often choose to dose their pet prior to leaving for the day based on a weather forecast or expected phobic stimulus occurrence. This is especially helpful when panic attacks in response to noise or thunderstorms are severe in intensity, involving self-traumatization or property damage when a pet is alone. Readministration of the medication will be dependent on the duration of the stimulus and the pharmacokinetics of the medication chosen (1,2,68). There is an urgent need for more controlled clinical trials of drug efficacy for specific phobias with panic attacks.

Behavioral Pharmacotherapy

Several injectable BZDs are available for combination use in restraint and anesthesia of companion animals. However, these have little practical application to behavioral pharmacotherapy in phobic companion animals with panic attacks. The oral BZDs that are currently available and have shown some benefit include diazepam, chlorazepate, and alprazolam. Oxazepam is primarily used as an appetite stimulant in cats (91) but may offer a safer alternative in geriatric pets, especially cats. Oxazepam is preferred in elderly human patients at reduced dosages, as it is only metabolized through glucuronide conjugation and does not form any additional active metabolites.

DIAZEPAM

Diazepam is a commonly used BZD in veterinary medicine. Its metabolites, including nordiazepam (desmethyldiazepam), temazepam, and oxazepam all have some clinical activity. Hence, serum levels of diazepam itself have little correlation with efficacy. After oral diazepam dosing, approximate serum half-lives are 1.3 to 5 hours in the dog, 5.5 to 20 hours in the cat, and 7 to 22 hours in the horse, compared with 20 to 50 hours in humans. Approximate serum half-lives for nordiazepam, diazepam's active metabolite, include 2.9 to 4.1 hours in the dog and 21.3 hours in the cat, compared with 30 to 200 hours in humans (78,89,92). In humans, plasma protein binding for diazepam is 99% (81); in the dog, it has been reported to be 94 to 96% (92), and in the horse, 87% (78). Conversion of diazepam to nordiazepam is less pronounced following intravenous dosing than after oral administration (89).

Despite a reported tendency to increase excitability in otherwise calm dogs and providing minimal reduction in excitability in excitable dogs, diazepam has proven more effective than chlorpromazine in reducing fear (71,76). The short half-life in dogs makes diazepam a drug of limited practical use in this species due to the need for frequent dosing, every 3 to 6 hours. With isolated or as-needed use for short-term phobic situations, however, a short half-life may be beneficial, because side effects wear off much faster than those of more traditional tranquilizers.

A dose range of 0.1 to 0.5 mg/kg has been used successfully in the treatment of thunderstorm phobias in dogs. However, dosage adjustment based on the dog's response may be necessary (1,2). With a potential for paradoxical excitement or hyperactivity (2,76), owners should always be present for the first few doses. Daily doses given orally every 8 hours have been shown to produce steady-state concentrations of nordiazepam that can be clinically effective. This requires higher doses of diazepam, on the order of 1 to 2 mg/kg (89,92). At these doses, steady-state serum concentrations of 1 to 2 μg/mL of nordiazepam were obtained (92).

The sedative effects of diazepam are usually only transient, and patients typically overcome them within a few days. Maximum daily doses should probably not exceed 40 mg (13). A newer sustained-release preparation of diazepam may be more effective than short-acting preparations (60). Diazepam has shown no effect on disposition (friendliness) in dogs (76), and, as with any BZD, should not be used in aggressive patients. It has been suggested that diazepam be contraindicated in greyhounds and related breeds due to reports of hyperesthesia, ataxia, struggling, and CNS excitation (89).

Similarities between both cats and humans have been reported in response to BZDs (93). More excitable or outgoing cats required higher doses of BZDs to normalize neurotic behavior than withdrawn neurotic cats. Neurotic behavior in cats was described as cats being restless, depressed, uncooperative, and having dilated pupils; it also included piloerection, vocalization, urination, and phobic reactions. These behaviors were normalized by the oral BZD chlordiazepoxide at 6 to 10 mg/kg or diazepam at 3 to 6 mg/kg. Increased activity was noted in the food-reward box in cats treated with these medications, despite the presence of an air blast (phobic stimulus) (93). Whether this is an anxiolytic effect or due to the appetite stimulant property (94) of these drugs in cats was not addressed. Amnesia and excessive friendliness have been reported in cats on diazepam; however, these are welcome attributes when treating a cat fearful of strangers or veterinary visits. With a longer half-life in cats than in dogs, usual feline doses are 1 to 2 mg per cat every 12 hours, and it is advised that every-12-hour doses not exceed 5 mg per cat (68,69).

While depth perception problems may result in difficulties for jumping cats (95), other side effects of diazepam in this species include oversedation, ataxia, bradycardia, and respiratory depression. Many of these side effects resolve within 3 to 4 days of the initiation of therapy (69).

Recent reports of a rare, idiopathic, often fatal, fulminant hepatic necrosis in this species (96) have led to more limited use of oral diazepam in cats. Fulminant hepatic necrosis tends to occur 7 to 9 days after beginning administration and the pathogenesis is unknown but suspected to be due to diazepam's metabolite, nordiazepam (97). At least four different brands have been implicated (98). This reaction seems to be idiosyncratic at normal doses rather than a toxic reaction to overdosing. Metabolic screening of circulating liver enzymes is indicated after 8 to 10 doses if pharmacotherapy is to be continued. If the metabolite, nordiazepine, is involved in the reaction, clorazepate would also be a poor choice in cats. Neither alprazolam nor oxazepam has active metabolites, so they may be preferred in this species when BZD therapy is necessary.

In pet birds, diazepam can be empirically dosed as 1.25 to 2.5 mg per 4 oz of drinking water for psychogenic feather-picking when anxiety is suspected as a contributing factor (99). Depending on the amount of seed, pellets, or fruit in the diet, however, water consumption can vary, and this is not a very exact way of dosing an individual psittacine. In addition, many suspensions have a bitter taste, and this may reduce the standard water intake for an individual bird. It is therefore probably best to consider formulating individual capsules when prolonged treatment is required. Reports of success are currently only anecdotal, and studies are needed to determine pharmacokinetics, dosing, and efficacy data in the variety of avian species commonly kept as companion animals.

CLORAZEPATE

Clorazepate has a short half-life in humans, less than 6 hours, although it is converted to an active metabolite, nordiazepam, which has a half-life of more than 20 hours (77). A sustained-delivery formulation has the convenience of less frequent dosing in humans and may be more effective in companion animals while promoting client compliance (60,69). Pharmacokinetics after single dosing in dogs, however, revealed no difference in blood levels of the major active metabolite, nordiazepam, after regular-release and sustained-delivery formulations of clorazepate (100). If therapeutic drug monitoring is attempted for BZDs like clorazepate, serum-separating blood collection tubes should be avoided. Compared to non–serum-separating tubes, the values were 35% less at 96 hours when stored at 20 to 22°C (101).

Clorazepate has been successful for the treatment of fear in dogs at 0.5 to 1.2 mg/kg every 12 to 24 hours (2,55,102). Dosage guidelines for the sustained-delivery formulation are 22.5 mg for large dogs, 11.25 mg for medium dogs, and 5.6 mg for small dogs, given every 12 to 24 hours. Dosage adjustment based on the dog's response may be necessary (1).

Clorazepate has been associated with hepatic failure in dogs, so hepatic function needs to be monitored soon after initiation of therapy (60). Clorazepate may increase serum alkaline phosphatase and serum cholesterol levels, but the clinical significance of these changes is unclear (103). Clorazepate is contraindicated in patients with significant liver dysfunction or acute narrow-angle glaucoma (103).

In a case series of four thunderstorm phobic dogs treated with clorazepate, mixed results were reported (28). Of three of the dogs with moderate phobic severity, two showed a good response initially. The third dog did not respond at all, although it later had a good response to imipramine and maintained this response after more than 1 year of therapy. The fourth dog, which had a severe phobia, was reported to show a fair response to treatment. A preliminary study on thunderstorm phobic dogs comparing the sustained-delivery form of clorazepate with a combination of phenobarbital and propranolol suggests better efficacy for clorazepate (34).

ALPRAZOLAM

Alprazolam is a triazolam analog of the BZDs. While all BZDs are apparently equally efficacious, alprazolam has replaced diazepam as the most frequently used anxiolytic in humans (77). A change to alprazolam's shorter half-life, 5 to 11 hours, means less accumulation and less sedation and interference with normal functioning. It does, however, require more frequent dosing and has greater potential for withdrawal symptoms (77).

Interdose rebound anxiety is more common with shorter half-life BZDs like alprazolam. This rebound effect may contribute to ongoing symptomatology and can foster a sense of dependence on the medication to control symptoms. The effects of shorter-acting BZDs like alprazolam may also wear off overnight, which may lead to nocturnal or early morning panic.

Regular and frequent dosing is important with alprazolam and, in some instances, long-acting drugs may be more appropriate. In humans, there has been recent interest in clonazepam for this reason (77). Clonazepam is relatively potent in comparison to other BZDs, having ten times the antianxiety effect of diazepam. It also produces less sedation (57). Plasma protein binding for alprazolam is approximately 70%. Alprazolam does not form an active metabolite as is common with other BZDs (81).

Alprazolam is labeled for use in treating humans with PD (77). It is reported to be useful for anxiety disorders primarily associated with motor tension, autonomic hyperactivity, and vigilance and scanning signs (81). Studies seeking to examine correlations between plasma concentration and treatment response have demonstrated that individual variation exists in how each patient metabolizes alprazolam. Also, individual dosing adjustments are critical for patient improvement with minimum side effects (104).

Alprazolam appears to have a wide therapeutic range that has yet to be explored in companion animals. While the majority of humans respond at between 2 and 6 mg/day, the recommended initial starting dose in patients with PD is 1 to 1.5 mg/day divided every 6 to 12 hours, with an increase of 1 mg every 3 days to a point of maximum benefit or dose-limiting side effects (90). When sedation is experienced, it usually subsides within 7 to 10 days. Patients are instructed to avoid abrupt termination of their drug trial so as not to have withdrawal symptoms or rebound anxiety (90). In a double-blind, placebo-controlled study in psychiatric patients, comparing alprazolam to high-dose buspirone, alprazolam produced a rapid and sustained improvement in panic attacks, anxiety, phobias, and disability and was superior to buspirone and placebo. Alprazolam, in those human patients who responded, was dosed at 5.2 ± 2.6 mg (SD) (105). It is suggested not to exceed 4 mg/day in elderly (35) or adolescent (13) patients. Relapse of panic attacks is higher when the alprazolam is tapered off over only 2 weeks. It is now suggested to taper this drug over at least 6 to 10 weeks to be more useful clinically (90). More prolonged, slow alprazolam tapers (e.g., 12–16 weeks) can reduce the incidence of withdrawal from 35% to 5–7% (90,106).

Pharmacokinetic studies in companion animals are lacking, but Overall (95) has indicated a half-life for alprazolam in dogs of approximately 12 hours, with peak levels obtained in 1 to 2 hours. Dosages for dogs demonstrate a wide therapeutic range, 0.02 to 0.25 mg/kg every 8 to 12 hours (70,72), and it has been suggested that the total daily dose does not exceed 4 mg (72). The most significant side effects in dogs are drowsiness and mild, transient incoordination. Many human patients discontinue alprazolam use because they experience dizziness.

A case study of six dogs with thunderstorm phobia indicated variable results with alprazolam (28). One dog with mild phobia had an excellent response for over 6 months. Two dogs with moderate phobia responded well initially. Of three dogs with severe phobic reactions, one did not respond at all, one responded poorly, and one showed a good response. Treatment with propranolol was tried in two cases following alprazolam, with results rated as poor. Imipramine was tried in the the dog that did not respond to alprazolam and produced no beneficial effect.

Alprazolam has been advocated for use in fearful cats at doses of 0.125 to 0.25 mg per cat every 12 hours (68,72). Typical indications include situational phobias involving car rides, home visitors, or veterinary examinations. The short-term amnesia and excessive friendliness seen as side effects in this species are beneficial in these scenarios, especially in those cats whose panic includes frantic escape behavior or aggression. Doses are recommended to be given 20 to 30 minutes prior to transportation. While the excessive friendliness response can be quite dramatic, this author has seen few cats respond this way to an initial, single dose. Several doses are more typically necessary to produce this effect.

A weekend therapeutic trial is often most practical to assess a cat's response to alprazolam. An initial dose of 0.125 mg is given Friday night, and general activity is monitored for at least 2 hours. If no or limited response is seen, 0.25 mg is planned for Saturday every 12 hours and Sunday every 12 hours, such that the owner can be home to monitor the cat after each dose. The trial can be stopped when an acceptable response is noted or after the fifth dose. The author has routinely stopped the trial after three to five doses, but higher doses or longer therapy may reveal more responders. Responders appear less reactive or, more typically, are quite affectionate and outgoing, seeking human attention. The established protocol for each cat can be utilized as needed when fearful situations are anticipated. Continued use can be considered for cats exposed to extended visits by relatives, especially when young or loud children are involved. Liver parameters have been monitored on follow-up appointments following prolonged alprazolam therapy due to concerns about idiosyncratic hepatic necrosis, but no problems have yet been noted (Thompson SB, unpublished data, 1997). As indicated earlier, alprazolam is not metabolized into nordiazepam or any other active metabolite, as is the case with diazepam and clorazepate.

Neuroleptics

Mechanisms of Action

Neuroleptics are drugs that initially showed benefits in treating psychoses in humans, although not all modern antipsychotics are neuroleptics. Historically, phenothiazines were some of the first neuroleptics developed. Phenothiazines are commonly used in veterinary medicine for sedation and restraint. The principal central activity of neuroleptics is the blockade of dopamine receptors in the basal ganglia and limbic system, producing behavioral quieting (70). Phenothiazines act as dopamine antagonists at the dopamine excitatory receptor, and most phenothiazine derivatives increase dopamine turnover in the brain by blocking presynaptic dopamine receptors (85). They are believed to depress the reticular activating system and brain regions that control thermoregulation, basal metabolic rate, emesis, vasomotor tone, and hormonal balance (107). Most phenothiazines exert some degree of ganglionic blockade (89). They also cause stimulation of extrapyramidal motor pathways and have been shown to have anticholinergic, antihistaminic, and antiserotonergic actions (108).

Pharmacokinetics

Acepromazine is one of the most potent phenothiazines available. It has replaced chlorpromazine, as it seems to cause fewer problematic side effects than chlorpromazine in clinical use and is generally the first choice phenothiazine in veterinary medicine (89). Acepromazine is metabolized in the liver, with both conjugated and unconjugated metabolites excreted in the urine (85). Limited pharmacokinetic studies are available in cats and dogs.

During the time that phenothiazines are taking effect (initial 30 minutes), the animal should not be disturbed. An exaggerated arousal reaction is most likely during this time (89). Onset of action in noted by changes in facial expression, as ptosis occurs and the nictitating membrane is relaxed and protruded. The first indication of posterior ataxia is present at this time. Lethargy and reduced motor activity will be present and a drop in temperature occurs (85). While some effect is seen around 15 minutes after oral dosing, maximal effect is not usually achieved until 1 hour after administration (109). This effect is maintained for 3 to 4 hours and may still be present after 7 hours in some dogs (85). Duration of action can range from 4 hours in a healthy animal to more than 24 hours after high doses in a debilitated animal (109). Consistency of the sedative effect of phenothiazines is poor, and marked variation in individual animals can be expected (89); this is especially true after oral dosing in cats and dogs (109). Increasing the dosage does not usually help. Higher dose rates, although not likely to increase sedation, are likely to increase duration of action (89,109). Antidiarrheal mixtures including kaolin/pectin and bismuth subsalicylate and antacids interfere with gastrointestinal absorption of oral phenothiazines. Concurrent use of propranolol with phenothiazines will cause increased blood levels of both drugs (107).

Side Effects and Limitations

Common side effects of acepromazine include sedation, ataxia, and hypotension. Paradoxical external reactions and prolonged after effects have been reported in horses, cats, and occasionally dogs that have been treated with phenothiazines. Effects related to its various mechanisms of action must be monitored in individual patients. Overdosage can result in loss of placing reflexes, paresis, or catalepsy (108). Acepromazine causes increased central venous pressure, a vagally induced bradycardia, and transient sinoatrial arrest. Sudden collapse within 5 to 10 minutes—manifest as apnea, bradycardia, and then unconsciousness—has been reported in a few case reports in dogs when acepromazine was given intramuscularly at standard doses of 0.55 mg/kg (85). The bradycardia is usually negated by the reflex increased heart rate due to falling arterial blood pressure (107).

Giant breeds and greyhounds may be very sensitive to the drug, while terrier breeds are somewhat resistant to its effects (107,109). Acepromazine may cause syncope in brachycephalic breeds. Boxers are reportedly very sensitive to the hypotensive and bradycardic effects of acepromazine and even small doses should be used cautiously in this breed (107,110).

Acepromazine has hematologic side effects including thrombocytopenia and thrombocytopathia (109). A dose-dependent decrease in hematocrit has been demonstrated in the horse and dog 30 minutes after dosing, and this is likely due to increased splenic sequestration of red blood cells. Acepromazine may discolor the urine to a pink or red-brown color; however, this is not considered abnormal (107). Phenothiazines can cause hyperglycemia in many species, and this is believed to be due to release of epinephrine from the adrenal medulla and inhibition or blockade of the effect of insulin in the tissues (85). Acepromazine has limited usefulness in cattle because it may cause ruminal engorgement with accompanying respiratory compromise (89).

Prolonged treatment with neuroleptics can result in tardive side effects. An early indication of overdosage with chronic therapy is the occurrence of a fine tremor that is present at rest but disappears with movement. Additional side effects can include dysphagia, continuous restlessness, agitation, insomnia, and seizures. Such effects warrant reduced dosages or discontinuation of therapy (108). The major side effects of long-term use are cardiovascular disturbances, especially hypertension, and extrapyramidal signs such as ataxia, muscle tremors, and incoordination (67).

Phenothiazines can also potentiate the action of hypnotics, narcotics, anesthetics, and analgesics (108). Phenothiazines cause stimulation of extrapyramidal motor pathways and can lower the convulsive threshold. They are contraindicated in patients with a history of seizures and animals exposed to organophosphates (85). Caution has been urged in several unique patient populations: patients with renal impairment (109); young animals or outdoor animals exposed to harsh weather (because of the drug's hypothermic action) (107); weak, debilitated, geriatric, cardiac, or hypovolemic patients (85); and pregnant animals, as high doses have resulted in cleft lip and cleft palate in mice (although this may not have been a direct drug effect). At high doses, phenothiazines have been shown to block release of follicle-stimulating hormone and luteinizing hormone, resulting in blocking of ovulation and suppression of the estrous cycle. Phenothiazines have also been shown to inhibit the release of oxytocin, melanocyte-stimulating hormone, and antidiuretic hormone. They can also increase prolactin levels and cause galactorrhea (85).

Acepromazine should be used cautiously when restraining aggressive dogs because they are more reactive to noises and startle when under its influence. Also, the level and duration of tranquilization varies, rendering an aggressive animal more unpredictable (69).

Clinical Use

A single dose of a phenothiazine causes the following typical changes in behavior: decreased motor activity and exploratory behavior with unchanged spinal reflexes; impairment of motor coordination; and diminished response to non-nociceptive stimuli, including auditory or tactile stimuli (i.e., the response to painful stimuli does not seem to be impaired). There is also indifference and decreased responsiveness to the environment, a depression of operant behavior and conditioned reflexes, suppression of conditioned or spontaneously occurring emotional responses, and a taming effect in vicious or agitated animals. Other effects include hypotension with a compensatory tachycardia, raised threshold for arousal evoked by indirect stimuli, a potent antiemetic effect in dogs at the chemoreceptor trigger zone within the medulla, and antipyretic and hypothermic effects due to a depletion of catecholamines and depression of the hypothalamus (108).

Phenothiazines are commonly used in veterinary medicine to aid in the management of fearful dogs, although they are not drugs of choice in managing fear or phobic behavior because they have poor anxiolytic activity and produce marked sedation. Sedation to the point of disorientation and ataxia is frequently necessary before the behavioral component of the fear response is adequately attenuated. While owners have reported that phenothiazines help suppress the frantic responses of thunderstorm phobic dogs during storms, the high doses required also caused disorientation and ataxia, and usually the dogs still appeared frightened (2). Despite this, some dogs with high-intensity fear responses may need heavy sedation, as it is the only effective treatment to prevent self-trauma or property damage. Dogs with less intense phobias should initially be given a less sedating anxiolytic, prior to treatments that produce heavy sedation (1).

Behavior modification techniques are necessary to modify the phobic or anxiety disorder so that these medications may eventually be discontinued (68). Acepromazine may reduce responses to a conditioned stimulus such as a veterinarian's presence but not an unconditioned stimulus like needle pain (68,71). Dose ranges of 1 to 3.3 mg/kg every 8 to 12 hours have been necessary when the need for heavy sedation necessitates the use of acepromazine (68,89,107). Usually it is necessary to repeat doses every 6 to 8 hours to maintain tranquilization (85). As-needed dosing may also be an option when a phobic stimulus can be anticipated or when medication is needed only when an owner is away in cases where owner presence moderates the dog's phobic severity. Newer, high-potency neuroleptics may be an option in the future, once clinical trials are performed and therapeutic ranges are determined (60). These should produce less sedation, although they still may carry increased risk of extrapyramidal side effects.

Chlorpromazine at an oral dosage of 3 to 6 mg/kg resulted in reduced neurotic behavior in cats in response to air blasts as a conditioned phobic stimulus, although the improvement was less than that attributed to BZDs and barbiturates (93). In cats, acepromazine has been recommended as a tranquilizer at a dose of 0.8 to 1.1 mg/kg orally as needed (111). Acepromazine has been recommended for anxiety in primiparous queens during kindling, especially in queens that are human-dependent. Normal parturition can be restored in some queens by administering acepromazine (112). A dose of 1 to 3 mg/kg orally as needed (68,89) will cause deep sedation that rarely is acceptable to most cat owners. Other therapuetic options include BZDs, which are not contraindicated in aggressive states in this species, or antihistamines for milder anxious states.

In horses, acepromazine can reduce excitability so that an animal can be easily handled, and it has been used to provide tranquilization for travel in a trailer. The standard dose is 2 to 4 mg/45 kg, with the drug administered 30 to 45 minutes prior to travel. Medications can be buried in a piece of apple to facilitate administration (85). A paste formulation, for oral use, is available for horses (89). Horses on acepromazine retain auditory and visual acuity, so loud sounds and rapid movements should be avoided. Priapism or penile prolapse occasionally occurs following phenothiazine administration, as has been noted with acepromazine use in horses. This drug should not be given to stallions used as breeding animals to avoid the possibility of permanent paralysis of the retractor penis muscle; acepromazine use is not recommended in stallions per manufacturer labeling. Horses should not be ridden within 36 hours of treatment (85,89,109), making this drug one of little practical value for any persistent or unanticipated phobic occurrences. Other side effects in horses include excitement, restlessness, sweating, trembling, tachypnea, tachycardia, and, rarely, seizures and recumbency (107).

Azapirones

Mechanism of Action

Azapirones, like buspirone, are anxiolytic agents that differ structurally from the BZDs and phenothiazines. The mechanism for buspirone's anxiolytic activity is not well understood although it does have a high affinity for serotonin (5-HT) receptors in the CNS. The anxiolytic effect is thought to be due to an agonist action at 5-HT1A presynaptic and postsynaptic receptors (113). Buspirone appears to have mixed agonist/antagonist properties on dopaminergic receptors (114). It does not bind to GABA receptors and increases rather than decreases the rate of firing of the locus coeruleus (1,113).

Pharmacokinetics

Buspirone is metabolized by the liver to several metabolites, including an active metabolite, 1-pyrimidinyl-piperazine (1-PP). 1-PP does not appear to have significant clinical effects (13). These metabolites are excreted primarily in the urine. Antianxiety effects are often noticed after about 2 weeks (68). Buspirone's onset of action is gradual, and full effects may not be realized for up to 4 or more weeks (60).

Side Effects and Limitations

Common side effects in humans include gastrointestinal upset, dizziness, headaches, and insomnia (13). Bradycardia, muscle cramps, and stereotypic behavior have also been observed (72). Unlike BZDs, buspirone has no significant muscle relaxant, sedative, hypnotic, or anticonvulsive properties, is not associated with withdrawal phenomena, and has little, if any, abuse potential (13). Buspirone also has a wide margin of safety with no reported cases of fatal overdose. Paradoxical responses have been reported in some animals. Aggression may become a problem in previously low-ranking cats on buspirone in multicat households (86). Caution is urged in the presence of significant renal or hepatic impairment. While not proven safe during pregnancy, toxicity studies in rabbits and rats receiving more than thirty times the recommended dose have failed to show any teratogenicity. Buspirone should not usually be used with a monoamine oxidase inhibitor (MAOI), as hypertension could occur (114). Buspirone does not appear to potentiate the CNS depressant effects of BZDs or amitriptyline (13) and may lend itself to combination therapy.

Clinical Use

Buspirone appears to be equally efficacious in the treatment of generalized anxiety disorder when compared to BZDs. Clinical trials for social phobia and panic disorder in humans have shown only a mild to moderate benefit with buspirone (113,115,116). It appears that buspirone reduces anxiety levels, especially anticipatory anxiety, in PD patients, without significantly influencing or blocking situation-specific panic attacks. Buspirone may therefore likely be a useful adjunctive anxiolytic agent in selected patients rather than a primary treatment or a drug of first choice (116).

Dose ranges for dogs are 0.5 to 2.0 mg/kg every 8 to 24 hours (60) or 10 to 15 mg per dog every 8 to 12 hours (55). Buspirone appears to be effective in treating some companion animal behavior disorders, particularly those that are fear related (55). Buspirone appears to be beneficial in the treatment of low-intensity fear, but it appears inadequate for high-intensity phobic responses (1). Buspirone has been used successfully to treat fear of humans in dogs and cats, and it appears effective in smoothing the transition of semiferal animals into a social environment (60). Signs associated with thunderstorm phobia can be reduced but not eliminated with buspirone (60). Dogs with separation anxiety often do quite well with buspirone treatment (68). The author has obtained better responses with buspirone than amitriptyline when comorbid noise phobias are involved. Dogs with separation anxiety that is controlled on amitriptyline often relapse when thunderstorms, fireworks, or other noise stimuli recur.

Buspirone may help cats with mild anxious situational phobias or when transitioning from stray to household family member. Reported doses include 2.5 to 7.5 mg per cat every 12 hours. Many cats appear more outgoing, to people and other cats, once effective buspirone levels are achieved. Low-ranking cats from multicat households may display aggressive spats (68,72,86).

Beta-Blockers

Mechanism of Action
Beta-blockers may selectively block one or both beta-1 and beta-2 adrenergic receptors in the myocardium, bronchi, and vascular smooth muscle depending on the pharmacokinetics of the specific agent (117). Many of the autonomic symptoms of fear, such as rapid heart rate, sweating, and trembling, are the result of beta-adrenergic activity. Propranolol's exact mode of action as an anxiolytic is unknown but may include activity at both central and peripheral beta-1 adrenergic sites (13). Other pharmacologic effects for propranolol, a beta-1 and beta-2 blocker, include increased airway resistance and increased uterine activity (117).

Pharmacokinetics
Propranolol, atenolol, and pindolol are the most common beta-blockers used in veterinary medicine. Whereas atenolol is an exclusive beta-1-adrenergic blocking agent, pindolol is a mixed beta agonist/antagonist. Propranolol is principally metabolized by the liver and, due to a rapid first pass effect, has a very short half-life in dogs, approximately 0.77 to 2 hours (117). Cimetidine may inhibit the metabolism of propranolol and increase blood levels.

Side Effects and Limitations

Side effects of these drugs are minimal but can cause bradycardia and hypotension. Adverse effects can include lethargy, depression, hypoglycemia, and bronchoconstriction, and, rarely, syncope or diarrhea. Caution is urged in pets with significant renal or hepatic insufficiency. Preexisting bradycardia, hypotension, and heart failure are contraindications for propranolol use, as is bronchospastic disease (117). Pindolol may cause urinary incontinence in some dogs due to an agonist effect on the internal sphincter of the bladder (60). Hypotensive effects are enhanced if pindolol is given with phenothiazines. To avoid exacerbating symptoms by stimulation of upshifted beta-receptors (117), therapy should be withdrawn gradually in patients who have been receiving a beta-blocker chronically.

Clinical Use

The potential to attenuate the fear response through use of beta-blockers has resulted in clinical use in both animals and humans (1). In humans, beta-blockers are effective in selective types of anxiety, such as performance anxiety (stage fright), but the majority of evidence shows that beta-blockers are no more effective than placebos in the treatment of panic (90). Although beta-blocking drugs have generated considerable interest, their usefulness for phobic disorders seems limited. Reasons for this include their minimal effect on panic attacks—they appear less effective than BZDs and do not seem to enhance the effects of behavior modification (57).

Propranolol has limited effectiveness in thunderstorm phobic dogs, although it may be suitable for dogs with mild phobias. The fear response to a thunder simulation appears to be only partially attenuated with propranolol (1). Propranolol doses are 0.5 mg/kg orally every 8 hours, and clinicians must monitor for bradycardia. Propranolol doses to aid in control of fearful behavior are 5 mg every 8 hours for small dogs, and 10 to 20 mg every 8 hours for large dogs (69). Pindolol doses are 0.125 to 0.25 mg/kg orally every 12 hours and can result in panting and urinary incontinence (60). In a case series of thunderstorm phobic dogs, seven were treated with propranolol with poor results (28). Five dogs had no response, and the other two showed only a poor or fair response. In dogs in which another drug was attempted to modify phobic severity, propranolol never performed better than the other drug options tried—alprazolam and clorazepate.

Another group of investigators, however, continues to promote the use of propranolol in treating anxious and phobic companion animals (118). Combination therapy in dogs has been advocated with propranolol at 2 to 3 mg/kg every 12 hours and phenobarbital at 2 to 3 mg/kg every 12 hours. Propranolol alone will control general agitation, tremors, and outdoor nervousness. The addition of phenobarbital seems to extend the anxiolytic control to include phobias and situational fears. Some cases have resulted in excellent control without panic, while others had minor residual pacing and hiding that most owners could tolerate (119). Another dosing regimen utilized is phenobarbital 15 mg per dog every 12 hours, combined with propranolol 10 mg per dog every 8 to 12 hours. This combination has, over a series of several months, produced very good results in dogs with specific fears and phobias (118). The investigators do not indicate whether the dose of propranolol eventually needs to be adjusted due to increased metabolism after hepatic enzyme induction by phenobarbital (117). A preliminary study in dogs (34) comparing the sustained-release formulation of clorazepate to the combination of propranolol with phenobarbital has indicated that clorazepate is better in the acute management of panic attacks due to thunderstorm phobias. Whether the combination therapy will improve these same dogs if given enough time has not yet been reported.

Although as-needed therapy strategies have not been widely studied, they may be useful in patients whose symptoms are predictable and relatively infrequent. In human patients whose autonomic symptoms predominate over their cognitive symptoms, beta-blockers may be the most appropriate agent for as-needed therapy. Guidelines for determining the appropriate dose of a beta-blocker for as-needed treatment in social phobia include the following:

1. Determine a pulse rate before and after 5 minutes of strenuous exercise.
2. Administer propranolol or atenolol.
3. Repeat pulse measurement as in step 1, 1 hour after drug administration. If the pulse rate increases more than 10 beats per minute with exercise after the beta-blocker, the dose is too low.
4. Repeat steps 1–3 the next day with a higher dose.

Some patients require therapeutic doses of propranolol almost three times the standard initial dosing to achieve adequate blockade (30). This protocol, or minor modifications of it, may have applications to individual patient scenarios in companion animal phobias. This program may prove more beneficial in obtaining an optimal therapeutic dose when contrasted to standard guidelines using a drop in baseline heart rate of 5 to 10 beats per minute (90).

Limited use has been reported in cats, but propranolol at a dose of 0.25 mg/kg as needed has been tried (70,73). Combination therapy with propranolol at 5 mg per cat every 8 to 12 hours and phenobarbital 7.5 mg per cat every 12 hours has been reported to produce very good results in a few phobic cats when used over several weeks (118).

Other Options

ANTIHISTAMINES

Antihistamines have been used occasionally for their sedative properties to assist with car travel or to assist with animals that are restless at night; however, most panic attacks are too severe to be controlled by antihistamines. They are associated with a lowered seizure threshold and excessive drowsiness and are not routinely used in adolescent anxiety disorders (13). While side effects typically relate to sedation and their anticholinergic effects, tolerance to sedation usually develops quickly (70), and antihistamines rarely help with managing companion animal phobias.

BARBITURATES

Barbiturates are beneficial in controlling excessive vocalization in cats (73). Barbiturates do not seem to provide sufficient antianxiety benefits to manage most moderate to severe panic reactions. As with phenothiazines, heavy sedation may be indicated in some animals when severe panic attacks result in self-trauma or property destruction (2). This will usually require dosing at the high range routinely used to control seizures: 2 to 6 mg/kg every 12 hours or as needed in dogs, and 1 to 3 mg/kg every 12 to 24 hours or as needed in cats (73,120). Phenothiazines are still preferred in patients with no known seizure history, as phenobarbital is a controlled drug and may cause hepatic damage if used long term. Low-dose therapy in combination with propranolol, however, may provide acceptable outcomes in some anxious or phobic pets (118,119). Further controlled studies and comparison studies are needed.

PROGESTINS

Progestins have a very nonspecific depressive effect on the CNS, with variable effects on behavior centers in the hypothalamus and limbus (69,121). This can have calming benefits when dealing with anxiety (71). The availability of other medications having less potential for side effects has permitted veterinarians to delegate this medication to the back shelf. Progestins should be drugs of last resort when all other rational therapy considerations have failed or when an injectable, long-acting, depot formulation is the only viable pharmacotherapeutic option. Side effects are often worse in females (vs males) and dogs (vs cats). Side effects can include paradoxical arousal, mammary neoplasia, pyometra, blood dyscrasias, and diabetes (122,123). Better options in behavior management and pharmacotherapy are now limiting the necessity of progestin use (see Chapter 10).

ANTIDEPRESSANTS

Heterocyclic antidepressants, including amitriptyline, clomipramine, doxepin, nortriptyline, and imipramine, are gaining use in veterinary medicine for a variety of behavior disorders (60,68–73). Individual drugs vary widely in their specificity for blocking the uptake of norepinephrine and 5-HT, which gives them their central effects. Side effects for these drugs often vary and can reflect their antihistaminic and anticholinergic properties as well. These drugs have a narrow therapeutic index, so considerations of any of these medications must take into account the widely differing pharmacologic profiles of these drugs (124,125). Imipramine in particular may be indicated, as it is one of the first choice medications used to treat humans with panic disorder and anxiety disorders (57,90,126). Combination therapy with imipramine and behavior modification enhances the likelihood that patients will respond markedly to treatment (127). Nortriptyline has fewer anticholinergic side effects compared to imipramine yet similar clinical indications and treatment profiles in humans. Clomipramine may also show benefit for animals with panic attacks and phobia, not just for separation anxiety and compulsive, stereotypic disorder (60). Gradual increases in doses are necessary to avoid the high incidence (20–30% in humans) of amphetamine-like stimulation that can occur when starting on these medications. Initial doses are often well below therapeutic ranges and require incremental dose increases every 2 to 4 days (90). Ongoing studies are needed to evaluate their benefit in chronic management of phobic animals.

SELECTIVE SEROTONIN REUPTAKE INHIBITORS

Selective serotonin reuptake inhibitors (SSRIs) block presynaptic neuronal uptake of 5-HT, may increase 5-HT output, and may change postsynaptic receptor sensitivity (128). All these serve to enhance the central effects of serotonin. SSRIs have been effective in the treatment of PDs, and they may be superior to heterocyclic antidepressants because of their broader spectrum of efficacy in many anxiety disorders (90). SSRIs have minimal to no effects on other neurotransmitters and have a high safety profile with minimal side effects. Overstimulation may occur if patients are begun on standard therapeutic doses, so subtherapeutic dosages are usually initiated. Side effects are limited and usually do not include sedation. Gastrointestinal signs including anorexia, diarrhea, and nausea may occur, and some patients may respond with increased anxiety, agitation, restlessness, or insomnia (125,128). Although recent veterinary pharmacotherapy reviews (60,70,72) include SSRIs as therapy options for anxiety and phobias, controlled studies of efficacy are lacking.

MONOAMINE OXIDASE INHIBITORS

Monoamine oxidase inhibitors (MAOIs) modify the regulation of monoamine content in the nervous system. Therapeutic action appears to be a result of amine accumulation and secondary adaptive mechanisms. This results in a reduction in the number of beta-adrenoceptors, alpha-1 and alpha-2-adrenoceptors, and 5-HT1 and 5-HT2 receptors (129). MAOIs, in particular phenelzine, have shown good efficacy in treating panic and anxiety disorders in humans and have already become the most established agent used in the treatment of social phobia (30). Nighttime insomnia and daytime lethargy seem to be the most significant limiting side effects (90). Some patients cannot tolerate the imposition of tyramine dietary restrictions, as beer, wine, and cheese are not allowed (129). An irreversible monoamine oxidase-B inhibitor (selegiline or L-deprenyl), which is free of dietary restrictions, is being used in veterinary medicine for treatment of cognitive dysfunction and sleep disorders in older dogs (34,72,73). (See Chapter 13.)

OTHER ANXIOLYTIC MEDICATIONS

A few other drugs are worth mentioning. Trazodone and nefazodone possess unique antianxiety and behavioral calming effects and have benign side-effect profiles. In humans, these are often used as a single nighttime dose with other antidepressants, such as SSRIs, to aid in sleep induction (125). They may provide another therapeutic option for some companion animal phobias. Meprobamate, with its tendency to produce drowsiness, sluggishness, and impaired mental function, may be of benefit in companion animals that fail other pharmacotherapy trials (68,71).

References

1. Shull-Selcer EA, Stagg W. Advances in the understanding and treatment of noise phobias. Vet Clin North Am Small Anim Pract 1991;21:353–367.
2. Voith VL, Borchelt PL. Fears and phobias in companion animals. Comp Cont Ed 1985;7:209–218.
3. Tuber DS, Hothersall D, Peters MF. Treatment of fears and phobias in dogs. Vet Clin North Am Small Anim Pract 1982;12:607–623.
4. Hart BL. Fear and emotional reactions in dogs. In: Hart BL, Hart LA. Canine and feline behavioral therapy. Philadelphia: Lea & Febiger, 1985:56–69.
5. Hothersall D, Tuber DS. Fears in companion dogs: characteristics and treatment. In: Keehn JD, ed. Psychopathology in animals: research and clinical implications. New York: Academic Press, 1979:239–255.
6. Wright JC, Nesselrote MC. Classification of behavior problems in dogs: distribution of age, breed, sex and reproductive status. Appl Anim Behav Sci 1987;19:169–178.
7. Voith VL. Applied animal behavior and the veterinary profession: a historical account. Vet Clin North Am Small Anim Pract 1991;21:203–206.
8. Danneman PJ, Chodrow RE. History taking and interviewing techniques. Vet Clin North Am Small Anim Pract 1982;12:587–592.
9. Hart BL. Medical interview and case history assessment in behavioral therapy. In: Hart BL, Hart LA. Canine and feline behavioral therapy. Philadelphia: Lea & Febiger, 1985:14–25.
10. Hunthausen W. Collecting the history of a pet with a behavior problem. Vet Med 1994;89:954–959.
11. Crowell-Davis SL, Houpt KA. Techniques for taking a behavioral history. Vet Clin North Am Equine Pract 1986;2:507–518.
12. Burghardt WF Jr. Behavioral medicine as a part of a comprehensive small animal medical program. Vet Clin North Am: Small Anim Pract 1991;21:343–352.
13. Kutcher SP, Reiter S, Gardner DM, Klein FG. The pharmacotherapy of anxiety disorders in children and adolescents. Psychiatr Clin North Am 1992;15:41–67.

14. Russell PA. Fear-evoking stimuli. In: Sluckin W, ed. Fear in animals and man. New York: Van Nostrand Reinhold, 1979:86–124.
15. Archer J. Behavioral aspects of fear. In: Sluckin W, ed. Fear in animals and man. New York: Van Nostrand Reinhold, 1979:56–84.
16. Neville PF, Walker R. Management of separation problems (anxiety, frenzy, panic, and rage) in dogs. Proc North Am Vet Conf 1996;23–24.
17. Ursin H. Neurophysiology of behavior. In: Anderson RS, ed. Nutrition and behaviour in dogs and cats. Oxford: Pergamon Press, 1984:139–146.
18. Mayes A. The physiology of fear and anxiety. In: Sluckin W, ed. Fear in animals and man. New York: Van Nostrand Reinhold, 1979:24–55.
19. Pincus HA, Henderson B, Blackwood D, et al. Trends in research in two general psychiatric journals in 1969–90; research on research. Am J Psychiatry 1993;150:135–142.
20. Borchelt PL, Voith VL. Classification of animal behavior problems. Vet Clin North Am Small Anim Pract 1982;12:571–585.
21. Wright JC. The effects of differential rearing on exploratory behavior in puppies. Appl Anim Ethol 1983;10:27–34.
22. American Psychiatric Association. Diagnostic and statistical manual of mental disorders, 4th ed. Washington, DC: American Psychiatric Association, 1994.
23. Overall KL. Neurochemistry and neurobiology of separation anxiety and aggression. Proc North Am Vet Conf 1997;11:33–39.
24. Uhde TW, Nemiah JC. Anxiety disorders (anxiety and phobic neuroses). In: Kaplan HI, Sadock BJ, eds. Comprehensive textbook of psychiatry, 5th ed. Baltimore: Williams & Wilkins, 1989:952–984.
25. Stein MB, Uhde TW. Biology of anxiety disorders. In: Schatzberb AF, Nemeroff CB, eds. Textbook of psychopharmacology. Washington, DC: The American Psychiatric Press, 1995:501–521.
26. Butler RW, Braff DL, Rausch J, et al. Physiological evidence of exaggerated startle response in a subgroup of Vietnam veterans with combat-related posttraumatic stress disorder. Am J Psychiatry 1990;147:1308–1312.
27. Shalev AY, Orr SP, Peri T, et al. Physiologic responses to loud tones in Israeli patients with posttraumatic stress disorder. Arch Gen Psychiatry 1992;49:870–875.
28. Shull EA. Analysis and treatment of noise phobias. Presentation notes from the 131st Annual Convention of the American Veterinary Medical Association. San Francisco, CA July 9, 1994.
29. Adams GJ, Johnson KG. Behavioural responses to barking and other auditory stimuli during night-time sleeping and waking in the domestic dog (Canis familiaris). Appl Anim Behav Sci 1994;39:151–162.
30. Social phobias: current evidence favours MAOI's. Drug Ther Perspect 1996;7:10–13.
31. Meyers JK, Weissman MM, Tischler GL, et al. Six-month prevalance of psychiatric disorders in three communities. Arch Gen Psychiatry 1984;41:959–967.
32. Robins LN, Heltzer JE, Weissman MM. Lifetime prevalence of specific psychiatric disorder in three sites. Arch Gen Psychiatry 1984;41:949–959.
33. Brunner F. The application of behavior studies in small animal practice. In: Fox MW, ed. Abnormal behavior in animals. Philadelphia: Saunders, 1968:398–449.
34. Houpt KA, Lindell EM. Separation and panic disorders in older dogs. Convention notes from the 133rd Annual Convention of the American Veterinary Medical Association Louisville, KY 1996;337–338.
35. Garvey MJ. Panic disorder: guidelines to safe use of benzodiazepines. Geriatrics 1993; 48:49–58.
36. Rachman S. The conditioning theory of fear-acquisition: a critical examination. Behav Res Ther 1977;15:375–387.

37. Di Nardo PA, Guzy LT, Jenkins JA, et al. Etiology and maintenance of dog fears. Behav Res Ther 1988;26:241–244.

38. McNally RJ, Steketee GS. The etiology and maintenance of severe animal phobias. Behav Res Ther 1985;23:431–435.

39. Di Nardo PA, Guzy LT, Bak RM. Anxiety response patterns and etiological factors in dog-fearful and non-fearful subjects. Behav Res Ther 1988;26:245–251.

40. Murphree OD, Dykman RD, Peters JE. Genetically determined abnormal behavior in dogs: results of behavioral tests. Cond Reflex 1967;2:199–205.

41. Landsberg, GM. The distribution of canine behavior cases at three behavior referral practices. Vet Med 1991;86:1011–1018.

42. Voith VL, Wright JC, Danneman PJ. Is there a relationship between canine behavior problems and spoiling activities, anthropomorphism, and obedience training? Appl Anim Behav Sci 1992;34:263–272.

43. Voith V. Clinical animal behavior. Cal Vet 1979;June:21–25.

44. Chapman BL, Voith VL. Behavioral problems in old dogs: 26 cases (1986–1987). J Am Vet Med Assoc 1990;196:944–946.

45. Johnson MR, Lydiard RB. The neurobiology of anxiety disorders. Psychiatr Clin North Am 1995;18:681–725.

46. Uhde TW, Tancer ME, Gurguis GNM. Chemical models of anxiety: evidence for diagnostic and neurotransmitter specificity. Int Rev J Psychiatry 1990;2:367–384.

47. Gorman JM, Liebowitz MR, Fyer AJ, et al. A neuroanatomical hypothesis for panic disorder. Am J Psychiatry 1989;146:148–161.

48. Reiman EM, Raichle ME, Robins E, et al. The application of positron emission tomography to the study of panic disorder. Am J Psychiatry 1986;143:469–477.

49. Nordahl TE, Semple WE, Gross M, et al. Cerebral glucose metabolic differences in patients with panic disorder. Neuropsychopharmacology 1990;3:261–272.

50. George M, Ballenger J. The neuroanatomy of panic disorder: the emerging role of the right parahippocampal region. J Anxiety Disorders 1992;6:181–182.

51. Rapee RM, Brown TA, Antony MM, et al. Response to hyperventilation and inhalation of 5.5% carbon dioxide-enriched air across the DSM-III-R anxiety disorders. J Abnorm Psychol 1992;101:538–552.

52. Verburg C, Griez E, Meijer J. A 35% carbon dioxide challenge in simple phobia. Acta Psychiatr Scand 1994;90:420–423.

53. Tuber DS, Hothersall D, Voith VL. Animal clinical psychology: a modest proposal. Am Psychol 1974;29:762–766.

54. Hart BL. General use of conditioning procedures. In: Hart BL, Hart LA. Canine and feline behavioral therapy. Philadelphia: Lea & Febiger, 1985:207–230.

55. Houpt KA. Miscellaneous behavioral disorders. In: Houpt KA. Domestic Animal Behavior, 2nd ed. Ames, IA: Iowa State University Press, 1991; 332–345.

56. Voith VL. Principles of learning. Vet Clin North Am Equine Pract 1986;2:485–506.

57. Beaver BV. Fear of loud noises. Vet Med/Small Anim Clinician 1983;333–334.

58. Noyes R Jr, Chaudry DR, Domingo DV. Pharmacologic treatment of phobic disorders. J Clin Psychiatry 1986;47:445–452.

59. Hart BL, Cooper LL. Integrating use of psychotropic drugs with environmental management and behavioral modification for treatment of problem behavior in animals. J Am Vet Med Assoc 1996;209:1549–1551.

60. Dodman NH, Shuster L. Pharmacologic approaches to managing behavior problems in small animals. Vet Med 1994;89:960–969.

61. Sheehan DV, Ballenger J, Jacobsen G. Treatment of endogenous anxiety with phobic, hysterical, and hypochondriacal symptoms. Arch Gen Psychiatry 1980;37:51–59.

62. Zitrin CM, Klein DF, Woerner MG, et al. Treatment of phobias: comparison of imipramine hydrochloride and placebo. Arch Gen Psychiatry 1983;40:125–138.

63. Hart BL, Cliff KD. Interpreting published results of extra-label drug use with special reference to reports of drugs used to correct problem behavior in animals. J Am Vet Med Assoc 1996;209:1382–1385.

64. Voith VL, Borchelt PL. Fear of thunder and other loud noises. Chicago: Veterinary Learning Systems, 1991.

65. Voith VL, Borchelt PL. The fearful dog . . . easing its fright. Chicago: Veterinary Learning Systems, 1991.

66. Voith VL, Borchelt PL. Strangers and the family dog. Chicago: Veterinary Learning Systems, 1991.

67. Hart BL. Psychoactive drugs and behavioral therapy. In: Hart BL, Hart LA. Canine and feline behavioral therapy. Philadelphia: Lea & Febiger, 1985:249–264.

68. Marder AR. Psychotropic drugs and behavioral therapy. Vet Clin North Am Small Anim Pract 1991;21:329–342.

69. Overall KL. Practical pharmacological approaches to behavior problems. In: Behavioral Problems in Small Animals. Ralston Purina Company, 1992:36–51.

70. Simpson, BS. Psychopharmacology for pets: indications and side effects. Convention notes from the 133rd Annual Convention of the American Veterinary Medical Association Louisville, KY 1996;599–608.

71. Voith VL. Possible pharmacological approaches to treating behavioural problems in animals. In: Anderson RS, ed. Nutrition and behaviour in dogs and cats. Oxford: Pergamon, 1984:227–234.

72. Overall KL. Introduction to psychotropic drugs. Proc North Am Vet Conf 1997;11:40–44.

73. Hunthausen WL, Lansberg GM. A practitioner's guide to pet behavior problems. American Animal Hospital Association, 1995.

74. Plumb DC. Veterinary drug handbook—pocket edition, 2nd ed. Ames, IA: Iowa State University Press, 1995.

75. Rehm WF, Schatzmann U. Pharmacological properties of benzodiazepines in animals. In: Van Miert, Asjpam, Bogaert MG, Debackere M, eds. Comparative veterinary pharmacology, toxicology and therapy. Lancaster, UK: MTP Press Limited, 1985:13–23.

76. Hart BL. Behavioral indications of phenothiazine and benzodiazepine tranquilizers in dogs. J Am Vet Med Assoc 1985;186:1192–1194.

77. Ballenger JC. Benzodiazepines. In: Schatzberg AF, Nemeroff CB, eds. Textbook of psychopharmacology. Washington, DC: The American Psychiatric Press, 1995:215–230.

78. Plumb DC. Drug monographs. In: Plumb DC. Veterinary drug handbook—pocket edition, 2nd ed. Ames, IA: Iowa State University Press, 1995:197–201.

79. Krueger KE. Peripheral-type benzodiazepine receptors: a second site of action for benzodiazepines. Neuropsychopharmacology 1991;4:237–244.

80. Bruhwyler J, Chleide E. Comparative study of the behavioral, neurophysiological, and motor effects of psychotropic drugs in the dog. Biol Psychiatry 1990;27:1264–1278.

81. Callahan AM, Fava M, Rosenbaum JF. Drug interactions in psychopharmacology. Psychiatr Clin North Am 1993;16:647–671.

82. Preskorn SH, Burke MJ, Fast GA. Therapeutic drug monitoring: principles and practice. Psychiatr Clin North Am 1993;16:611–641.

83. Dellefield K, Miller J. Psychotropic drugs and the elderly patient. Nur Clin North Am 1982;17:303–318.

84. Glassman R, Salzman C. Interactions between psychotropic drugs: an update. Hosp Community Psychiatry 1987;38:236–242.

85. Booth NH. Psychotropic agents. In: Booth NH, McDonald LE, eds. Veterinary pharmacology and therapeutics, 5th ed. Ames, IA: Iowa State University Press, 1982:321–352.

86. Hart BL, Eckstein RA, Powell KL, Dodman NH. Effectiveness of buspirone on urine spraying and inappropriate urinations in cats. J Am Vet Med Assoc 1993;203:254–258.

87. Roy-Byrne PP, Sullivan MD, Cowley DS, Ries RK. Adjunctive treatment of benzodiazepine discontinuation syndromes: a review. J Psychiatr Res 1993;27(suppl 1):143–153.

88. Pollack MH, Smoller JW. The longitudinal course and outcome of panic disorder. Psychiatr Clin North Am 1995;18:785–801.

89. Lees P. Sedatives, anticonvulsants, central muscle relaxants and analgesics. In: Brander GC, Pugh DM, Bywater RJ, Jenkins WL, eds. Veterinary applied pharmacology and therapeutics, 5th ed. London: Bailliere Tindall, 1991:328–354.

90. Roy-Byrne P, Wingerson D, Cowley D, Dager S. Psychopharmacologic treatment of panic, generalized anxiety disorder, and social phobia. Psychiatr Clin North Am 1993;16:719–735.

91. Macy DW, Ralston SL. Cause and control of decreased appetite. In: Kirk RW, ed. Current veterinary therapy. X. Small animal practice. Philadelphia: Saunders, 1989:18–24.

92. Frey HH, Loscher W. Pharmacokinetics of anti-epilepsy drugs in the dog: a review. J Vet Pharmacol Ther 1985;8:219–233.

93. Yen HCY, Krop S, Mendez HC, Katz MH. Effects of some psychoactive drugs on experimental 'neurotic' (conflict induced) behavior in cats. Pharmacology 1970;3:32–40.

94. Macy DW, Gasper PW. Diazepam-induced eating in anorexic cats. J Am Anim Hosp Assoc 1985;21:17–20.

95. Overall KL. State of the art: advances in the pharmacological therapy for behavioral disorders. TNAVC 1994 Proceedings of the North American Veterinary Conference 1994; 43–51.

96. Center SA, Elston TH, Rowland PH, et al. Fulminant hepatic failure associated with oral administration of diazepam in 11 cats. J Am Vet Med Assoc 1996;209:618–625.

97. Trepanier LA. Avoiding adverse drug reactions in cats. Feline Proceedings of the 1996 Practitioner's Symposium of the American Board of Veterinary Practitioners Chicago, IL 1996;307–318.

98. Messinger LM. Therapy for feline dermatoses. Vet Clin North Am Small Anim Pract 1995;25:981–1005.

99. Gould WJ. Caring for pet birds' skin and feathers. Vet Med 1995;90;53–63.

100. Brown SA, Forrester SD. Serum disposition of oral clorazepate from regular-release and sustained-delivery tablets in dogs. J Vet Pharmacol Ther 1991;14:426–429.

101. Boothe DM, Simpson G, Foster T. Effects of serum separation tubes on serum benzodiazepine and phenobarbital concentrations in clinically normal and epileptic dogs. Am J Vet Res 1996;57:1299–1303.

102. Voith VL. Behavioral disorders. In: Ettinger SJ, ed. Textbook of veterinary internal medicine, 3rd ed. Philadelphia: Saunders, 1989:227–238.

103. Plumb DC. Drug monographs. In: Plumb DC. Veterinary drug handbook—pocket edition, 2nd ed. Ames, IA: Iowa State University Press, 1995:163–164.

104. Lesser IM, Lydiard RB, Antal E, et al. Alprazolam plasma concentrations and treatment response in panic disorder and agoraphobia. Am J Psychiatry 1992;149:1556–1562.

105. Sheehan DV, Raj AB, Harnett-Sheehan K, et al. The relative efficacy of high-dose buspirone and alprazolam in the treatment of panic disorder: a double blind placebo-controlled study. Acta Psychiatr Scand 1993;88:1–11.

106. Pecknold JC, Swinson RP, Kuch K, et al. Alprazolam in panic disorder and agoraphobia: discontinuation effects. Arch Gen Psychiatry 1988;45:429–436.

107. Plumb DC. Drug monographs. In: Plumb DC. Veterinary drug handbook—pocket edition, 2nd ed. Ames, IA: Iowa State University Press, 1995:1–5.

108. Kakolewski JW. Psychopharmacology: clinical and experimental aspects. In: Fox MW, ed. Abnormal behavior in animals. Philadelphia: Saunders, 1968:523–543.

109. Debuf Y. Drugs acting on the nervous system. In: Debuf Y, ed. The veterinary formulary: handbook of medicines used in veterinary practice, 2nd ed. London: The Pharmaceutical Press, 1994;197–224.

110. Martin RJ. Small animal therapeutics. London: Wright, 1989:91.
111. Boothe DM. Drug therapy in cats: recommended dosing regimens. J Am Vet Med Assoc 1990;196:1845–1850.
112. Beaver BV. Feline behavior: a guide for veterinarians. Philadelphia: Saunders, 1992:15–62.
113. Dourish CT, Hutson PH, Curzon G. Putative anxiolytics 8-OH-DPAT, buspirone and TVX Q 7821 are agonists at 5-HT$_{1A}$ autoreceptors in the raphé nuclei. TIPS 1986;212–214.
114. Plumb DC. Drug monographs. In: Plumb DC. Veterinary drug handbook—pocket edition, 2nd ed. Ames, IA: Iowa State University Press, 1995: 94–96.
115. Schneider R, Saoud J, Campeas R, et al. Buspirone in social phobia. J Clin Psychopharmacol 1993;13:251–256.
116. Robinson SD, Shrotriya RC, Alms DR, et al. Treatment of panic disorder: nonbenzodiazepine anxiolytics, including buspirone. Psychopharmacol Bull 1989;25:21–26.
117. Plumb DC. Drug monographs. In: Plumb DC. Veterinary drug handbook—pocket edition, 2nd ed. Ames, IA: Iowa State University Press, 1995:592–594.
118. Neville PF, Walker R. Treatment of phobias in dogs and cats. TNAVC 1996 Proceedings 1996;25–27.
119. Walker R, Fisher J. Notes on propranolol and phenobarbitone as an adjunct to behaviour therapy. Presentation notes from Association of Pet Behaviour Counsellors, November 1994.
120. Plumb DC. Drug monographs. In: Plumb DC. Veterinary drug handbook—pocket edition, 2nd ed. Ames, IA: Iowa State University Press, 1995:537–540.
121. Hart BL. Behavior modification through hormonal manipulation. In: Hart BL, Hart LA. Canine and feline behavioral therapy. Philadelphia: Lea & Febiger, 1985:231–248.
122. Romatowski J. Use of megestrol acetate in cats. J Am Vet Med Assoc 1989;194:700–702.
123. Weikel JH Jr, Nelson LW, Reno FE. A four-year evaluation of the chronic toxicity of megesterol acetate in dogs. Toxicol Appl Pharmacol 1975;33:414–426.
124. Shanley K, Overall K. Rational selection of antidepressants for behavioral conditions. Vet Forum 1995;11:30–34.
125. Simpson BS, Simpson DM. Behavioral pharmacotherapy. Part 1: antipsychotics and antidepressants. Comp Cont Ed 1996;18:1067–1081.
126. Taylor CB. Treatment of anxiety disorders. In: Schatzberb AF, Nemeroff CB, eds. Textbook of psychopharmacology. Washington, DC: The American Psychiatric Press, 1995;641–656.
127. Mavissakalian M. Differential effects of imipramine and behavior therapy on panic disorder and agoraphobia. Psychopharmacol Bull 1989;25:27–29.
128. Tollefson GD. Selective serotonin reuptake inhibitors. In: Schatzberg AF, Nemeroff CB, eds. Textbook of psychopharmacology. Washington, DC: The American Psychiatric Press, 1995:161–182.
129. Krishman KRR. Monoamine oxidase inhibitors. In: Schatzberg AF, Nemeroff CB, eds. Textbook of psychopharmacology. Washington, DC: The American Psychiatric Press, 1995:183–193.

III COMPULSIVE BEHAVIOR

7 Basic Mechanisms of Compulsive and Self-Injurious Behavior

Louis Shuster

Nicholas H. Dodman

For 22 years, a polar bear in the Calgary Zoo has spent 70% of its day pacing back and forth in its enclosure. At each turn, it displays a sudden facial twitch and emits a huffing cough (1). Such mindless, repetitive actions are referred to as *stereotypies* or *compulsive behaviors*. There used to be a greater distinction between stereotypies and compulsions than there is presently, but the notion of a spectrum of obsessive-compulsive disorders in humans and the neuro-ethologic approach toward the understanding of these conditions have led some of us to regard the terms as virtually synonymous (2). The basis of the neuroethologic approach is that species-typical naturalistic ("hard-wired") survival-oriented behaviors can be expressed repetitively under certain circumstances. According to this theory, behaviors expressed compulsively could be derived from predation, ingestion, grooming, locomotion, and procreative activities.

Some persistent compulsions, such as paw-licking in dogs and feather-picking in birds, can lead to physical lesions and manifest as self-injurious behavior (SIB). Self-injurious behavior is a symptom of dysfunction and not a disease per se. Although obsessive-compulsive disorder (OCD) in humans and compulsive disorders in animals may lead to self-injury, the damage inflicted is incidental rather than purposeful. This is in contrast to the deliberate self-harm form of SIB that is prevalent in mentally retarded and institutionalized human patients and certain apparently more purposeful SIBs that affect animals (2).

Many species exhibit deliberate self-harm. For example, rodents that have been subjected to sciatic nerve damage will often resort to autotomy, perhaps because of some alteration in sensation (3). Many animals auto-amputate a limb if caught in a leghold trap. Some horses will purposely bite their own flanks, sometimes necessitating surgical correction of the wounds inflicted (4). Primates in captivity may engage in self-biting and neurotic excoriative behavior, and some escalate this self-directed behavior to the level of autocastration or enucleation by eye gouging (5).

What drives these behaviors? Are they expressions of (obsessive) compulsive disorder? The answers to these questions are not simple, but some forms of deliberate self-harm may represent compulsive behavior based on aggression. Indeed it would be curious if all other naturalistic behaviors except aggression could be manifested as compulsive behaviors. Some human OCD sufferers do have obsessions involving aggression, but ostensibly they do not spill over into aggressive acts and/or compulsions. If aggression is the form that OCD takes and there is no obvious target for that aggression, auto-aggression may lead to self-injury.

Human SIB is known to occur with greatest frequency in institutional settings where isolation and sensory deprivation are imposed. This is also true for some animal forms of SIBs (e.g., self-mutilating horses and captive primates). Mental retardation and severe psychological trauma, leading to borderline personality disorder, may also lead to deliberate self-harm in humans. In such cases, SIB may be due to social isolation, which will have an impact similar to physical isolation. There may be no direct equivalent in animals, though some dogs that have been mistreated when young do become extremely aggressive. Sometimes tail-chasing in dogs and cats is associated with tailbiting. This behavior has been variously described as an opioid-mediated stereotypy, a seizure-linked behavior, and a compulsive behavior (6). The presumed involvement of opioids in SIB is not surprising in light of the role of opioids in the propagation of aggression (see Chap. 1).

Are all forms of SIB related to OCD? Probably not. Lesch-Nyhan syndrome in humans has a clear genetic and metabolic basis (7). Digital self-mutilation in an inbred strain of Pointer dogs, which also has a genetic basis, is atypical as a compulsive behavior (8). On the other hand, SIB does appear to involve neurotransmitters identical to those associated with classic OCD (vide infra). Also, the same main classes of drugs that are used for the management of OCD are effective in SIB.

Etiology

As described in detail in Chapters 8 and 9, compulsive behaviors stem from innate behaviors that have become displaced and autonomous, persisting as fixed motor sequences. Normal precursory behaviors include grooming, foraging, feeding, predation, fear/avoidance, and sexual behaviors. A common impetus for the development of compulsive behaviors seems to be the stress of an impoverished or otherwise anxiety-provoking environment. For example, the polar bear in the Calgary Zoo began to pace when it was removed from its parents and placed in a separate enclosure (1). It stopped pacing 20 days later when it was returned to its parents' enclosure, but it resumed pacing in the same enclosure after another 2 months, even in its parents' presence. This case illustrates the impact of environmental stressors on the development of compulsive behaviors.

It has been postulated that compulsive behavior is one way of coping with stress (9). Wiepkema et al (10) found that calves displaying stereotypic tongue movements had less abomasal damage than those that did not. However, preventing mice from engaging in stereotypic wire-gnawing had no effect on hormonal indices of stress (11). There is a possibility that stereotypies may decrease stress more effectively while they are developing than after they have become established (12). The changing nature of stereotypies over time is illustrated by altered pharmacologic responsiveness during their development (12,13).

NEURAL MECHANISMS

Different approaches have pointed to the involvement of three main neurotransmitter systems in compulsive and self-injurious behaviors; specifically, dopaminergic, serotonergic, and opioidergic pathways have been implicated.

Dopamine

The involvement of dopamine and the nigrostriatal system in stereotypies is evidenced by experiments in which 6-hydroxydopamine was used to lesion dopaminergic nerve endings in the striatum of newborn or adult rats. The

Table 7.1. Response of self-biting horses to various drug treatments

		Interval (hr)	Self-biting attempts	Head tosses	Vocalizations	Kicks
Control mean		0–1	18.7	2.2	2.8	20.2
Drug	**Dose (mg/kg)**	**Percent of control response**				
Detomidine	0.02	0–1	10	0	18	2
Morphine	0.75	3–4	206	138	237	16
Naltrexone	0.75	1–2	14	26	85	12
Acepromazine	0.04	1–2	6	6	11	3
Buspirone	0.5	1–2	14	6	102	32
D-amphetamine	0.4	1–2	234	79	264	240
Haloperidol	0.004	1–2	13	0	50	23
Cocaine	0.75	0–1	47	80	232	135
Apomorphine	0.06	0–1	292	216	210	52
Clomipramine	1.0	2–3	52	10	70	69

Note: All values are the mean for eight horses, except for clomipramine, which was administered to five horses for 3 weeks. The postinjection time interval chosen for scoring was the one showing the greatest change from control values. The control mean is based on five separate determinations following IV injection of saline, 10 mL. These experiments were supported by a grant from the Tourette Syndrome Association, Inc, 42-40 Bell Boulevard, Bayside, NY 11361-2874.

resulting postsynaptic supersensitivity caused increased stereotypy and SIB following the injection of dopamine agonists such as apomorphine (14,15) (Figure 7.1). Dopaminergic supersensitivity, with resultant stereotypy, has also been induced by pretreatment of intact animals with a dopamine blocker such as haloperidol (16). In the clinical arena, certain compulsive behaviors in cats, birds, and humans are improved following treatment with dopamine antagonists (17–19). In addition, we have found that acepromazine and haloperidol reduce Tourette-like SIB in horses (Table 7.1).

Further support for the role of dopamine in repetitive behavior comes from the finding that OCD symptoms are exacerbated by chronic treatment with dopamine agonists (20). The main dopaminergic pathways travel from the brain stem to the basal ganglia and parts of the limbic system. Basal ganglia and limbic structures have received attention as brain regions involved in OCD psychopathology. Imaging studies, however, have produced inconsistent results (21). What evidence there is points to hyperactivity in orbitofrontal-basal

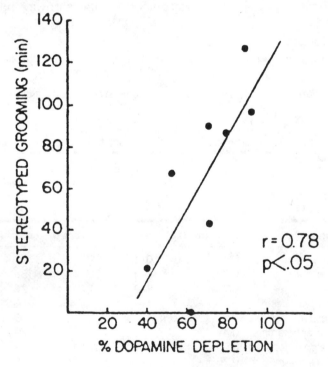

Figure 7.1.
Correlation between striatal dopamine depletion and stereotypic grooming induced by subcutaneous injection of apomorphine into rats that had received intrastriatal injections of 6-hydroxydopamine. Apomorphine was injected 10 days after chemical lesioning, and dopamine was assayed at least 8 days after the last drug test. (Reproduced by permission from Hartgraves SL, Randall PK. Dopamine agonist-induced stereotypic grooming and self-mutilation following striatal dopamine depletion. Psychopharmacology 1986;90:358–363.)

ganglionic-thalamic pathways in human OCD subjects (22), but these findings have yet to be substantiated in animals with compulsive behaviors.

Serotonin

An important role for serotonin (5-HT) in compulsive behaviors is suggested by a positive response of various compulsive disorders in humans and animals to treatment with 5-HT reuptake inhibitors, such as clomipramine and fluoxetine (2,23,24). The polar bear previously discussed completely stopped its compulsive pacing after 84 days of treatment with fluoxetine (Prozac) (1) (Figure 7.2). Bull Terriers that compulsively chase their tails and birds that compulsively pull out their feathers also respond positively to treatment with 5-HT reuptake inhibitors (6,25,26). The reduction of SIB in horses by buspirone and clomipramine is illustrated in Table 7.1.

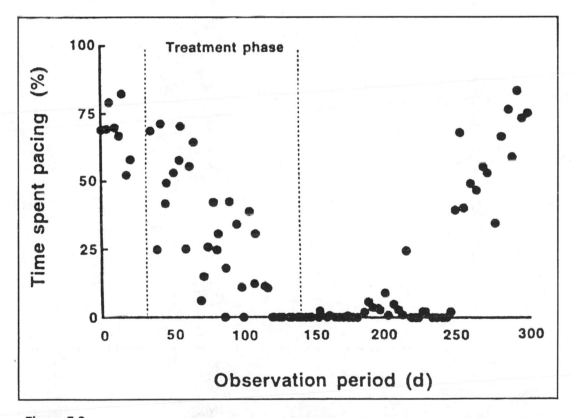

Figure 7.2.
The effect of fluoxetine administration on pacing by a captive polar bear. Oral fluoxetine was administered daily from day 33 to day 140. The dose of fluoxetine varied between 0.62 and 1.32 mg/kg. Behavior was recorded for 9-hour periods with a video camera. (Reproduced by permission from Poulsen EMB, Honeyman V, Valentine PA, Teskey GC. Use of fluoxetine for the treatment of stereotypical pacing behavior in a captive polar bear. *J Am Vet Med Assoc* 1996;209:1470–1474.)

Serotonergic dysregulation, particularly in the dorsal raphe nucleus (DRN), or the DRN's targets in basal ganglia and cortex, may be instrumental in the propagation of many forms of OCD. Pharmacologic challenges and treatment outcome studies have indicated that changes in the DRN's inhibitory influence on basal ganglionic circuitary may correlate with alterations in OCD symptoms (19).

Opioids

Some compulsive behaviors in animals and SIB in humans respond to treatment with opioid antagonists, suggesting opioidergic involvement in these behaviors (27,28). Opioid receptors are found closely associated with dopaminergic and serotonergic neurons, and are distributed in regions such as the limbic system, hypothalamus, striatum (specifically, the head of the caudate nucleus), and periaqueductal gray matter. The association is more than simply anatomic, however, as dopaminergic and serotonergic systems interact func-

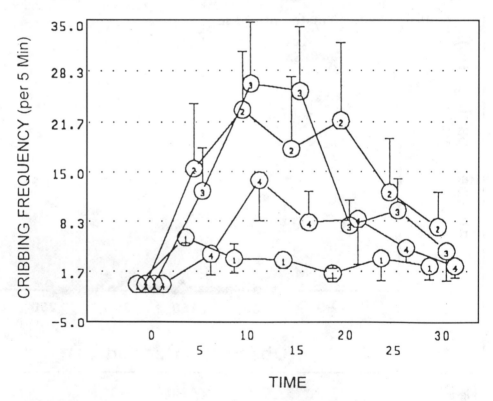

Figure 7.3.

Cribbing rate (mean ± SEM) of five horses before ① and after the feeding of sweet-feed ②, 16% protein pellets ③, or alfalfa pellets ④. (Reproduced by permission from Gilham SB, Dodman NH, Shuster L, et al. The effect of diet on cribbing behavior and plasma beta endorphin in horses. Appl Anim Behav Sci 1994;41:147–153.)

tionally, with opioids facilitating dopaminergic effector systems and 5-HT acting as the "brakes" (24,29).

One compulsive behavior that has received considerable attention in terms of opioidergic involvement is cribbing. This oral compulsion is readily induced in susceptible horses by feeding them a small amount of sweet-feed (grain mixed with molasses). Pellets containing 16% protein are just as effective as sweet-feed in promoting cribbing, while alfalfa pellets produce only a slight increase in the cribbing rate (30) (Figure 7.3). A plausible explanation for the interrelationship of feeding and cribbing is that both behaviors involve activation of narcotic receptors. Sweet and palatable foods are known to release

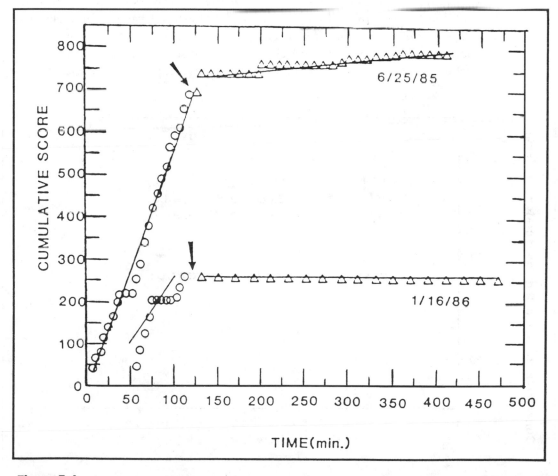

Figure 7.4.
The effects of naltrexone on cribbing frequency. The horse received an IV injection of naltrexone 0.04 mg/kg on 6/25/85 and a 0.4 mg/kg injection on 1/16/86 (*arrows*). (Reproduced by permission from Dodman NH, Shuster L, Court MH, Dixon R. Investigation into the use of narcotic antagonists in the treatment of a stereotypic behavior pattern (crib-biting) in the horse. Am J Vet Res 1987;48:311–319.)

endogenous opioids from the hypothalamus (31), thereby increasing pain thresholds (32) and the potency of morphine (33). Narcotic antagonists, such as naloxone and naltrexone, inhibit ingestion, especially of sweet foods, in many different species (34). If cribbing is reinforced because it releases endogenous opioids, then blocking narcotic receptors in the brain should abolish this reinforcement. Several antagonists of mu receptors prevent cribbing when injected intravenously (27) (Figure 7.4). Also, exogenous mu agonists should stimulate cribbing in susceptible horses; such stimulation has been observed (35) (Becker T, Dodman NH, Shuster L, unpublished data, 1992).

Limbic and striatal opioid receptors may be involved in the motor and emotional effects of opiates (36). Dopamine appears to be instrumental in the locomotor effects of opiates, once again supporting the concept of an opioid-dopamine interaction (35). Oral stereotypies evoked by dopamine agonists in rats that were pretreated chronically with haloperidol were completely prevented by naloxone (37). Other compulsions related to eating or grooming, such as acral lick in dogs (38) (Fig. 7.5), flank-sucking in dogs (39), wool-sucking in cats (39), chain-biting in pigs (40), also respond to narcotic antago-

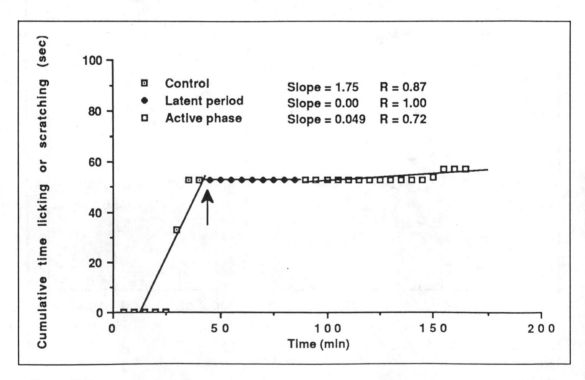

Figure 7.5.
The effect of nalmefene on self-licking or self-chewing by a dog with lick granuloma. At the time indicated nalmefene, 1 mg/kg, was injected SC. (Reproduced by permission from Dodman NH, Shuster L, White SD, et al. Use of narcotic antagonists to modify stereotypic self-licking, self-chewing, and scratching behavior in dogs. J Am Vet Med Assoc 1988;193:815–819.)

nists but not to the same extent as cribbing. Naltrexone decreases self-biting in horses (see Table 7.1).

Basis for Treatment

ENVIRONMENTAL MODIFICATION

If the impetus for compulsive behaviors and SIB is assumed to be environmental stress, then treatment should include modification of the environment or improved management aimed at minimizing stress. Enriching the environment of chain-biting sows has been demonstrated to decrease their compulsive behaviors (41), and exercise and dietary alterations diminished SIB in a flank-biting stallion (42). However, attempts to enrich the environment of the Calgary Zoo polar bear failed to diminish its stereotypic pacing (1). It is obviously not practical to provide the wide range of territory that polar bears enjoy in the wild. Furthermore, the longer that stereotypic behavior has been performed, the more resistant it is to change (12,13). It is therefore often necessary to supplement environmental and behavior modification strategies with pharmacologic therapy.

PHARMACOTHERAPY

One aim of pharmacotherapy is to block the rewarding effects of the deviant behavior. For example, if cribbing leads to activation of narcotic receptors, then acute administration of a narcotic antagonist should eliminate reinforcement of this behavior while the drug is present. To produce lasting improvement, however, it is usually necessary to modify specific receptors that subserve particular behaviors, and such modification may take weeks or even months.

Dopamine plays an important role in OCD, Tourette's syndrome, and SIB in humans. Patients with these conditions often describe a buildup of inner tension that is relieved by what seems to be an impulsive, mindless behavior. It could be argued that such behavior may lead to "reward" in the form of dopamine release, either directly or via the release of enkephalins. However, usual doses of dopamine blockers are sometimes ineffective in curtailing such behaviors, and higher doses are often associated with unacceptable levels of sedation (39).

Another approach is to enhance serotonergic neurotransmission, thus modulating other dependent systems. Serotonin-reuptake inhibitors (SRIs) are the most universally effective pharmacologic treatments available for compulsive behaviors. They do, however, have some limitations, not the least of which is variability in the response of individual patients. Although SRIs are extremely effective in some patients, other patients are merely controlled, while others are virtually nonresponsive to this treatment. In addition, the majority of patients receiving SRIs for treatment of OCD require long-term therapy, and side effects can be troublesome in some cases.

Based on the efficacy of SRIs, it can be argued that OCD somehow involves a deficiency of 5-HT that is countered by 5-HT reuptake inhibition. On the other hand, 5-HT's role in OCD may be simply modulation of other neurotransmitter systems that have gone awry. Because some repetitive motor behaviors activate 5-HT systems, Jacobs (43) believes that OCD patients engage in compulsive behaviors to self-medicate with 5-HT. If this were true, 5-HT reuptake inhibition, by raising 5-HT levels, would relieve OCD patients of the need to engage in compulsive behaviors in order to generate 5-HT.

NEUROTRANSMITTER INTERACTIONS

The role of multiple neurotransmitters in OCD remains enigmatic. Why are 5-HT-enhancing drugs generally effective in classic human OCD and animal compulsive behaviors? Why does cribbing respond to treatment with opioid antagonists? Why do human OCDs with a comorbid tic disorder respond to dopamine antagonist augmentation of SRI treatment (44)? Why does feather-picking in psittacine birds respond to treatment with dopamine antagonists (18), whereas classic human OCD does not? The answers to these questions are to be found by applying a neuroethologic approach toward an understanding of compulsive disorders (26). According to this approach, the behavior displayed in OCD is a species-specific, "hard-wired" behavior pattern necessary for survival of the animal. Typical behaviors giving rise to the many possible manifestations of OCD include grooming, predation, consummatory behavior, and sexual behavior. These behaviors rely on different neural pathways and neural substrates for their propagation, and this diversity may explain the different responsiveness of the various forms of OCD to pharmacologic intervention. For example, endogenous opioids are intimately involved in the propagation and reward of consummatory behaviors (31,45). It can be extrapolated from these observations that opioid antagonists might be useful for the alleviation of compulsions related to consummatory behaviors. These agents have been demonstrated to be effective treatments for psychogenic polydipsia in psychiatric inpatients (46), cribbing in horses (27), and flank-sucking in dogs (39).

Because opioids facilitate offensive aggression (see Chap. 1) and are released in response to stress and injury (47), opioid antagonists should be effective treatments for deliberate self-harm, a form of SIB, in humans and other animals. Once again this is borne out by what has been found in humans (28,48,49) and horses (50; Shuster L, Dodman NH, Kinney L, unpublished data, 1994) (Figure 7.6).

Locomotor behaviors involve dopaminergic activation (35,51). In case studies, the dopamine agonist apomorphine was found to exacerbate weaving,

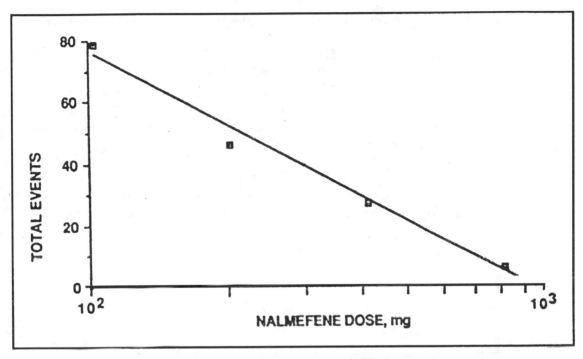

Figure 7.6.
The effect of different doses of nalmefene on a stallion with SIB. Self-biting attempts by the muzzled horse were counted on different days for 4 hours after 1 M administration of nalmefene. (Reproduced by permission from Dodman NH, Shuster L, Court MH, Patel J. Use of a narcotic antagonist (nalmefene) to suppress self-mutilative behavior in a stallion. J Am Vet Med Assoc 1988;192:1585–1586.)

a compulsive behavior that is an abbreviated form of fence running (Dodman NH, Shuster L, unpublished data, 1988). Nigrostriatal dopamine is instrumental in skeletal muscle activity, but mesolimbic dopamine may also be involved in propagating motor compulsions by providing reward and reinforcement (29). Dopamine antagonists should be effective in reducing locomotor compulsions in animals, but to date these agents have not found much application for this purpose. One reason might be their tendency to produce sedation, a side effect most animal owners find unacceptable. As dopamine is involved in grooming, retrieval, licking/chewing, and self-mutilation (14,52,53), dopamine antagonists should be effective in reducing compulsive behaviors with such components. Feline psychogenic alopecia (25) and feather-picking in birds (18) both respond to therapy with dopamine antagonists.

Many different forms of OCD have been found to respond to treatment with SRIs, probably because serotonin has a wide range of modulatory functions in different parts of the brain (20). Serotonin is involved in facilitating skeletal motor function, aggression, pain perception, sexual behavior, and mood (43,54) (see also Chap. 1). Serotonin's wide range of activity is mediated by numerous receptor subtypes, with different receptors controlling different functions.

Perhaps compulsive behaviors generate 5-HT, stabilizing mood or generating fleeting gratification. For example, serotonergic neurons are activated during repetitive oral-buccal movements such as chewing/biting and grooming (55). This hypothesis, if confirmed, would explain the overall efficacy of 5-HT-enhancing drugs in regulating OCD but does not account for individual differences in response. Some behaviors may be more powerfully modulated by serotonergic systems than others, or there may be individual differences in the sensitivity of 5-HT receptors. Another peculiarity is the long latent period before maximal response to treatment with SRIs. Downregulation of presynaptic receptors controlling 5-HT release may be necessary for the full

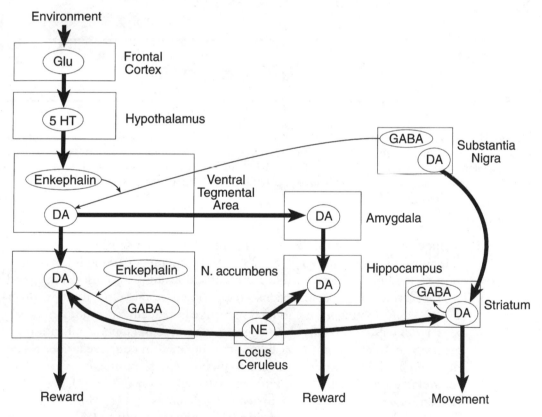

Thick Lines: Stimulation or release
Thin Lines: Inhibition

Figure 7.7.
Neuroanatomic and neurochemical substrates that lead to reward and movement. Glu = glutamate; 5-HT = serotonin; DA = dopamine; GABA = gamma-amino butyric acid; NE = norepinephrine. (Adapted from Blum K, Cull JC, Braverman ER, Comings DE. Reward deficiency syndrome. Am Scientist 1996;84:132–145.)

effect of SRIs to become apparent (56). In the future, it may be possible to select a specific 5-HT receptor agonist to treat a particular OCD with more dependable results. Currently, the 5-HT1D receptor is receiving some attention with regard to human OCD (57), implying that this pathway is most intimately involved in affective and perhaps motor aspects of classic human OCD.

The interaction of dopamine, 5-HT, and enkephalins in the basic circuitry that underlies compulsive behaviors is illustrated in Figure 7.7. There is functional integration of so-called pleasure centers with the nigrostriatal system that controls movement, and the mesolimbic-mesocortical system that plays an important role in mood and emotion (29). Superimposed modulation of these pathways is provided by norepinephrine, which increases reward and alertness, and corticotropin-releasing hormone (CRH), which influences responses to stress and to several different neurotransmitters (58). As can be seen in Figure 7.7, stimulation of narcotic receptors increases the release of dopamine by blocking the inhibitory effect of gamma-aminobutyric acid (GABA). Narcotic antagonists prevent drug-induced increases in extracellular dopamine in the nucleus accumbens and corpus striatum (59).

Heterogeneity and Genetic Determinants

Most behavior disorders in both human and animal patients have one characteristic in common: no individual drug treatment is effective for more than 60% of the affected population (60). It may be necessary to employ two or more SRIs in succession or to engage in various augmentation strategies to produce a clinically useful effect in any one patient. In view of the contribution of environment, heredity, and duration of the disorder, such heterogeneity of response might be anticipated. Also, as can be seen in Figure 7.7, the same compulsive behavior may result from reduced serotonergic activity in one patient, and increased dopaminergic or opioid activity in another.

Elucidation of genetic determinants of specific behaviors may prove helpful in establishing their etiology and determining suitable therapy. Evidence is accumulating for strong genetic involvement in OCD and Tourette syndrome in humans (61). Self-biting in horses (62) and wool-sucking in cats (25) also appear to be strongly influenced by heredity. In examining the familial basis of behavior disorders in animals it is important to take into account learning by example and the influence of environment.

Analysis of behavior in transgenic animals is a promising new approach that is presently limited almost entirely to mice. Initial reports suggest that single genes controlling 5-HT receptors (63,64), dopamine receptors (65,66), narcotic receptors (67), monoamine oxidase (68), and nitric oxide synthase (69) can all affect behavior.

Mice in which 5-HT_{1B} receptors have been knocked out are more aggressive than wild-type mice (63). Their decreased latency to attack has been compared to increased impulsive behavior observed in primates with a central 5-HT deficit (70). Mice missing 5-HT2C receptors suffer from spontaneous epileptic seizures, which are often preceded by repetitive grooming of the snout. They also display increased appetite and weight gain that is not suppressed by the 5-HT agonist meta-chloro-phenylpiperazine (MCPP) (64).

Mice lacking D1 dopamine receptors are growth retarded and display normal locomotor activity but markedly reduced stereotypic rearing behavior (71). There is a striking decrease in dynorphin synthesis and in hyperactivity and stereotypy after cocaine administration to these same mice (72). Inactivation of D2 dopamine receptors yields a murine model of parkinsonism (73). Dopamine D3 receptor knockout mice display both increased locomotion and rearing (66). From these indirect observations it might be concluded that D1 and D2 receptors facilitate some stereotypic behaviors, while D3 receptors may have an inhibitory function.

There are, however, certain problems in applying information gained from transgenic models to the clinical situation. Development of knockout mice takes place without the specific protein produced by the gene that has been eliminated, so that they may die in utero or be born defective. On the other hand, there can be compensation to produce a phenotype that is almost normal. For example, mice in which the gene for hypoxanthine-guanine-ribosyltransferase (HGPRT) has been inactivated do not display the SIB characteristic of human patients with Lesch-Nyhan syndrome (74).

One way to circumvent this problem is to produce conditional knockouts. By linking a gene for a neurotransmitter receptor to a tetracycline-controlled promoter, it is possible to produce mice in which expression of the receptor is abolished only when the animal is given tetracycline (75). Behavior can then be studied before and after tetracycline administration, so that each animal develops normally and also serves as its own control.

Another way to control gene expression in adult animals is to inject antisense oligodeoxynucleotides into the brain. This procedure has been used to block the expression of the dopamine D2 receptor (76). The main drawback, in addition to the need for repeated intracerebral injections, is that blockade of gene expression is usually incomplete (77). However, this technique has the advantage of being potentially usable in domestic animals as well as rodents.

Conclusion

There is clearly a great deal still to be learned about the etiology of compulsive/stereotypic behaviors in veterinary as well as human patients. The many different approaches previously discussed have provided important insights into the propagation of such behaviors, though integration and consolidation of the findings are still required. Neuropharmacologic and genetic evidence points to the role of specific receptors for 5-HT, dopamine, and perhaps opioids in the development and maintenance of these aberrant behaviors. Neuroimaging studies and neurophysiologic studies in humans support the involvement of brain regions rich in these receptors (21). A neuroethologic approach toward the understanding of OCD and the recent recognition of a range of compulsive behaviors, in the form of obsessive-compulsive spectrum disorders, have paved the way for a broader biologic understanding of compulsive behaviors. This approach helps to reconcile some of the previously diverging data, such as the different pharmacologic responsiveness of various forms of OCD.

We can learn much about specific components of OCD from laboratory models of OCD and from human clinical trials, but veterinary clinical models could contribute significantly toward furthering this understanding. The polar bear mentioned at the beginning of this chapter illustrates the role of an impoverished (restricted) environment in the development of OCD, ethologic constraints on the compulsive behavior expressed, and the potential value of 5-HT enhancement in therapy of this disorder.

References

1. Poulsen EMB, Honeyman V, Valentine PA, Teskey GC. Use of fluoxetine for the treatment of stereotypical pacing behavior in a captive polar bear. J Am Vet Med Assoc 1996; 209:1470–1474.
2. Dodman NH, Moon-Fanelli AA, Mertens PA, et al. Veterinary models of obsessive-compulsive disorder. In: Hollander E, Stein DJ, eds. Obsessive-compulsive disorder. New York: Marcel Dekker, 1997 (in press).
3. Wiesenfeld Z, Hallin RG. Continuous naloxone administration via osmotic minipump decreases autotomy but has no effect on nociceptive threshold in the rat. Pain 1983;16:145–153.
4. Houpt KA. Self-directed aggression: a stallion behavior problem. Equine Pract 1983;5:6–8.
5. Kraemer GW, Clarke AS. The behavioral neurobiology of self-injurious behavior in rhesus monkeys. Prog Neuropsychopharmacol Biol Psychiatry 1990;14:5141–5168.
6. Moon-Fanelli AA, Dodman NH. Phenomenology, development, and pharmacotherapy of compulsive tail chasing in 18 terrier breed dogs: a survey and prospective open trial of clomipramine. J Am Vet Med Assoc 1997 (in Press).
7. Lloyd KG, Hornykiewicz O, Davidson L, et al. Biochemical evidence of dysfunction of brain neurotransmitters in the Lesch-Nyhan syndrome. N Eng J Med 1981;305:1106–1111.
8. Cummings JF, de Lahunta A, Winn SS. Acral mutilation and nociceptive loss in English pointer dogs: a canine sensory neuropathy. Acta Neuropathol 1981;53:119–127.
9. Wechsler B. Coping and coping strategies: a behavioral view. Appl Anim Behav Sci 1995;43:123–134.
10. Wiepkema PR, van Hellemand KK, Roessingh P, Romberg H. Behavior and abomasal damage in individual veal calves. Appl Anim Behav Sci 1987;18:257–268.
11. Würbel H, Stauffacher M. Prevention of stereotypy in laboratory mice: effects on stress physiology and behavior. Physiol Behav 1996;59:1163–1170.
12. Kennes D, Odberg FO, Bouquet Y, DeRycke PH. Changes in naloxone and haloperidol effects during the development of captivity-induced jumping stereotypy in bank voles. Eur J Pharmacol 1988;153:19–24.
13. Cronin GM. The development and significance of abnormal stereotyped behaviors in tethered sows. PhD thesis, Agricultural University of Wageningen, 1985.

14. Criswell H, Mueller, Breese ER. Priming of D_1-dopamine agonist following repeated administration to neonatal 6-OHDA-lesioned rats. J Neurosci 1989;9:125–133.

15. Hartgraves SL, Randall PK. Dopamine agonist-induced stereotypic grooming and self mutilation following striatal dopamine depletion. Psychopharmacology 1986;90:358–363.

16. Tarsy D, Baldessarini RJ. Behavioral supersensitivity to apomorphine following chronic treatment with drugs which interfere with the synaptic function of catecholamines. Neuropharmacology 1974;13:927–940.

17. Cools AR, Van Rossum JM. Caudal dopamine and stereotypy behavior of cats. Arch Int Pharmacodyn Ther 1970;187:163–173.

18. Iglauer F, Rasim R. Treatment of psychogenic feather picking in birds with a dopamine antagonist. J Small Anim Pract 1993;34:564–566.

19. Stein DJ, Hollander E. Low dose pimozide augmentation of serotonin reuptake blockers in the treatment of trichotillomania. J Clin Psychiatry 1992;53:123–126.

20. Grove G, Coplan J, Margolin L, Hollander E. The neuroanatomy of serotonin (5HT) dysregulation in obsessive-compulsive disorder. CNS Spect 1996;1:16–22.

21. Hoehn-Saric R, Benkelfat C. Structural and functional imaging in obsessive compulsive disorder. In: Hollander E, Zohar J, Marazitti D, Olivier B, eds. Current insights in obsessive-compulsive disorder. New York: John Wiley & Sons, 1994:183–211.

22. Brody AL, Saxena S. Brain imaging in obsessive-compulsive disorder: evidence for involvement of frontal-subcortical circuitry in the mediation of symptomatology. CNS Spect 1996;1:27–41.

23. Rapoport JL, Ryland DH, Kriete M. Drug treatment of canine acral lick. An animal model of obsessive-compulsive disorder. Arch Gen Psychiatry 1992;49:517–521.

24. Feinberg M. Clomipramine for obsessive-compulsive disorder. Am Fam Physician 1991;43:1735–1738.

25. Moon-Fanelli AA, Dodman NH, O'Sullivan RL. Veterinary models of compulsive self-grooming: parallels with trichotillomania. In: Christenson GA, Stein DJ, eds. Trichotillomania. 1997: In Press.

26. Dodman NH, Olivier B. In search of animal models of obsessive-compulsive disorder. CNS Spect 1996;1:10–15.

27. Dodman NH, Shuster L, Court MH, Dixon R. Investigation into the use of narcotic antagonists in the treatment of a stereotypic behavior pattern (crib-biting) in the horse. Am J Vet Res 1987;48:311–319.

28. Herman BH, Hammock MK, Arthur-Smith A, et al. Naltrexone decreases self-injurious behavior. Ann Neurol 1987;22:550–552.

29. Blum K, Cull JC, Braverman ER, Comings DE. Reward deficiency syndrome. Am Scientist 1996;84:132–145.

30. Gilham SB, Dodman NH, Shuster L, et al. The effect of diet on cribbing behavior and plasma beta endorphin in horses. Appl Anim Behav Sci 1994;41:147–153.

31. Dum J, Gramsch C, Herz A. Activation of hypothalamic β-endorphin pools by reward induced by highly palatable food. Pharmacol Biochem Behav 1983;18:443–447.

32. Blass E, Fitzgerald E, Kehoe P. Interactions between sucrose, pain and isolation distress. Pharmacol Biochem Behav 1987;26:483–487.

33. Roane DS, Martin RJ. Continuous sucrose feeding decreases pain threshold and increases morphine potency. Pharmacol Biochem Behav 1990;35:225–229.

34. Levine AS, Billington CJ. Opioids—are they regulators of feeding? Ann NY Acad Sci 1989;575:209–220.

35. Shuster L, Dodman NH, D'Allesandro T, Zuroff S. Reverse tolerance to the stimulant effects of morphine in horses. Equine Vet Sci 1984;4:233–236.

36. Lader M. Introduction to psychopharmacology. Kalamazoo, MI: The Upjohn Company, 1980:109.

37. Pollock J, Kornetsky C. Naloxone prevents and blocks the emergence of neuroleptic-mediated oral stereotypic behavior. Neuropsychopharmacology 1991;4:245–249.

38. Dodman NH, Shuster L, White SD, et al. Use of narcotic antagonists to modify stereotypic self-licking, self-chewing, and scratching behavior in dogs. J Am Vet Med Assoc 1988;193:815–819.

39. Dodman NH, Shuster L. Pharmacologic approaches to managing behavior problems in small animals. Vet Med 1994;Oct:960–969.

40. Cronin GM, Wiepkema PR, Van Ree JM. Endogenous opioids are involved in abnormal stereotyped behaviors of tethered sows. Neuropeptides 1985;6:527–530.

41. Petersen V, Simonsen HB, Lawson LG. The effect of environmental stimulation on the development of behavior in pigs. Appl Anim Behav Sci 1995;45:215–224.

42. McClure SR, Chaffin MK, Beaver BV. Nonpharmacologic management of stereotypic self-mutilative behavior in a stallion. J Am Vet Med Assoc 1992;200:1975–1977.

43. Jacobs BL. Serotonin and behavior: emphasis on motor control. J Clin Psychiatry 1991;52:17–23.

44. McDougle CJ, Goodman WK, Price LH. Dopamine antagonists in tic-related and psychotic spectrum obsessive compulsive disorder. J Clin Psychiatry 1994;53:24 31.

45. Morley JE, Levine AS. The pharmacology of eating behavior. Annu Rev Pharmacol Toxicol 1985;25:127–146.

46. Nishikawa T, Tsuda A, Tanaka M, et al. Involvement of the endogenous opioid system in the drinking behavior of schizophrenic patients displaying self-induced water intoxication: a double blind placebo controlled study with naloxone. Clin Neuropharmacol. 1996;19:252–258.

47. Szekely JI. Opioid peptides and stress. Crit Rev Neurobiol 1990;6:1–12.

48. Bystritsky A, Strausser BP. Treatment of obsessive-compulsive cutting behavior with naltrexone. J Clin Psychiatry 1996;57:423–424.

49. Smith KC, Pittlekow MR. Naltrexone for neurotic excoriations. J Am Acad Dermatol 1989;20:860–861.

50. Dodman NH, Shuster L, Court MH, Patel J. Use of a narcotic antagonist (nalmefene) to suppress self-mutilative behavior in a stallion. J Am Vet Med Assoc 1988;192:1585–1586.

51. Hurd YL, Weiss F, Koob GF, et al. Cocaine reinforcement and extracellular dopamine overflow in rat nucleus accumbens: an in vivo microdialysis study. Brain Res 1989;498:199–203.

52. Korsgaard S, Povlsen UJ, Randrup A. Effects of apomorphine and haloperidol on "spontaneous" stereotyped licking behavior in the Cebus monkey. Psychopharmacology 1985;85:240–243.

53. Giordano AL, Johnson AE, Rosenblatt JS. Haloperidol-induced disruption of retrieval behavior and reversal with apomorphine in lactating rats. Physiol Behav 1990;48:211–214.

54. Jacobs BL, Azmitia EC. Structure and function of the brain serotonin system. Physiol Rev 1992;72:165.

55. Jacobs BL, Fornal CA. Activity of brain serotonergic neurons in the behaving animal. Pharmacol Rev 1991;43:563–578.

56. Shader RI, Fogelman SM, Greenblatt DJ. Newer antidepressants: hypotheses and evidence. J Clin Psychopharmacol 1997;17:1–3.

57. Dolberg OT, Iancu I, Sasson Y, Zohar J. The pathogenesis and treatment of obsessive-compulsive disorder. Clin Neuropharmacol 1996;19:129–144.

58. Owens MJ, Nemeroff CB. Physiology and pharmacology of corticotropin releasing factor. Pharmacol Rev 1991;43:425–473.

59. Schad CA, Justice JB Jr, Holtzman SG. Different effects of δ- and μ-opioid receptor antagonists on the amphetamine-induced increase in extracellular dopamine in striatum and nucleus accumbens. J Neurochem 1996;67:2292–2299.

60. Hollander E. Is there a distinct OCD spectrum? CNS Spect 1996;1:17–26.

61. Wolf SS, Jones DW, Knable MB, et al. Tourette syndrome: prediction of phenotypic variation in monozygotic twins by caudate nucleus D_2 receptor binding. Science 1996;273:1225–1227.

62. Dodman NH, Normile JA, Shuster L, Rand W. Equine self-mutilation syndrome (57 cases). J Am Vet Med Assoc. 1994;204:1219–1223.

63. Sadou F, Amara DA, Dierich A, et al. Enhanced aggressive behavior in mice lacking 5-HT_{1B} receptor. Science 1994;265:1875–1878.

64. Tecott LH, Sun LM, Akana SF, et al. Eating disorder and epilepsy in mice lacking 5-HT_{2C} serotonin receptors. Nature 1995;374:542–546.

65. Mortalla R, Xu M, Tonegawa S, Graybiel AM. Cellular responses to psychomotor stimulants and neuroleptic drugs are abnormal in mice lacking D_1 dopamine receptor. Proc Nat Acad Sci USA 1996;93:14928–14933.

66. Accili D, Fishburn CS, Drago J, et al. A targeted mutation of the D_3 dopamine receptor gene is associated with hyperactivity in mice. Proc Nat Acad Sci USA 1996;93:1945–1949.

67. Matthes HWD, Maldonado R, Simonin F, et al. Loss of morphine induced analgesia, reward effect and withdrawal symptoms in mice lacking the μ-opioid-receptor gene. Nature 1996;383:819–823.

68. Cases O, Seif I, Grimsly J, et al. Aggressive behavior and altered amounts of brain serotonin and norepinephrine in mice lacking MAOA. Science 1995;268:1763–1766.

69. Nelson RJ, Demas GE, Huang DL, et al. Behaviorial abnormalities in male mice lacking neuronal nitric oxide synthase. Nature 1995;378:383–386.

70. Hen R. Mean genes. Neuron 1996;16:17–21.

71. Drago J, Gerfen CR, Lachowitz JE, et al. Altered striatal function in a mutant mouse lacking D_{1A} dopamine receptors. Proc Nat Acad Sci USA 1994;91:12564–12568.

72. Xu M, Hu XT, Cooper DC, et al. Elimination of cocaine-induced hyperactivity and dopamine-mediated neurophysiological effects in dopamine D_1 receptor mutant mice. Cell 1994;79:945–955.

73. Balk JH, Picetti R, Saalrdi A, et al. Parkinson-like locomotor impairment in mice lacking dopamine D_2 receptors. Nature 1995;377:424–428.

74. Kuehn MR, Bradley A, Robertson EJ, Evans MJ. A potential animal model for Lesch-Nyhan syndrome through introduction of HPRT mutations into mice. Nature 1987;326:295–298.

75. Furth PA, St. Onge L, Böger H, et al. Temporal control of gene expression in transgenic mice by a tetracycline-responsive promoter. Proc Nat Acad Sci USA 1994;91:9302–9306.

76. Zhou LW, Zhang SP, Quin ZH, Weiss B. In vivo administration of an oligo-deoxynucleotide antisense to the D_2 dopamine receptor messenger RNA inhibits D_2 dopamine receptor-mediated behavior and the expression of D_2 receptors in mouse striatum. J Pharmacol Exp Ther 1994;268:1015–1023.

77. Lucas JJ, Hen R. New players in the 5HT receptor field: genes and knockouts. Trends in Pharmacol Sci 1995;16:246–252.

Pharmacologic Treatment of Compulsive Disorder

8

U.A. Luescher

Stereotypies have been defined as behaviors that are repetitive, performed in constant form, and serve no obvious purpose (1,2). This definition is purely descriptive, however; that is, it defines signs of a disorder rather than the disorder itself (3).

Stereotypies have been reported in most farm animals (4) as well as in companion animals (5). It is generally suggested that stereotypies develop under inadequate environmental conditions inducing stress and that they indicate reduced animal welfare (6,7). However, because by definition stereotypy is a sign and not a diagnosis, the causes and expression of stereotypies vary greatly (2).

Some stereotypic behavior in companion animals has been likened to the compulsions of human patients with obsessive-compulsive disorder (OCD) (8). OCD is a common human psychiatric disorder, with an estimated lifetime prevalence of 2.5% in the United States (9). "Obsessive" refers to intrusive thoughts that the patient wishes to suppress, and compulsions are the accompanying, ritualistic behaviors (10). Because we do not have access to an animal's subjective experiences, and because there likely are neurobiologic differences between human OCD and the syndrome in animals, the use of the term *compulsive disorder* (CD) has been proposed for use in animals (3,11).

Stereotypic behavior may be an expression of CD in animals (12). Stereotypic behavior of companion animals includes licking or chewing specific parts of the body, hallucinatory behavior such as fly-snapping, whirling, pacing, freezing, rhythmic barking, wool-sucking, and self-mutilation (5). Disorders of this type represent approximately 3.5% and 6% of the canine and feline behavior caseload at the Ontario Veterinary College, respectively. Stereotypic behavior in horses includes cribbing, stall-walking, weaving, wood-chewing, tongue-playing, and self-mutilation (13). It has been hypothesized that these behaviors, too, may be an expression of compulsive disorder (14). The prevalence of stereotypic behavior in Thoroughbred horses has been estimated at 2% (15), and for horses in Southern Ontario at around 10% (16).

This chapter concentrates on compulsive disorder in companion animals and, to a lesser degree, in horses, as these are the only species for which pharmacologic treatment is feasible.

Etiology

Naturally occurring, environmentally induced stereotypies are commonly believed to be caused, or to have been caused, by some form of conflict or frustration (6). They are thought to be displayed initially in a specific context as a reactive abnormal behavior or conflict behavior (17), but with repeated or chronic conflict can then generalize to other contexts, i.e., they emancipate from their original cause (1,18). They are also believed to evolve gradually from more variable behavior to short sequences of a few simple behavioral elements (19).

Case histories of CDs in dogs and cats sometimes closely reflect this concept. In other cases, however, owners maintain that their dog or cat started to display the stereotypic behavior one day, without any identifiable initiating cause, and since its onset performed it in many different contexts and at a consistent rate. It has to be borne in mind, though, that recall bias can be a problem when trying to assess the early development of a behavior, whose origins may go back months or even years. In any case, once established, the highly ritualistic behaviors are displayed in various contexts which cause excitement in the dog or cat, or in contexts in which there is little external stimulation but presumably relatively high neurologic arousal (owners often comment that their dog seems to need to perform the stereotypic behavior in order to be able to settle down).

There also has been much speculation about the exact causes of stereotypic behavior in horses, and some research has established quantitative relationships between environmental and management factors and the prevalence of various stereotypies (14,20). However, it is unlikely that the factors identified are causal; instead, they more likely modulate the rates of already existing stereotypies. Without much-needed longitudinal studies, accounts of the etiology of stereotypies in companion animals and horses have to remain anecdotal and speculative.

Genetic predisposition for CD has been postulated based on clinical experience in dogs and cats (11). Similarly in horses, evidence of a genetic influence of stereotypy performance has been presented (15), as well as the effect of breed, sex, and age on various equine stereotypic behaviors (14).

Diagnosis

Diagnostic approaches to CD have been described elsewhere in detail (21,22). However, definite diagnostic criteria have not been established, mainly due to the absence of a biologic marker for the condition.

Diagnostic approaches vary according to the degree of confidence placed in behavioral histories. While some may be inclined to diagnose CD primarily by exclusion of medical and other behavioral conditions, this author believes that CDs have developmental and situational characteristics that permit a diagnosis based on minimal medical data and a thorough behavioral history.

The minimal data required to diagnose CD includes: 1) a physical examination, with a basic neurologic exam; 2) a complete blood cell count; 3) a chemistry profile; and 4) urinalysis. Depending on the behavior, additional diagnostic tests may need to be performed. For example, in cases of stereotypic grooming or self-mutilation, physical trauma, dermatologic lesions, and some neurologic conditions will have to be evaluated and excluded.

A detailed behavioral history is of paramount importance. It should include general information on breed (there are breed predispositions for specific compulsive behaviors), sex, age, developmental experiences (e.g., socialization), and general management (type of training and punishment, type and amount of exercise, etc.) of the patient. Questions should be asked to determine the basic temperament of the animal (e.g., fearfulness, excitability, aggressivity). Specific information related to the problem behavior must include:

1. A detailed description of the patient's behavior immediately before, during, and after an episode (the client should be asked to supply a videotape of the behavior).
2. The exact circumstances in which the behavior is typically performed, including the eliciting stimuli.
3. The location, and people or other animals present.
4. The behavior of the owner or of other animals present just prior to the behavior, and their reaction(s) to the animal performing the behavior.
5. The duration and frequency of bouts of the behavior.
6. The ease or difficulty with which the behavior can be interrupted.

This information should be gathered for the problem as it exists, as well as for the initial bouts of stereotypy performance. The animal's age when the problem started and, in particular, any changes over time in the parameters listed above should be noted. The owner should also be questioned about any attempts to treat the problem (e.g., punishment, change in management), as these often aggravate and/or perpetuate the problem.

Reported diagnostic differentials include normal responses to acute conflict or frustration (e.g., to separation), operantly conditioned behavior (e.g., attention-seeking behavior or behavior reinforced by subsequent feeding), psychomotor seizures (23), tumors, encephalitis, hydrocephalus (24), nerve damage resulting in paresthesia (e.g., degenerative lumbosacral stenosis) (25), dermatologic conditions (e.g., skin allergies), anal gland infection, trauma, metabolic disease, hyperkinesis, and some infectious diseases (3,11,21,22).

Pathophysiology

It has long been known that large doses of dopaminergic drugs, such as amphetamine or apomorphine, induce stereotypic behavior in rodents and in humans. Pharmacologically induced stereotypies have been studied as a model for schizophrenia. Much of our knowledge of the pathophysiology of CD in animals is based on studies of pharmacologically induced stereotypies. The appropriateness of using such models for the study of spontaneous or environmentally induced stereotypies has been reviewed in detail (26). The fact that pharmacologically induced stereotypies are aggravated by stress and environmentally induced stereotypies are enhanced by amphetamine seems to indicate that stereotypies of both pathogeneses have much in common (26). However, differences between the two classes of stereotypies have been recognized in pigs (27,28).

Involvement of dopamine in spontaneous stereotypies has been shown indirectly by demonstrating the inhibitory effect of the dopamine antagonist, haloperidol, on stereotypy performance in voles (29) and pigs (30). Furthermore, treatment of human OCD patients with the serotonin reuptake inhibitor (SRI), clomipramine, not only reduced OCD symptoms but also the level of the dopamine metabolite, homovanillic acid (HVA), in CSF (31), presumably because of the inhibitory effect of serotonin (5-HT) on nigrostriatal dopaminergic neurons (32). Addition of a dopamine antagonist to clomipramine treatment has proven beneficial in some patients with OCD and a comorbid chronic tic disorder; dopamine antagonist monotherapy, however, is not usually effective in reducing compulsive rituals in OCD patients (33).

Two different brain dopamine systems have been implicated in stereotypy performance. Dopamine injected into the caudate nucleus produced stereotypic behavior in cats (34). The *nigrostriatal dopamine system* containing the nucleus caudatus seems to mediate mainly oral stereotypic behavior, whereas stimulation of the *mesolimbic dopamine system*, including the nucleus accumbens, results in increased locomotion (26). Some consider this response to represent stereotypy as well (35). In apomorphine-induced stereotypy in rats, locomotion appears first (or at lower doses of apomorphine) and oral stereotypies later (or at higher doses of apomorphine) (35).

The neurotransmitters that have received the most attention in studies of farm animal stereotypies are the beta-endorphins. This may be because their involvement in stereotypy supports the view that repetitive behaviors indicate reduced welfare (36). Interest in beta-endorphins was sparked by the finding that the beta-endorphin receptor blocker, naloxone, reduced stereotypic behavior in sows (37,38). Subsequently, narcotic antagonists were used successfully to treat cribbing and self-mutilation in horses (39,40). Narcotic antagonists also have been shown to have therapeutic effects on stereotypic behavior in dogs (41–43).

However, the role of beta-endorphins in the development and maintenance of stereotypic behavior is unclear. From studies on bank voles, it was suggested that beta-endorphins may be important only in recently acquired stereotypies but not in well-established ones: The inhibiting effect of naloxone on stereotypies declined sharply after 4 months and had disappeared at 6 months after the development of the stereotypy (29). A decrease in the effectiveness of naloxone with time since the onset of the stereotypy was also observed in pigs (38). Further, the beta-endorphin plasma levels of cribbing horses were not elevated after a cribbing episode, and their pain sensitivity (an indirect measure of beta-endorphin release) actually increased while they were cribbing (44).

Serotonin has been implicated in human OCD because it has been found that drugs inhibiting 5-HT reuptake, such as clomipramine, are effective in reducing obsessive-compulsive symptoms (45–47). Recently, following the recognition that stereotypies have similarities with human OCD (8), 5-HT has received attention as a neurotransmitter of importance in animal stereotypic behavior. Pharmacologic stimulation of 5-HT receptors in rodents results in the 5-HT syndrome, which includes, among other signs, stereotyped head weaving and reciprocal forepaw treading. The stereotypic behaviors induced by 5-HT receptor stimulation are probably dopamine dependent (48), demonstrating an interaction between the brain 5-HT and dopamine systems (32). Direct evidence of 5-HT involvement in spontaneous stereotypy has been presented. The 5-HT metabolite 5-hydroxyindoleacetic acid (5-HIAA) was found to be at reduced levels in the caudate nucleus of stereotyping vs nonstereotyping bank voles (49). SRIs were found effective for treatment of acral lick dermatitis in dogs (8,50) and are now generally recommended as the drugs of choice for the treatment of CD in companion animals (5,11,12,51). However, the mechanism of 5-HT involvement in OCD is not known (47).

Treatment

Behavior therapy is one of the cornerstones of treatment for OCD (52). In human OCD patients, behavior therapy includes graded exposure to the eliciting situation and response prevention (53,54).

CD in animals is usually caused by an environmentally induced conflict or frustration. Therefore, manipulation of the environment to remove the conflict is the first step in treatment. A program of behavior modification is then put in place, including providing consistent animal-handler interaction, renunciation of punishment, and, if necessary, desensitization and counterconditioning. Behavioral treatment of CD has been reviewed in detail elsewhere (11).

Pharmacologic treatment is an adjunct to the behavioral treatment of CD. No drugs have been proven effective through randomized, controlled clinical trials except for serotonin reuptake blockers in the treatment of lick-granuloma (11). The following discussion of drugs considered useful for treating CD is largely based on information from human medicine and clinical experience in animals.

DRUGS ACTING ON DOPAMINE RECEPTORS

Drugs of interest that interact with the dopaminergic system are the antipsychotic or neuroleptic drugs, including haloperidol, pimozide, and phenothiazines. Neuroleptics reduce initiative, interest in the environment, and the manifestation of emotion or affect; intellectual functions are retained. Unconditioned escape and avoidance behaviors are not affected, but conditioned avoidance may be reduced (55). Spontaneous motor activity is diminished (56).

There should be no ataxia at clinical doses. However, low-potency antipsychotics such as acepromazine have a marked sedative effect. High-potency antipsychotics such as fluphenazine are not sedative at clinical doses but are more likely to produce extrapyramidal side effects such as tremor, rigidity, hypersalivation, bradykinesia, and motor restlessness. With higher doses, the risk of seizures increases. Hypotension, hyperthermia, sedation, arrhythmias, and dermatologic reactions are other potential side effects (56).

Neuroleptics act primarily on D2 receptors. After oral administration, there is extensive first-pass metabolism, and in plasma these drugs are highly protein bound. Neuroleptics are lipophilic and therefore their elimination from the organism is slow. They are metabolized in the liver and are excreted in urine and bile. The metabolites are generally not active compounds (56). The role of neuroleptics in the treatment of behavior problems in animals is limited.

Haloperidol

For haloperidol, the median lethal dose in dogs is 90 mg/kg orally, or 18 mg/kg when given intravenously. At 6 mg/kg/day and 12 mg/kg/day for 12 months, decreased weight gain and liver toxicity were observed. At 12 mg/kg/day for 12 months, side effects included convulsions, tremors, and emesis (55). An appropriate dose rate of haloperidol for the treatment of CD in companion animals has not been established. This author has used haloperidol only in a few dogs, at a dose of 1 to 2 mg PO bid, invariably with undesirable effects. Haloperidol has been used experimentally in cats, at a dose of 0.1 to 0.2 mg/kg, to counteract dopamine-induced stereotypy (34). Haloperidol might be considered as an augmenting agent in cases that are refractory to SRI monotherapy (33,57).

Pimozide

Pimozide, a drug similar to haloperidol, appears to be a fairly specific blocker of central dopamine receptors. It has marked cardiovascular side effects and may cause blood dyscrasia. After oral administration in capsules, median lethal dose for dogs is given as approximately 40 mg/kg. In dogs, application of doses as low as 0.16 mg/kg orally produced side effects including catalepsy and mild sedation. Chronic doses of 0.5 mg/kg resulted in muscle tremors and mammary and gingival dysplasia. At 3 mg/kg orally, weight loss also occurred (58). No dose rates have been established for dogs, but with side effects appearing at relatively low doses, the use of pimozide in dogs appears to be limited.

Phenothiazines

Among the phenothiazines, the high-potency drugs with little sedative effect are of some interest. However, phenothiazines are not specific agents and interact with various neurotransmitter systems other than dopamine (e.g., 5-HT and norepinephrine). They also have antihistaminic and anti-tryptaminergic properties. Extrapyramidal side effects limit their long-term use (56).

Long-acting formulations of phenothiazines, such as fluphenazine enanthate or decanoate, may be of interest for the treatment of animals that are difficult or impossible to dose orally. If such preparations are to be used, an appropriate dose should first be established with a short-acting compound. Therapeutic doses of fluphenazine in companion animals have yet to be established.

DRUGS INTERACTING WITH OPIOID RECEPTORS

Opioid antagonists have been of interest for the treatment of CD ever since their effectiveness in reducing stereotypies in sows was demonstrated (37,38). Opioid antagonists include naloxone, naltrexone, and nalmefene. Their effect is mostly on mu opioid receptors, although they are also antagonists at kappa and delta receptors (59). Their use is limited because of their short half-lives, and in most cases, parenteral administration route.

Naloxone

The opioid antagonist most often used in research on stereotypic behavior is naloxone. Unfortunately, if given orally, it is almost completely metabolized (conjugated with glucuronic acid) in the liver before reaching the systemic circulation. If given intravenously, it is also cleared very quickly. Its clinical effect after intravenous administration lasts for 1 to 4 hours in humans (59). Intramuscular administration produces a more prolonged effect. Naloxone causes virtually no side effects, although cardiovascular effects and seizures have been reported when naloxone has been used postoperatively to reverse opioid anesthesia in human patients (60). In dogs, a half-life of about 70 minutes has been established after intravenous application of naloxone (61).

Naloxone has been effective in the temporary relief of compulsive tail-chasing in a dog (41). A single dose of 0.2 mg injected subcutaneously stopped a 7-month-old male Bull Terrier from chasing its tail for approximately 3 hours. Because of the parenteral route and the short-lived clinical effect, the use of naloxone for the treatment of CD is limited.

Naltrexone

Naltrexone is a more potent opioid antagonist than naloxone and, when administered orally, has a clinical effect that lasts 24 to 72 hours in humans. Oral naltrexone has been recommended for use in companion animals because of a presumed long half-life in these species. However, after intravenous injection of naltrexone in dogs, half-life was reported as about 47 to 85 minutes—similar to that of naloxone (61)—and considerably less than the 10.5 hours reported for humans (62). In humans first-pass metabolism of naltrexone is extensive (about 60–95%), but the first metabolite (6-beta-naltrexol) is an active opiate antagonist as well, with a half-life of approximately 13 hours. In dogs, however, naltrexone is not metabolized to 6-beta naltrexol, but conjugated and excreted in urine and bile (62).

Naltrexone may cause hepatocellular injury at higher doses (i.e., five times the therapeutic dose in humans). It has therefore been suggested that naltrexone not be used in patients with liver damage (63). However, at clinical doses, even long-term treatment with naltrexone for 10 to 36 months did not result in signs of liver damage (64).

In dogs, naltrexone was about 26% protein bound in the plasma. Emesis, salivation, mild tremors, and muscular weakness were observed when dogs were given 50 mg/kg/day subcutaneously, but not at 2 mg/kg/day and 10 mg/kg/day subcutaneously for 28 days. Median lethal dose was not determined for the dog, but it is over 130 mg/kg orally (63).

Clinical dose of naltrexone for companion animals is given as 2.2 mg/kg/day (43) and up to 4.4 mg/kg/day orally (65). In one study, eleven dogs with stereotypic self-licking, chewing, or scratching were injected subcutaneously with naltrexone 1 mg/kg, or nalmefene 1 to 4 mg/kg (42). In seven of the dogs, stereotypic behaviors were reduced or suppressed for at least 90 minutes. In an open-label trial, dogs with acral lick dermatitis were given 2.2 mg/kg orally once or twice per day. This resulted in cessation or substantial decrease in the amount of licking and re-epithelization of the lesion in 7 of the 11 dogs (43). One dog treated for compulsive tail-chasing with naltrexone, 2 mg/kg orally every 6 hours, developed intense generalized pruritus, which subsided when the dose was reduced to 1 mg/kg every 6 hours (66).

Nalmefene

Narcotic antagonists have been used experimentally to reduce crib-biting in horses (39). Naloxone was injected intravenously in one horse at 0.02 to 0.04 mg/kg, which suppressed cribbing for an average duration of 20 minutes, after an average latent period of 18 minutes. Three horses were administered naltrexone intravenously at 0.04 to 0.4 mg/kg. Cribbing in these horses was greatly reduced or suppressed completely for 1.5 to 7 hours, after a latent period of up to 45 minutes. Nalmefene given intramuscularly or subcutaneously to five horses at 0.08 to 0.1 mg/kg was effective for 1.5 to almost 7 hours. Sustained-release formulations extended that time to several days in some cases, but such compounds are not available commercially.

Hydrocodone

The use of an opioid agonist has also been suggested for the treatment of CD. Hydrocodone has been used orally at 0.25 mg/kg for the treatment of canine acral lick dermatitis, with complete remission of licking in one and partial remission in two of the three treated dogs (67).

DRUGS ACTING ON SEROTONIN SYNAPSES: SEROTONIN REUPTAKE INHIBITORS

On stimulation, a serotonergic neuron releases 5-HT into the synapse. Serotonin acts as a neurotransmitter, binding to postsynaptic 5-HT receptors as well as to presynaptic and somatodendritic autoreceptors. Reaction with postsynaptic receptors causes stimulation of the postsynaptic neuron, while binding to autoreceptors provides negative feedback inhibiting further 5-HT release. A proportion of the 5-HT released is taken up again into the presynaptic neuron, the site of 5-HT metabolism. Inhibitors of 5-HT reuptake allow 5-HT to accumulate in the synapse. Because this accumulation is dependent on further firing of the presynaptic neuron and there is a negative feedback via autoreceptors, the concentration of 5-HT in the synapse does not exceed three to five times the normal value (68).

Compounds that inhibit the reuptake of biogenic amines, and thus their degradation in the presynaptic neuron, are believed to potentiate the actions of these amines. However, while the anxiolytic effect of 5-HT reuptake blockers is almost immediate, their therapeutic effect on depression or OCD in humans may be delayed by several weeks. This indicates that the effect of 5-HT reuptake blockers on these conditions may not be due to the simple accumulation of neurotransmitter in the synapse, but possibly due to a whole cascade of other events initially triggered by the accumulation of neurotransmitter, including the ensuing changes in autoreceptor and postsynaptic receptor sensitivity and density (69). For example, autoreceptors desensitize as a consequence of chronic administration of an SRI, resulting in greater release of 5-HT while reuptake is still inhibited (68). In addition, 5-HT is released from varicosities or axonal swellings and is thought to act on outlying targets. Serotonin thus is not only a neurotransmitter, it is also a neuromodulator (70). The increase of 5-HT at the serotonergic synapse after application of an SRI therefore might not be as fundamental to its action in the treatment of CD as was previously believed. The study of the effect of reuptake inhibitors is complicated by the fact that their effect may be different for different brain regions (68).

SRIs are a heterogenous group and include the tricyclic antidepressant, clomipramine, and atypical antidepressants such as fluoxetine, paroxetine, and sertraline. While clomipramine has side effects in common with other tricyclics and, through its first metabolite chlordesipramine, also affects norepinephrine reuptake, the atypical antidepressants have a more benign side-effect profile in humans, as they are specific inhibitors of 5-HT reuptake (69).

Clomipramine

Clomipramine is the only tricyclic antidepressant with anti-obsessional activity in humans. Like the other tricyclic antidepressants, clomipramine has anticholinergic side-effects. It may affect micturition, cause gastrointestinal disturbances, and lower the seizure threshold. At high doses, it may produce sinus tachycardia, changes in cardiac conduction time, and cardiac arrhythmias, and has a mild hypotensive action. Clomipramine reduces or suppresses REM sleep and has some sedative properties. In laboratory animals, it has been demonstrated to produce irritability and aggressiveness (71).

Absorption after oral administration of clomipramine is rapid. The plasma half-life in humans is approximately 21 hours; 96 to 97% of the drug is transported protein bound in the plasma. The use of clomipramine is contraindicated in human patients with a history of myocardial infarction, acute congestive heart failure, liver or kidney damage, blood dyscrasias, glaucoma, or cardiovascular disorder. Clomipramine is also contraindicated in hyperthyroid patients and in those receiving thyroid medication (71).

In humans, it is suggested that the patient's blood pressure be measured before initiating treatment, and that it be measured repeatedly in patients susceptible to lowered blood pressure or postural hypotension. Because clomipramine has caused ECG abnormalities, ECGs should be performed frequently in patients with heart disease during long-term treatment (71).

In patients with liver disease, periodic monitoring of hepatic function is recommended. Clomipramine may cause transient elevation of liver enzymes in healthy individuals. Leukocyte and differential blood cell counts are recommended for patients treated long term. Abrupt discontinuation of treatment may result in withdrawal symptoms (71).

Clomipramine should not be given together with a monoamine oxidase inhibitor, anticholinergic agent, or with antihistamines. Caution must be exercised when clomipramine is used in conjunction with selective serotonin reuptake inhibitors (SSRIs), neuroleptics, or benzodiazepines, as these drugs increase the plasma concentration of clomipramine (71).

Clomipramine is relatively nontoxic. When dogs were treated daily for 8 days at 12.5, 50, and 100 mg/kg orally, death occurred only at 100 mg/kg. Spermatogenesis was disturbed at 50 and 100 mg/kg (71).

Goldberger and Rapoport (8) used clomipramine in a single-blind trial for the treatment of acral lick dermatitis in dogs. The control treatment was desipramine. The dose of clomipramine was increased, as tolerated, from 1 mg/kg to a maximum of 3 mg/kg PO sid. Six out of nine dogs showed a reduction in licking as rated by the owner on a scale from 1 to 10. The dose of 3 mg/kg PO sid was subsequently recommended for treatment of compulsive disorder in dogs (65,72,73). For cats, the dose of clomipramine has yet to be substantiated; this author employs 1 mg/kg PO sid. A significant reduction in stereotypic motor behavior in three dogs was reported when clomipramine was used at a dose of 3 mg/kg PO bid for several months, in combination with counterconditioning (12).

There is some evidence that clomipramine is metabolized more quickly in dogs than in humans (74). A pharmacokinetic trial of clomipramine in dogs has just been completed and may provide some basis for determining an appropriate dose rate (Hewson CJ, personal communication, 1997). It has to be borne in mind, though, that the plasma values for clomipramine may not reflect brain levels (69). A randomized, double-blind, crossover trial using 3 mg/kg PO bid on dogs with CD is currently under way at the University of Guelph.

Side effects seen in our clinic include sedation, gastrointestinal problems in dogs, and urinary retention in cats. To reduce the chance for gastrointestinal signs, the drug should be given with food. Urinary retention and sedation appear to be dose related.

Fluoxetine

Among the specific 5-HT reuptake blockers, fluoxetine is the one most commonly used in companion animals. Fluoxetine specifically inhibits the reuptake of 5-HT by blocking presynapic uptake channels. Because of its specificity, it does not react with muscarinic receptors and thus lacks the anticholinergic side effects of the tricyclics; because it does not interact with alpha-1 adrenergic receptors it does not cause sedation or hypotension; and because it is not an H1 histaminic receptor antagonist it does not cause drowsiness. In addition, fluoxetine does not bind with 5-HT receptors, gamma-aminobutyric acid (GABA) receptors, dopamine receptors, or opioid receptors, and it lacks the direct cardiovascular effects of tricyclics. Fluoxetine's first metabolite, norfluoxetine, is essentially as potent and as specific a 5-HT reuptake blocker as fluoxetine itself (75). Despite the differences between clomipramine and fluoxetine, clinical data proved them to be equally effective for the treatment of human OCD and to result in a similar incidence of side effects (76,77).

Despite marked first-pass metabolism, fluoxetine is suited for oral administration because of its active metabolite. It is well absorbed after oral administration, and peak plasma levels are reached in humans after about 6 to 8 hours. Fluoxetine is highly protein bound in the plasma. It is metabolized in the liver and its metabolites are eventually excreted by the kidney. Fluoxetine inhibits the enzyme involved in its own metabolism. In humans, the half-life of fluoxetine is 1 to 4 days after a single dose, and 4 to 6 days after multiple dosing; the half-life of the metabolite norfluoxetine is about 9 days. Steady-state plasma levels are attained after 4 to 5 weeks of drug administration, and it may take 1 to 2 months after cessation until the active drug has disappeared from the body. In humans, it is recommended that a patient be drug-free for 6 weeks after cessation of fluoxetine administration, before another drug that interacts with fluoxetine, such as a monoamine oxidase inhibitor, is given (78).

Side effects in humans include anxiety, nervousness, and insomnia in 10 to 15% of patients, as well as weight loss. Fluoxetine possibly reduces the seizure threshold, may cause cardiovascular reactions and allergic skin reactions, and may lead to inappropriate antidiuretic hormone secretion. Patients with diabetes may be difficult to regulate while being treated with fluoxetine. Concomitant use of fluoxetine and monoamine oxidase inhibitors is contraindicated. If fluoxetine is used with tricyclic antidepressants, the metabolism of the latter is slower and therefore their blood levels are elevated. Patients receiving fluoxetine together with tryptophan may experience adverse reactions (78).

In dogs, the bioavailability of fluoxetine is reported as 72%. In dogs given fluoxetine at 5 to 10 mg/kg PO for 15 days, the plasma half-lives of fluoxetine and norfluoxetine were 1 day and 2.1 to 5.4 days, respectively. The median lethal dose of fluoxetine is reported as more than 50 mg/kg in cats, and more than 100 mg/kg in dogs. Side effects in dogs given 5 to 50 mg/kg PO sid for 2 weeks included anorexia, mydriasis, and vomiting, and at the highest dose, ataxia and tremors, and a convulsion in one dog (78).

Three treatment trials were conducted comparing clomipramine with desipramine, fluoxetine with fenfluramine, and sertraline with placebo, respectively, in the treatment of canine acral lick dermatitis (50). Doses were 3 mg/kg for clomipramine, desipramine, and sertraline, and 1 mg/kg for fluoxetine and fenfluramine; each drug was given for 5 weeks. Clomipramine and fluoxetine produced similar clinical effects—an approximately 40% reduction of licking—as compared to their respective controls. Sertraline resulted in an approximately 20% reduction in self-licking. Side effects included lethargy, loss of appetite, diarrhea, and growling with clomipramine; and lethargy, loss of appetite, and hyperactivity with fluoxetine treatment (50).

In another study, one dog treated with fluoxetine, at approximately 0.5 mg/kg PO sid, exhibited dilated pupils and developed fibrogingival hyperplasia, possibly as a side effect of fluoxetine treatment. After several years of continued treatment, however, the dog did not develop renal or hepatic problems (79). Successful treatment of compulsive tail mutilation in a Bichon Frise with 1 mg/kg fluoxetine PO sid for 3 weeks has been reported (80). The recommended dose of fluoxetine for dogs and cats is 0.5 to 1 mg/kg PO sid (65,73,81).

Paroxetine/Sertraline

Paroxetine and sertraline have a similar action and side effect profile to fluoxetine. However, their metabolites are pharmacologically inactive, and their half-lives are shorter (82,83).

Dosing Caveats

This author usually uses SRIs for approximately 3 to 4 weeks after an effective dose has been established, before weaning the drug off gradually over 3 weeks. Only in very few of this author's cases was long-term drug administration recommended; the use of the drug was always accompanied by behavior modification.

As already mentioned, SRIs not only increase extracellular 5-HT, but also indirectly affect 5-HT receptors, reducing their density and sensitivity. If an SRI is suddenly discontinued, extracellular 5-HT decreases due to renewed reuptake into the presynaptic neuron and metabolism, but receptor density and sensitivity are still reduced. Therefore, a rebound effect is likely following abrupt discontinuation of the drug. Sixteen of 18 human patients with OCD experienced a recurrence of their symptoms when clomipramine was withdrawn over a 4-day period (84). A rebound effect has also been observed in dogs when clomipramine was discontinued abruptly (Hewson CJ, personal communication, 1997). It is therefore recommended that the drug be tapered gradually by decreasing dose but not dose frequency over a period of at least 3 weeks following treatment (11).

BUSPIRONE

In contrast to SRIs, the azapirone buspirone acts through its affinity for serotonin receptors. Buspirone is an agonist at 5-HT_{1A} autoreceptors, decreasing the synthesis and release of 5-HT. Buspirone also increases dopamine and noradrenaline turnover (56), and is used for symptomatic relief of excessive anxiety in patients with generalized anxiety disorder (85). It is not considered effective for treatment of OCD in humans (56) and was found to be ineffective as an adjuvant to fluoxetine therapy (86). Buspirone was an ineffective treatment for compulsive circling in a dog, and may even have exacerbated the problem in this case (79).

TRYPTOPHAN

In horses, drug treatment of behavior problems is often impractical and/or too expensive. However, instead of drugs, it may be possible to influence 5-HT metabolism with the nutritive amino acid, L-tryptophan (87). L-tryptophan is a 5-HT precursor, but it also increases other pharmacologically active substances (68). L-tryptophan competes with other large neutral amino acids for uptake into the brain (88), and its effect on brain 5-HT levels is thus dependent on the protein level in the diet (89,90). L-tryptophan at 0.05 mg/kg and 0.1 mg/kg reduced performance of a stereotypic head twist to about two-thirds in one horse (91). L-tryptophan has been recommended for the clinical treatment of equine compulsive behavior at 2 g/bid for a standard size horse (92).

Conclusion

The steps that should be taken in the clinical treatment of CD in companion aimals are outlined in Table 8.1.

If pharmacologic treatment yields no apparent effect, the dose should be increased. In view of the great individual variability in drug metabolism, dose increase is indicated before changing the drug. The usefulness and dosages of adjuvant drugs, such as clonazepam and haloperidol (93,94), given in conjunction with SRI treatment, have not been established for companion animals.

Treatment duration has to be considered. Treatment at an effective dose will need to be prolonged if signs recur during the gradual withdrawal of the drug.

Lastly, it has to be kept in mind that pharmacologic treatment alone cannot be expected to be successful. Appropriate changes in the patient's environment and an effective behavior modification strategy with good client compliance are a cornerstone of the treatment of CD.

Table 8.1.   Clinical treatment of compulsive disorder in companion animals

Diagnosis
Physical examination, with basic neurologic exam
CBC, profile, urinalysis
Possibly dermatologic or additional neurologic tests
Behavioral history

Behavioral Treatment
Identification and removal of cause of conflict
Possibly desensitization to situation causing conflict
Ignoring the animal most of the time to avoid inconsistent interaction and inadvertent
   reinforcement
Structured interaction (obedience training in dogs, regular quality time in cats)
Avoiding punishment
Regular exercise, at least twice a day (dogs)
Counterconditioning, if necessary

Pharmacologic Treatment
Clomipramine—Dogs: 1–3 mg/kg PO tid or 2–3 mg/kg PO bid
             —Cats: 1 mg/kg PO sid
                                     OR
Fluoxetine—Dogs and cats: 0.5–1 mg/kg PO sid (syrup form for small dogs and cats)

References

1. Ödberg FO. Abnormal behaviours (stereotypies). Proceedings of the First World Congress on Ethology Applied to Zootechnics. Madrid, Editorial Garsi, Industrias Graficas Espana, 1978:475–480.

2. Mason GJ. Stereotypies: a critical review. Anim Behav 1991;41:1015–1037.

3. Luescher UA. Conflict, stereotypic and compulsive behavior. Presented at the 131st Annual Meeting of the American Veterinary Medical Association, San Francisco, July, 1994.

4. Lawrence AB, Rushen J. Introduction. In: Lawrence AB, Rushen J, eds. Stereotypic animal behaviour: fundamentals and applications to welfare. Wallingford, CAB International, 1993:1–5.

5. Luescher UA, McKeown DB, Halip J. Stereotypic or obsessive-compulsive disorders in dogs and cats. Vet Clin North Am Sm Anim Pract 1991;21:401–413.

6. Wiepkema PR. Abnormal behaviours in farm animals: ethological implications. Neth J Zool 1985;35:279–299.

7. Dantzer R. Stress, stereotypies and welfare. Behav Proc 1991;25:95–102.

8. Goldberger E, Rapoport JL. Canine acral lick dermatitis: response to the antiobsessional drug clomipramine. J Am Anim Hosp Assoc 1991;27:179–182.

9. Karno M, Golding JM, Sorensen SB, et al. The epidemiology of obsessive-compulsive disorder in five U.S. communities. Arch Gen Psychiatry 1988;45:1094–1098.

10. American Psychiatric Association. Diagnostic and statistical manual of mental disorders, 4th ed. Washington, DC: American Psychiatric Association 1994:422–423.

11. Hewson CJ, Luescher UA. Compulsive disorder in dogs. In: Voith VL, Borchelt PL, eds. Readings in companion animal behavior. Trenton, NJ: Veterinary Learning Systems, 1996:153–158.

12. Overall KL. Use of clomipramine to treat ritualistic stereotypic motor behavior in three dogs. J Am Vet Med Assoc 1994;205:1733–1741.

13. Houpt KA, McDonnell SM, Ralston S. Equine stereotypies. In: Voith VL, Borchelt PL, eds. Readings in companion animal behavior. Trenton, NJ: Veterinary Learning Systems, 1996:159–166.

14. Luescher UA, McKeown DB, Halip J. Reviewing the causes of obsessive-compulsive disorders in horses. Vet Med 1991 (May); 527–530.

15. Vecchiotti GG, Galanti R. Evidence of heredity of cribbing, weaving, and stall-walking in thoroughbred horses. Livestock Prod Sci 1986;14:91–95.

16. Luescher UA, McKeown DB, Dean H. A cross-sectional study on compulsive behavior (stable vices) in horses. Proceedings of the 30th International Congress of the International Society for Applied Ethology, Guelph, Canada, August, 1996:22.

17. Hinde RA. Animal behavior, 2nd ed. New York: McGraw Hill, 1970:396–421.

18. Ödberg FO. Future research directions. In: Lawrence AB, Rushen J, eds. Stereotypic animal behaviour: fundamentals and applications to welfare. Wallingford: CAB International, 1993:173–192.

19. Cronin GM. The development and significance of abnormal stereotyped behaviours in tethered sows. Thesis, Wageringen University, 1985:19–50.

20. McGreevy PD, Cripps PJ, French NP, et al. Management factors associated with stereotypic and redirected behaviour in the Thoroughbred horse. Equine Vet J 1995;27:86–91.

21. Overall KL. Recognition, diagnosis, and management of obsessive-compulsive disorders, Part I. Canine Pract 1992;17:40–44.

22. Overall KL. Recognition, diagnosis, and management of obsessive-compulsive disorders, Part II. Canine Pract 1992;17:25–27.

23. Dodman NH, Knowles KE, Shuster L, et al. Behavioral changes associated with suspected complex partial seizures in Bull Terriers. J Am Vet Med Assoc 1996;208:688–691.

24. Blackshaw JK, Sutton RH, Boyhan MA. Tail chasing or circling behaviors in dogs. Canine Prac 1994;19:7–11.

25. Oliver JE, Lorenz MD. Handbook of veterinary neurology. Philadelphia: Saunders, 1993:156.

26. Cabib S. Neurobiological basis of stereotypies. In: Lawrence AB, Rushen J, eds. Stereotypic animal behaviour: fundamentals and applications to welfare. Wallingford: CAB International, 1993:119–146.

27. Terlouw EMC, DeRosa G, Lawrence AB, et al. Behavioural responses to amphetamine and apomorphine in pigs. Pharmacol Biochem Behav 1992;43:329–340.

28. Terlouw EMC, Lawrence AB, Illius AW. Relationship between amphetamine and environmentally induced stereotypies in pigs. Pharmacol Biochem Behav 1992;43:347–355.

29. Kennes D, Ödberg FO, Bouquet Y, DeRycke PH. Changes in naloxone and haloperidol effects during the development of captivity-induced jumping stereotypy in bank voles. Eur J Pharmacol 1988;153:19–24.

30. von Borell E, Hurnik JF. The effect of haloperidol on the performance of stereotyped behavior in sows. Life Sci 1991;49:309–314.

31. Altemus M, Swedo SE, Leonard HL, et al. Changes in cerebrospinal fluid neurochemistrty during treatment of obsessive-compulsive disorder with clomipramine. Arch Gen Psychiatry 1994;51:794–803.

32. Kelland MD, Freeman AS, Chiodo LA. Serotonergic afferent regulation of the basic physiology and pharmacological responsiveness of nigrostriatal dopamine neurons. J Pharmacol Exp Ther 1990;253:803–811.

33. McDougle CJ, Goodman WK, Price LH. Dopamine antagonists in tic-related and psychotic spectrum obsessive compulsive disorder. J Clin Psychiatry 1994;55:24–31.

34. Cools AR, van Rossum JM. Caudal dopamine and stereotyped behaviour of cats. Arch Int Pharmacodyn Ther 1970;187:163–173.

35. Teitelbaum P, Pellis SM, deVietti TL. Disintegration into stereotypy induced by drugs or brain damage: a microdescriptive behavioural analysis. In: Cooper SJ, Dourish CT, eds. Neurobiology of stereotyped behaviour. Oxford: Clarendon Press, 1990:169–199.

36. Ladewig J, dePassille AM, Rushen J, et al. Stress and the physiological correlates of stereotypic behaviour. In: Lawrence AB, Rushen J, eds. Stereotypic animal behaviour: fundamentals and applications to welfare. Wallingford: CAB International, 1993:97–118.

37. Cronin GM, Wiepkema PR, vanRee JM. Endorphins implicated in stereotypies of tethered sows. Experientia 1986;42:198–199.

38. Cronin GM, Wiepkema PR, vanRee JM. Endogenous opioids are involved in abnormal stereotyped behaviours of tethered sows. Neuropeptides 1985;6:527–530.

39. Dodman NH, Shuster L, Court MH, Dixon R. Investigation into the use of narcotic antagonists in the treatment of a stereotypic behavior pattern (crib-biting) in the horse. Am J Vet Res 1987;48:311–319.

40. Dodman NH, Shuster L, Court MH, Patel J. Use of a narcotic antagonist (nalmefene) to suppress self-mutilative behavior in a stallion. J Am Vet Med Assoc 1988;192:1585–1587.

41. Brown SA, Crowell-Davis S, Malcolm T, Edwards P. Naloxone-responsive compulsive tail chasing in a dog. J Am Vet Med Assoc 1987;190:1434.

42. Dodman NH, Shuster L, White SD, et al. Use of narcotic antagonists to modify stereotypic self-licking, self-chewing, and scratching behavior in dogs. J Am Vet Med Assoc 1988;193:815–819.

43. White SD. Naltrexone for treatment of acral lick dermatitis in dogs. J Am Vet Med Assoc 1990;196:1073–1076.

44. Lebelt D, Zanella AJ, Unshelm J. Changes in thermal threshold, heart rate, and plasma β-endorphin associated with cribbing behaviour in horses. Proceedings of the 30th International Congress of the International Society for Applied Ethology, 1996:28.

45. Rapoport JL. The neurobiology of obsessive-compulsive disorder. JAMA 1988;260:2888–2890.

46. Benkelfat C, Murphy DL, Zohar J, et al. Clomipramine in obsessive-compulsive disorder. Arch Gen Psychiatry 1989;46:23–28.

47. Insel TR, Zohar J, Benekelfat C, Murphy DL. Serotonin in obsessions, compulsions, and the control of aggressive impulses. Neuropharmacol Serotonin 1990;600:574–586.

48. Curzon G. Stereotyped and other motor responses to 5-hydroxytryptamine receptor activation. In: Cooper SJ, Dourish CT, eds. Neurobiology of stereotyped behavior. Oxford: Clarendon Press, 1990:142–168.

49. Vanderbroek I, Ödberg FO, Caemaert J. Microdialysis study of the caudate nucleus of stereotyping and non-stereotyping bank voles. Proceedings of the 29th International Congress of the International Society for Applied Ethology, 1995:245.

50. Rapoport JL, Ryland DH, Kriete M. Drug treatment of canine acral lick. Arch Gen Psychiatry 1992;49:517–521.

51. Simpson SB, Simpson DM. Behavioral pharmacotherapy. In: Voith VL, Borchelt PL, eds. Readings in companion animal behavior. Trenton, NJ: Veterinary Learning Systems, 1996:100–115.

52. Greist JH. Behavior therapy for obsessive compulsive disorder. J Clin Psychiatry 1994;55:60–68.

53. March JS. Cognitive-behavioral psychotherapy for children and adolescents with OCD: a review and recommendations for treatment. J Am Acad Child Adolesc Psychiatry 1995;34:7–18.

54. Abel JL. Exposure with response prevention and serotonergic antidepressants in the treatment of obsessive compulsive disorder: a review and implications for interdisciplinary treatment. Behav Res Ther 1993;31:463–478.

55. Product Monograph. Haldol, haloperidol tablets, solution and injection USP, antipsychotic agent. Don Mills, Ontario: McNeil Pharmaceutical Ltd, 1992.

56. Baldessarini RJ. Drugs and the treatment of psychiatric disorders, psychosis and anxiety. In: Harman JG, Goodman-Gilman A, Limbird LE, eds. Goodman & Gilman's the pharmacological basis of therapeutics, 9th ed. New York: McGraw Hill, 1996:399–430.

57. McDougle CJ, Goodman WK, Leckman JF, et al. Haloperidol addition in fluvoxamine-refractory obsessive-compulsive disorder. Arch Gen Psychiatry 1994;51:302–308.

58. Product Monograph. ORAP Pimozide tablets: antipsychotic. Stouffville, Ontario: McNeil Pharmaceuticals Ltd, 1990.

59. Reisine T, Pasternak G. Opioid analgesics and antagonists. In: Harman JG, Goodman-Gilman A, Limbird LE, eds. Goodman & Gilman's the pharmacological basis of therapeutics, 9th ed. New York: McGraw Hill, 1996:521–555.

60. Product Monograph. Pr Narcan injection: Naloxone Hydrochloride injection, USP, narcotic antagonist. Scarborough, Ontario: DuPont Pharmaceuticals, 1991.

61. Pace NL, Parrish RG, Lieberman MM, et al. Pharmacokinetics of naloxone and naltrexone in the dog. J Pharmacol Exp Ther 1979;208:254–256.

62. Garrett ER, el-Koussi AEA. Pharmacokinetics of morphine and its surrogates. V. Naltrexone and naltrexone conjugate pharmacokinetics in the dog as a function of dose. J Pharm Sci 1985;74:50–56.

63. Product Monograph. Revia, opioid antagonist. Mississauga, Ontario: DuPont Pharmaceuticals, 1995.

64. Sax DS, Kornetsky C, Kim A. Lack of hepatotoxicity with naltrexone treatment. J Clin Pharmacol 1994;34:898–901.

65. Marder AR. Psychotropic drugs and behavioral therapy. Vet Clin North Am Sm Anim Pract 1991:329–342.

66. Schwartz S. Naltrexone-induced pruritus in a dog with tail-chasing behavior. J Am Vet Med Assoc 1993;202:278–280.

67. Brignac MM. Hydrocodone treatment of acral lick dermatitis. Proceedings of the 2nd World Congress of Veterinary Dermatology, Montreal, Quebec, 1992.

68. Fuller RW. Minireview: Uptake inhibitors increase extracellular serontonin concentration measured by brain microdialysis. Life Sci 1994;55:163–167.

69. Baldessarini RJ. Drugs and the treatment of psychiatric disorders: depression and mania. In: Harman JG, Goodman-Gilman A, Limbird LE, eds. Goodman & Gilman's the pharmacological basis of therapeutics, 9th ed. New York: McGraw Hill, 1996:431–459.

70. Sanders-Bush E, Mayer SE. 5 hydroxytryptamine (serotonin) receptor agonists and antagonists. In: Harman JG, Goodman-Gilman A, Limbird LE, eds. Goodman & Gilman's the pharmacological basis of therapeutics, 9th ed. New York: McGraw Hill, 1996:249–263.

71. Product Monograph. Anafranil (clomipramine hydrochloride), antidepressant—antiobsessional. Mississauga, Ontario: Ciba-Geigy Pharmaceuticals, 1996.

72. Overall KL. Recognition, diagnosis, and management of obsessive-compulsive disorders, Part III. Canine Prac 1992;17:39–43.

73. Overall KL. Practical pharmacological approaches to behavior problems. In: Purina specialty review: behavioral problems in small animals. Ralston Purina Company, 1992:36–51.

74. Faigle JW, Dieterle W. The metabolism and pharmacokinetics of clomipramine. J Int Med Res 1973;1:281–290.

75. Fuller RW, Wong DT, Robertson DW. Fluoxetine, a selective inhibitor of serotonin uptake. Med Res Rev 1991;11:017–034.

76. Freeman CPL, Trimble MR, Deakin JFW, et al. Fluvoxamine versus clomipramine in the treatment of obsessive compulsive disorder: A multicenter, randomized, double-blind, parallel group comparison. J Clin Psychiatry 1994;55:301–305.

77. Greist JH, Jefferson JW, Kobak KA, et al. Efficacy and tolerability of serotonin transport inhibitors in obsessive-compulsive disorder. Arch Gen Psychiatry 1995;52:53–60.

78. Product Monograph. Prozac (fluoxetine hydrochloride) capsules and oral solution, antidepressant/antiobsessional/antibulimic. Scarborough, Ontario: Eli Lilly, 1996.

79. Overall KL. Animal behavior case of the month. J Am Vet Med Assoc 1995;206:629–632.

80. Melman SA. Case report: a tale of (tail) mutilation. Am Vet Soc Anim Behav Newsletter 1995:7–8.

81. McKeown DB, Luescher UA, Halip J. Stereotypies in companion animals and obsessive-compulsive disorder. In: Purina specialty review: behavioral problems in small animals. Purina Ralson Company, 1992:30–35.

82. Product Monograph. Paxil. Paroxetine (as paroxetine hydrochloride) tablets, antidepressant-antiobsessional-antipanic agent. Oakville, Ontario: SmithKline Beecham, 1995.

83. Product Monograph. Zoloft (sertraline hydrochloride), antidepressant. Kirkland, Quebec: Pfizer, 1995.

84. Pato MT, Zohar-Kadouch R, Zohar J, Murphy DL. Return of symptoms after discontinuation of clomipramine in patients with obsessive-compulsive disorder. Am J Psychiatry 1988;145:1521–1525.

85. Product Monograph. BuSpar (buspirone hydrochloride) tablets, anxiolytic. Montreal, Quebec: Bristol, 1993.

86. Grady TA, Pigott TA, L'Heureux F, et al. Double-blind study of adjuvant buspirone for fluoxetine treated patients with obsessive-compulsive disorder. Am J Psychiatry 1993;150:819–821.

87. Teff KL, Young SN. Effects of carbohydrate and protein administration on rat tryptophan and 5-hydroxytryptamine: differential effects on the brain, intestine, pineal, and pancreas. Can J Physiol Pharmacol 1988;66:683–688.

88. Fernstrom JD, Wurtman RJ. Brain serotonin content: physiological regulation by plasma neutral amino acids. Science 1972;178:414–416.

89. Hedaya RJ. Pharmacokinetic factors in the clinical use of tryptophan. J Clin Psychopharmacol 1984;4:347–348.
90. Colombo JP, Cervantes H, Kokoroyic M, et al. Effect of different protein diets on the distribution of amino acids in plasma, liver, and brain in the rat. Ann Nutr Metab 1992;36:23–33.
91. Bagshaw CS, Ralston SL, Fisher H. Behavioral and physiological effect of orally administered tryptophan on horses subjected to acute isolation stress. Appl Anim Behav Sci 1994;40:1–12.
92. McDonnell SM. Pharmacological aids to behavior modification in horses. Basel, Switzerland: Swiss Society for Equine Medicine, 1996.
93. Leonard HL, Topol D, Bukstein O, et al. Clonazepam as an augmenting agent in the treatment of childhood-onset obsessive-complusive disorder. J Am Acad Child Adolesc Psychiatry 1994;33:792–794.
94. Dominguez RA, Mestre SM. Management of treatment-refractory obsessive compulsive disorder patients. J Clin Psychiatry 1994;55(suppl 10):86–92.

Self-Injurious Behavior and Obsessive-Compulsive Disorder in Domestic Animals

Karen L. Overall

Ritualistic and stereotypic behaviors have long been recognized in veterinary medicine and may include some forms of tail-chasing and biting, flank-sucking (particularly in Doberman Pinschers), wool-sucking (primarily in Oriental breeds of cats), self-sucking and over-grooming, and fly-biting in small animals (1,2), wind-sucking and cribbing in horses, and chain-rooting and chain-chewing in pigs (3). Some of these conditions involve self-destructive behaviors that range from those that are minor to those that are profoundly mutilating. Parallel examples of stereotypic behaviors are found in human medicine (4–6). In the past decade, much progress has been made in the understanding and treatment of these conditions, many of which have been grouped in a classification known as obsessive-compulsive disorder in the *Diagnostic and Statistical Manual of Mental Disorders*, Fourth Edition (DSM-IV) (7).

Treatment has usually been geared toward stopping injury through physical restraint and control; hence, the use of cribbing collars in horses and Elizabethan collars in cats and dogs. Such devices prevent the animal from accomplishing the actual behavior but do nothing to diminish the desire to perform the behavior, as is demonstrated when the devices are removed. We now believe that these disorders are behavioral, rooted in a neurophysiologic abnormality.

This chapter focuses on self-mutilatory or self-injurious behavior (SIB) in dogs and cats, particularly that associated with obsessive-compulsive disorder (OCD). Dogs and cats have been selected to live in close social proximity with humans in a manner that did not require disruption of their innate social patterns (8,9). Accordingly, many behavior problems involving self-mutilation in domestic animals may be suitable as analogous behavioral models and homologous neurochemical models for similar conditions involving SIB in humans. In contrast, laboratory and zoo animals, particularly primates, are subjected to profoundly altered social and physical environments. This is also true for many herd or flock animals (e.g., horses, psittacine birds). SIB in flock and herd species may be a sequela to the environmental and behavioral alterations attendant with husbandry conditions but may not be representative of analogous disorders in humans for whom environmental stress appears to be correlated with worsening of SIBs but does not cause them.

Terminology

Diagnoses are not diseases; correlation is not causality. Conditions for which there is putative etiologic and pathophysiologic heterogeneity (multifactorial disorders) are complex, and nowhere is this more true than for anxieties and stereotypy (OCD). Diagnosis and treatment is therefore, by definition, complex. These conditions are among the most difficult behavior problems to diagnose and treat. There is probably no other area in behavioral medicine that is fraught with so much confusion and opinion. OCD and anxiety are closely related but may not be identical at the neurophysiologic level. Diagnoses related to anxiety operate at the level of the phenotypic or functional diagnosis, but treatment often addresses the neurophysiologic level alone. Phenotypic (i.e., functional, phenomenologic) diagnoses are open by various mechanistic interactions of all subsequent levels portrayed in (Table 9.1). Some of these more reductionistic levels can be tested using pharmacologic agents, should they be sufficiently specific (and this is rare), but few phenotypic diagnoses can be specifically tested using behavior modification. Tests of mechanistic hypotheses should focus on the specific level to be tested.

Table 9.1.   Mechanistic levels ("causality") to consider in any behavioral diagnosis

Level	Concern
1. Phenotype	Role of underlying broad genotype by environment interactions Role of phenomenologic diagnoses
2. Neuroanatomy	Role of localization of activity Role of neuroanatomic diagnoses
3. Neurophysiology/neurochemistry	Role of chemical/substrate interaction Role of most mechanistic pathophysiologic diagnoses
4. Molecular receptor	Role of gene regulation and interaction with substrate Role of most etiologic diagnostic refinements
5. Genotype	Role of heritability

Definitions

A list of accepted definitions as they are used here is found in Table 9.2. While these definitions are clear, the conditions for which they are relevant may be multifactorial and heterogeneous. Therefore, diagnosis may not be as simple or clear-cut as a definition. We do not yet understand the manner in which the levels cited in Table 9.1 interact to produce the problem—all we can evaluate is the phenotypic form in which interactions occur. Clear use of terminology can help to make apparent the parts of these phenotypic diagnoses that are consistent, so that we can understand and separate them from those that are more complex. This approach is enhanced by the use of minimum *necessary and sufficient* criteria for diagnosis, thus avoiding the problems in definition that arise when descriptions of a behavioral event use the same terms as does a diagnosis (10,11). Descriptions imply no underlying mechanism of function; whereas diagnosis, in its most discrete form, implies a mechanism of function. For example, the term "self-injurious behavior" can be used broadly as a description of any volitional behavior that causes self-mutilation or damage. It is a symptom or sign—not a disorder—so it is necessary and prudent to identify the underlying causative condition and to avoid empirical treatment (12–14). A diagnosis of "self-injurious behavior," on the other hand, is restricted to chronic, repetitive behavior that causes external trauma on a mechanical basis and that occurs in a mentally impaired individual (12,15,16). The repetitive, and in some cases stereotypic, nature of the behavior is one criterion for the condition, but using this description as a criterion is different from requiring that the patient have a disorder that uses the repetitive nature as a distinguishing feature. Similar forms of disorders involving repetitive behavior have been called *stereotypies* in animals, and under some conditions these meet the necessary and sufficient diagnostic criteria for a veterinary OCD.

The implementation of "necessary and sufficient" diagnostic criteria, using the terms as they are used in logical and mathematical applications, is a refinement over descriptive definitions of terms. The imposition of such criteria acts as qualitative, and potentially quantitative, exclusion criteria. They allow for uniform and unambiguous assessment of aberrant, abnormal, and undesirable behaviors. A *necessary criterion or condition* is one that must be present for the listed diagnosis to be made; a *sufficient criterion or condition* is one that will stand alone to singularly identify the condition. Sufficiency is an outcome of knowledge: The more we learn about the genetics, molecular response, neurochemistry, and neuroanatomy of any condition and its behavioral correlates (see Table 9.1), the more succinctly and accurately we are able to define a sufficient condition. Definition of necessary and sufficient criteria is not synonymous with a compendium of signs associated with the condition. The number of signs present and their intensity may be a gauge for the severity of the condition, or may act as a flag when there can be variable, nonoverlapping presentations of the same condition.

Table 9.2. Definitions

Abnormal behavior: Activities that show dysfunction in action and behavior (132).

Anxiety: The apprehensive anticipation of future danger or misfortune, accompanied by a feeling of dysphoria (in humans) and/or somatic symptoms of tension (vigilance and scanning, autonomic hyperactivity, increased motor activity, and tension). The focus of the anxiety can be internal or external.

Conflict: A motivational state in which tendencies to perform more than one type of activity are simultaneously present (133,134).

Displacement activity: An activity that is performed out-of-context, or "displaced," because the animal is "frustrated" in its attempt to execute another activity or to otherwise occupy itself. This is considerably less specific than redirected activity, which implies a substitution of behavior "in kind" but toward another target. In cases where displacement activity is involved, the activity may not be "in kind."

Frustration: A motivational state that arises when an animal is engaged in a sequence of behaviors that it is unable to complete because of physical or psychological obstacles in the environment (133).

Mental disorder: "Clinically significant behavior of psychological syndrome or pattern that occurs in an individual and that is associated with present distress (e.g., a painful symptom) or disability (i.e., impairment in one or more areas of functioning) or with a significantly increased risk of suffering death, pain, disability, or a loss of freedom" (7). Regardless of cause, the disorder is a "manifestation of a behavioral, psychological, or biologic dysfunction in the individual" (7). The most prevalent disorders in the human mental health arena are anxiety disorder; specifically, panic disorder, phobias, OCD, generalized anxiety, and posttraumatic stress syndrome (7).

Obsessive-compulsive disorder: An American Psychiatric Association classification of abnormal behaviors that have as characteristics recurrent and frequent thoughts or actions that are out-of-context with the situation in which they occur. These behaviors can involve cognitive or physical rituals and are deemed excessive (given the context) in duration, frequency, and intensity of the behavior. One of the hallmarks of this condition that distinguishes it from motor tics, etc., is that OCD behaviors follow a set of rules created by the patient. The condition in domestic animals is probably similar and analogous through descent, and probably includes stereotypies, self-directed behaviors, etc. Regardless, the behavior must be sufficiently pronounced and interfere with normal functioning.

Redirected activity: Direction of an activity away from the principal target and toward another, less appropriate target. This is usually best identified when the recognized activity is interrupted by the less appropriate target or by a third party, and, in contrast to displacement activity, redirected activity appears to be a substitution "in kind" of the interrupted behavior.

Stereotypy: A repetitive, relatively unvaried sequence of movements that have no obvious purpose or function, but that are usually derived from contextually normal maintenance behaviors (e.g., grooming, eating, walking) (1). Inherent to the classification of dysfunction is the fact that the behavior interferes with normal behavioral functioning.

Vacuum activity: An activity involving an instinctive, unconscious, or response behavior in the absence of the stimulus that would normally elicit that behavior. Such activity seemingly has no apparent, contextual, or useful purpose (e.g., tongue-rolling in ruminants that are neither eating nor ruminating).

For example, self-mutilation (or SIB in the broad sense) in animals has as its necessary conditions the barbering or removal of coat and/or abrasion, petechiation, or ulceration of any body part using teeth, claws, or an external substrate (i.e., rubbing against a wall). The sufficient condition specifies the repeated and consistent (often stereotypic) manifestations of these behaviors in the absence of any primary dermatologic or physiologic condition (11). In extreme situations, this condition is not associated with anxiety due to environmental stimuli (or lack thereof). Physiologic associations between sensation, pain, pruritus, anxiety, and perception probably become more complex the longer self-mutilation behaviors continue, rendering the physiologic or neurochemical separation of these conditions extremely difficult.

The necessary condition for OCD in animals is the presence of repetitive, stereotypic motor, locomotory, grooming, ingestive, or hallucinatory behaviors that occur out-of-context to their otherwise normal occurrence, or in a frequency or duration that is in excess of that required to accomplish an ostensible or actual goal. The sufficient condition specifies that these behaviors occur in a manner that interferes with the animal's ability to function normally in its social environment (11).

One can debate whether animals can obsess. Given their responses to these abnormal behaviors, it appears that they perceive and experience concern and so it seems likely that they can obsess. Such discussions need to account for divergent evolutionary histories for animals that rely heavily on structured language (e.g., humans) and those that do not (e.g., domesticated and nondomesticated animals) (17). For animals that have evolutionary histories exclusive of speech, obsession is still a possibility, although its manifestations may be different from those we have learned to expect in humans. Given this logic and the otherwise homologous and analogous nature of OCD in humans and animals, there is no reason to discard this terminology.

Separate from the obsession issue is relative intensity; that is, whether a behavior is considered excessive or a manifestation of OCD may be a matter of degree. Careful description and recording of behaviors and their durations could provide data that would permit evaluation of the extent to which such behaviors may lie on a continuum. Good histories and observation are important, as some peculiar forms of OCD may resemble seizure-like activity. By definition, some epileptic or seizure-like activity is stereotypic, which is one reason why the explicit and specific diagnosis category of OCD is preferable to that of stereotypy.

A careful consideration of these criteria indicate that 1) OCD could involve SIB (in a broad sense); 2) not all SIB should be due to OCD; 3) these conditions may be related neurochemically; and 4) when these conditions occur concomitantly (i.e., the manifestation of OCD involves self-mutilation) the causal mechanism may be different than when they occur separately.

Using these criteria, SIB can be broadly defined in animals as self-inflicted mutilation in the absence of any apparent localized pathology that would stimulate such behavior. It is difficult to distinguish SIB that is primary, meets the criteria for the diagnosis of SIB in humans (including the impaired cognition aspects), and is neurochemically self-reinforcing, from SIB that is secondary, and either a manifestation of OCD or simply a correlate of another recognized disorder. These distinctions are important if they affect treatment or if the underlying mechanisms driving them differ.

SIB in Humans: Descriptions and Proposed Neurochemical Mechanisms

There is no one specific psychiatric diagnosis that can be successfully applied to patients with SIB (18). SIB is commonly seen in humans with autism, mental retardation, Tourette syndrome, acute psychosis, Lesch-Nyhan syndrome, Prader-Willi syndrome, organic brain syndrome, borderline personality disorder, and schizophrenia (19,20). For humans with these diagnoses, the specific behaviors involved in SIB include head-banging, self-hitting, gouging (primarily of the eyes), hair-pulling (trichotillomania), skin-picking, pica, chewing of fingers, and rectal digging. The more profound variant of SIB, self-mutilatory behavior (SMB), involves biting off one's lips or fingers, self-enucleation of the eye, and autocastration (18). SIB has a variety of behavioral presentations and has been postulated to be due to a variety of neurochemical mechanisms. SIB is also common in situations involving anxiety associated with penal incarceration (21), and in this manifestation may be a good model for self-injury in laboratory and zoo animals. Few specific data can be used to test putative mechanistic hypotheses for any of the conditions previously listed, but specific findings from studies of Lesch-Nyhan syndrome, Prader-Willi syndrome, OCD, and autistic patients are relevant here.

LESCH-NYHAN SYNDROME

Behaviors that accompany human Lesch-Nyhan syndrome include spasticity and compulsive and stereotypic self-injury, particularly that involved in the chewing of fingers, lips, and oral tissues. Lesch-Nyhan syndrome is an X-linked enzyme deficiency and, as such, provides a good paradigm for understanding some of the neurochemical factors involved in self-mutilation. The pathology involved in Lesch-Nyhan syndrome is the result of aberrant purine metabolism due to a profound deficiency of hypoxanthine guanine phosphoribosyl-transferase (HPRT). As a result of this enzyme defect, uric acid production in affected individuals is increased dramatically; however, this defect does not appear to be linked directly to the injurious behavior.

Dopaminergic and serotonergic pathways have been shown to be abnormal in Lesch-Nyhan syndrome, although the mechanism for these abnormalities, which are unrelated to HRPT, is unclear. In an animal model of

Lesch-Nyhan syndrome, brain dopamine is reduced in neonatal and adult rats by lesioning with 6-hydroxydopamine (6-OHDA) (22,23). Neonatal rats do not exhibit spontaneous SIB, but do display it when challenged with levodopa (L-dopa) as adults; this SIB is blocked by dopamine D1 antagonists and stimulated by D1 agonists (22–24). Dopamine supersensitivity at the D1 rather than the D2 receptors has also been postulated to be the cause of SIB in Lesch-Nyhan syndrome (25), yet some D2-receptor blocking agents (neuroleptics) have met with variable treatment success. The favorable response to dopamine antagonists like sulpiride suggests that dopaminergic supersensitivity and hypothalamic dysregulation may be one mechanism operating in SIB. Low levels of homovanillic acid (HVA), a dopamine metabolite, have been reported for these patients (18,26).

Lesch-Nyhan patients have also been reported to have increased urinary levels of 5-hydroxyindoleacetic acid (5-HIAA), a serotonin, 5-hydroxytryptamine (5-HT) metabolite (18). A role for increased 5-HT turnover rates has been postulated based on this and on the transient efficacy of 5-HT precursors in alleviating SIB. The 5-HT hypothesis of SIB focuses on decreased brain 5-HT and its precursor 5-hydroxytryptophan (5-HTP), which temporarily decreases SIB associated with Lesch-Nyhan syndrome (27).

PRADER-WILLI SYNDROME

The behaviors seen in Prader-Willi syndrome (PWS) include self-injury (e.g., compulsive skin-picking and gouging), compulsive eating, hoarding, and explosive outbursts. The incidence of PWS with SIB is low, 1:10,000 to 1:25,000 live births. Infants with the condition fail to thrive, may not suckle, and are hypotonic at birth. After 2 years of age, these patients are hyperphagic, obese, and display cognitive and behavioral abnormalities (4,20). This profile illustrates the importance of understanding developmental patterns in the presentation of the condition and of age-dependent behavioral changes. These data are almost always lacking for animals with OCD. PWS is characterized by low CNS 5-HT levels. Like other conditions with OCD as a component, some of these patients will respond to some of the selective serotonin reuptake inhibitors (SSRIs) (e.g., clomipramine (28), fluoxetine (29), and fluvoxamine (30)).

OCD

Behaviors associated with human OCD are often nonspecific, may include those also seen in impulse disorders, and can include skin-picking, trichotillomania, and onychophagia (nail-biting) (20). Studies involving computed tomography (CT) have implicated the basal ganglia, particularly in the region of the caudate nucleus, as the anatomical focus of the disorder (31). Studies involving positron emission tomography (PET) that have evaluated cerebral glucose metabolism in childhood onset OCD after 1 year of pharmacotherapy indicated a decrease in the orbitofrontal regional cerebral glucose metabolism bilaterally, which correlated with two measures of OCD improvement (32). Changes in caudate nucleus metabolism have also been detected (33,34). Use of neurophysiologic indicator variables associated with OCD suggests regions that warrant further study (35).

Signs of OCD appear to be partially attributable to aberrant 5-HT metabolism, although some have postulated a tandem role for abnormal endorphin metabolism (36,37). Low baseline beta-endorphin levels were found in cribbing horses (38). This was postulated to be due to impaired beta-endorphin release associated with increases in opioid receptor activity. Increased beta-endorphin levels activate dopamine pathways and can enhance stereotypic behavior (39). The basal ganglia and limbic system have also been implicated in animal models of OCD (40). Excess dopamine in basal ganglia structures has been noted, as has a relative increase in the 5-HT metabolite 5-HIAA in the CSF. These patterns are potentially illuminating because 5-HT promotes behavioral suppression and extinction of rewarded responses— this effect is opposite to that of dopamine (41,42).

INFANTILE AUTISM

Infantile autism has been associated with increased platelet levels of 5-HT, decreased levels of aspartic acid, decreased levels of glutamine, decreased levels of glutamic acid, and decreased levels of gamma-aminobutyric acid (GABA) (43). Serotonin is increased (hyperserotonemia) in 33% of autistic children. Infantile autism is associated with decreased responsiveness to pain and self-destructiveness. These signs may be associated with moderate elevations of CSF endorphins (44).

These associations illustrate how important it is to 1) qualify and quantify the behaviors in question, and 2) to understand that relative amount, location, and direction of change of neurochemicals can all influence the form represented by "abnormal" behaviors. These conditions are not single gene mutations that cause a solitary and unambiguous shift in one neurochemical. They are all complex and may involve interaction of endorphinergic, dopaminergic, and serotonergic pathways.

SUMMARY OF SPECIFIC NEUROCHEMICAL FINDINGS

SIB, although present in a variety of human conditions involving cognitive impairment, is not a singular condition. Endogenous opioids, dopamine, and 5-HT are all believed to have roles in various forms of SIB. The extent to which they are important in a particular form of SIB may depend on the pathophysiology of the concomitant, and perhaps, primary diagnosis. With that caveat in mind, it is possible to summarize the broad roles postulated for these

Table 9.3. General patterns of neurochemical activity and the presence of SIB/OCD

Neurochemical	General effects of neurochemical on SIB/OCD	Effect of neurochemical agonist	Effect of neurochemical antagonist
Opioids	↑ CSF opioids → ↑ SIB ↓ plasma opioids → ↑ cribbing	↑ SIB	↓ SIB
Dopamine	↑ DA → ↑ SIB ↓ HVA (DA metabolite; ↓ turnover) in SIB	D1 agonists ↑ SIB	D1 antagonists ↓ SIB Reversal of TCA effect on OCD (↓ OCD) = ↑ or return of OCD
Serotonin	↓ CNS 5-HT in OCD ↑ HIAA (5-HT turnover) in OCD	↓ SIB/OCD Reuptake inhibitors ↓ SIB/OCD	NA

CNS = central nervous system; CSF = cerebrospinal fluid; DA = dopamine; HIAA = hydroxy-indoleacetic acid; HVA = homovanillic acid; 5-HT = serotonin; NA = not applicable; OCD = obsessive-compulsive disorder; SIB = self-injurious behavior; TCA = tricyclic antidepressants; ↑ = increased; ↓ = decreased.

neurochemicals in SIB in general. (See Table 9.3 for a tabular summary of these general patterns.)

Endogenous Opioids

A case can be made for ritualistic behaviors being mediated through endogenous opioid receptors (36,37,45–48). There have been two major mechanistic hypotheses put forth regarding endogenous opioids. The first postulates that decreased sensitivity to pain is associated with increased basal activity of endogenous opioids (28,37,49,50). Such patients may have increases in the number, affinity, or activity of endorphin receptor sites. The second hypothesis postulates that the injurious behaviors serve to "downregulate" the reactivity of the receptors, resulting in an "addiction" to the painful stimuli (28,51). Plasma metencephalin concentrations are elevated in humans with SIB (29), but beta-endorphins are decreased in horses that crib (38), suggesting that the issue might be one of relative receptor regulation and cell metabolism.

The availability of opioid agonists and antagonists permits some testing of hypotheses related to endorphin mechanisms. For some patients, endorphin levels may be increased in blood, but not in CSF, which suggests that increased endorphin metabolism may be implicated (37). Should this be the case, morphine, an exogenous opioid agonist, should stimulate endorphin receptors producing an exaggerated response. Naloxone and naltrexone are relatively pure opioid blocking agents: The former is administered by injection and has a duration of 1 to 4 hours; the latter is administered orally and lasts up to 24 hours in humans (the half-life in dogs is approximately 85 minutes). Naloxone blocks central opioid receptors and should afford relief from stereotypic signs if opioid receptors are involved in propagating the behavior. If naloxone does *not* block the response, the etiology of the behavior probably does not involve over-activation of the opioid pathway. Naltrexone has been successfully used to block self-mutilative behavior in the horse (45) and dog (48). However, it was also reported to induce pruritus in one canine case, potentially complicating patient assessment (52).

A caveat to this logic may be necessary: Peripheral and central responses are not equivalent. Foot-shock in rats results in a five- to sixfold increase in beta-endorphin plasma levels and similar increases in adrenocorticotropic hormone (ACTH) plasma levels, but this physiologic increase in beta-endorphins induced by stress does not increase brain endorphin (53).

Dopamine

High levels of dopamine correlated with SIB and antagonists, specifically D1 antagonists, appear to block SIB, which is stimulated in lesioned rats by D1 agonists (24). Rats that are deprived of social stimuli and develop OCD-like motor and grooming behaviors experienced a restoration of normal behavior when treated with the tricyclic antidepressants amitriptyline or desipramine (54). Subsequent administration of a dopamine antagonist reversed this response, suggesting a functional increase in activity associated with dopamine synthesis as a potential mechanism of action for the OCD (54). This response also suggests that the effects of dopamine and 5-HT are not independent.

Serotonin

The 5-HT system is a mediator of learned and sustained fear responses in animals and humans (27,55,56). Selective serotonin (or serotonin-specific) reuptake inhibitors (SSRIs) commonly used to treat fears include fluoxetine, fluvoxamine, and zimelidine. The tricyclic antidepressant, clomipramine, a nonspecific "referential" serotonin reuptake inhibitor that also affects norepinephrine reuptake, is also employed for this purpose. Fluoxetine and buspirone (a partial 5-HT agonist) may also be useful in fear-based conditions if they act to ablate the *initial* stimulus (i.e., one associated with 5-HT) that induces the endorphin cascade (57). SRIs and 5-HT agonists act to decrease ritualistic activity, including those associated with SIB. Central levels of 5-HT and its precursors are decreased in SIB, while overall 5-HT turnover is increased (18,56).

SIB in Animals

Behaviors involved in most self-injurious and stereotypic behavior, whether or not they meet the criteria for a diagnosis of OCD, are relatively nonspecific. This is a risk inherent in phenotypic, phenomenologic diagnoses. Accordingly, before considering any conditions that involve primary self-mutilation or OCD involving self-injury, it is important to rule out other behavioral conditions that could involve self-injury as a nonspecific sign.

HISTORY

To understand the extent to which self-mutilation or SIB may be involved in OCD, it is important to get an accurate history of the actual behavior the animal is exhibiting. (An outline of the salient features in the clinical history is given in Table 9.4.) The history should include data about changes in the trajectories of the behaviors (i.e., better; worse; no change in content of the behavior, but longer individual bouts) with time, and with any treatments.

MEDICAL ISSUES

Diseases that could cause signs of repetitious and stereotypic behavior associated with SIB include, but are not restricted to, those caused by metabolic, neoplastic, traumatic, and infectious disease, including tick-borne pathogens (e.g., Lyme disease, *Ehrlichia*, Rocky Mountain spotted fever). In the absence of any abnormalities in ancillary physical signs, blood work, titers, radiographs, and bone marrow biopsies, it is likely that the self-injurious or stereotypic behavior does not have an underlying medical cause.

BOREDOM

Boredom is an often touted but seldom demonstrated cause for such behaviors. It may be presumed to occur when animals are confined, receive little human attention or animal interaction, have minimal sensory stimulation, and have

Table 9.4.   Behavioral history for SIB

Sex, breed, and age of animal (breed predispositions)
Age of onset of condition/complaint
Duration of condition/complaint
Description of actual behavior
Frequency of condition/behavior (hourly, daily, weekly, monthly)
Duration of average bout (seconds, minutes, hours)
Range of duration of bouts
Any changes in pattern, frequency, intensity, and bout duration
Any correction measures tried and the response (possibly none)
Any activities that stop the behavior (e.g., animal collapses)
24-hour schedule of pet and client
Pet's familial history
Anything else that the client thinks is relevant

decreased exercise. However, it is almost impossible to define boredom rigorously. For pet dogs and cats, a diagnosis of boredom is anthropomorphic and often an oversimplification of the stresses that come to bear.

ATTENTION-SEEKING BEHAVIOR

Behavioral diagnoses of attention-seeking behavior and anxiety can be difficult to distinguish and may share features in common with other disorders, including OCD (2,58–61). Animals quickly learn that if they are not getting the desired attention from positive, quiet behaviors, they can usually get it from behaviors the owners find less acceptable in dogs, including jumping, barking, howling, and swatting at the owner. Attention-seeking behavior can include spinning, tail-chasing, chewing, sucking, fly-biting, and limb- and foot-licking (58).

Attention-seeking behavior is fairly easy to treat and to dismiss as a cause of self-injury. First, this behavior should not be performed in the client's absence. Second, if the behavior is truly related to attention-seeking, ignoring it by not reacting should greatly diminish it. It is critical to couple this response with calm, loving attention when the animal is quiet. Sometimes, because the interaction between client and pet has become so stressful, the client's tendency is to ignore the animal when it finally ceases the behavior. If these simple behavior modification techniques do not work, the animal is probably not seeking attention by performing the behavior. Banishment may not extinguish the behavior if a pattern has been established. Instead, it may provoke more intense, but relatively transient, attention-seeking behaviors like chewing, biting, scratching, and sucking. If this exaggerated response does not diminish on repeated application of the aforementioned paradigm, it is unlikely that the mutilatory behaviors, however mild, are associated with attention-seeking behavior.

GENERALIZED ANXIETY

Generalized, nonspecific anxiety has as its necessary and sufficient conditions the consistent exhibition of increased autonomic hyperactivity, increased motor activity, and increased vigilance and scanning that interferes with a normal range of social interaction in the absence of any provocative stimuli. Implicit in this diagnosis is that the signs of the anxiety can be nonspecific and variable, and that their presence is correlated with an endogenous state of heightened reactivity. Some anxious animals will chase their tail, lick their feet, and chew and suck themselves or fabrics. Previous injury to an extremity may result in chasing or attacking that region. These animals are often neurologically normal. Anxiety-related responses have been reported in cats. Beaver (62) reported a seasonal hair loss in a 4.5-year-old spayed Burmese; the hair loss occurred only when the cat could see cats outside. While anxiety facilitates

SIBs and other manifestations of OCD, the behaviors exhibited in this context may not meet the rigid criteria outlined for self-mutilation or for OCD. Whether licking or chewing that is a manifestation of generalized anxiety is merely an early step on the continuum of SIB associated with OCD is unclear.

SIB AND OCD

OCD is probably responsible for an unknown proportion of companion animal behavioral conditions involving self-mutilation. Most of the compulsive behavioral conditions described (e.g., acral lick granuloma/dermatitis; fly-biting; flank-sucking; tail-chasing, -sucking, and -mutilation) might be better characterized as symptoms of underlying abnormalities. Viewing these conditions from this perspective may lead to improved treatment of these intractable conditions and new ways to view these behavioral complaints.

Given that at least 2 to 3% of the human population is estimated to suffer from OCD, the proportion in the animal population should be greater because genetic variation is canalized both by the development of breeds and by specific breeding practices like line-breeding. In a study designed to evaluate the effect of the environmental (i.e., type of neighbor) versus the genetic components of stereotypic behavior in mink, stereotypic behavior developed based on heritability, regardless of the social environment (63). The possibility that OCD, or the tendency to develop a stereotypy is heritable is also hinted at by the reports of tail-chasing in dogs. Bull Terriers, Australian Cattle Dogs, Terriers, and German Shepherds are overreported in the group of tail-chasing dogs when compared with other breeds (64).

OCD in animals has been divided into three groups of behaviors: conflict, vacuum, and stereotypy (37,65). Two of the behavior patterns most frequently attributed to conflict and frustration are aggression and displacement activities (65). Both aggression and displacement activities have their roots in anxiety. Traumatic, cataclysmic events may be associated with the development or suppression of anxiety-related behaviors and OCD (3). The most common motor abnormalities—including those involved in grooming—involve changes in the frequency, intensity, or context of the behavior. The extent to which the condition is detrimental can be evaluated by the relative proportions of "normal" vs "abnormal" behaviors (66).

Some SIB and OCD behaviors have been thought to be "coping" behaviors related to the stresses of confinement. Laboratory rats exhibit environmentally induced stereotypies, as do macaques (67). Some of these stereotypies may be associated with facilitation of social interaction; for example, auto-grooming stereotypies are more frequently exhibited by rats that are social subordinates (68). Piglets that have been deprived of suckling and that exhibit stereotypic nibbling have altered brain dopamine levels and, perhaps, altered metabolism (69). In pigs, one sees abnormal chewing, nibbling, and sucking of the ears, tail, preputium, claws, and other body parts in early weaned animals (3–5 weeks), but not in normally weaned ones (8–10 weeks) (70). Feather-picking/plucking in birds and stereotypies in veal calves have been regarded as attempts to decrease environmental tension (71,72). Veal calves that can suck on inanimate objects or can tongue roll have been found to have a decreased incidence of abomasal ulcers (72).

Viewed critically, however, these stereotypies do not provide self-medication in the sense that they "fix" the animal: ulcers and tongue rolling are both sequelae of distress that are not seen in free-ranging animals. "Self-medication" here involves the substitution of one anxiety-related consequence for another. There is little evidence for either an adaptive function for OCD, particularly when it involves SIB, or for the assertion that OCD allows animals to discharge tension. Instead, positive feedback of sensory stimulation on an underlying control system may result in progressive sensitization of the neurologic system (73). Such an explanation would account for the variation in presentation of the signs and history of development of conditions associated with SIB and OCD.

OCDs in humans frequently appear in adolescence and continue through mid-life (74). Symptoms may be worse or more pronounced in stressful or anxiety-producing circumstances. It has been hypothesized that there is a genetic and heritable component to the condition, as it appears to run in some families (74). The same pattern is true for animals exhibiting SIB and OCD; animals may therefore be excellent models for studying analogous conditions in humans, and may provide insight into the heritability of such conditions. Two conditions, feline hyperesthesia and canine acral lick dermatitis, that occur endogenously in domestic cats and dogs may be particularly relevant for discussions of SIB, its associations with OCD, and its putative underlying neurochemical mechanisms.

Feline Hyperesthesia, Overgrooming, and Self-Mutilation

Feline hyperesthesia syndrome has been variously called rolling skin syndrome, neuritis, twitchy cat disease, and atypical neurodermatitis (75). The behaviors demonstrated in this "condition" include: 1) those mimicking estrus; 2) biting at the tail, flank, anal, or lumbar areas, sometimes with resultant barbering or self-mutilation; and 3) skin rippling and muscle spasms or twitching (usually dorsally), often accompanied by vocalization, running/jumping, hallucinations, and self-directed aggression. Not all cats exhibiting these behaviors self-mutilate, but those that do can exhibit a gamut of mutilation ranging from excessive licking, to plucking (trichotillomania), barbering, and biting and chewing that leads to skin lesions. Regardless of the degree of the behavioral change, clients report that it is extremely difficult to distract the cat from the behavior. Furthermore, the behavioral sequence appears to be multidirectional: Cats might twitch and then focus on a part of the body to lick or chew; or they might be grooming, start to twitch, and then exhibit more furious behaviors.

The environmental and social cues or stressors that have been associated with this disorder range from those that are readily apparent (e.g., food allergies, the addition of another cat, the addition or loss of a human with attendant changes in attention) to indiscernible or, perhaps, nonexistent exogenous cues. The cues or changes that are perceived by the cat may truly be endogenous. Addressing these types of behaviors does not simply involve enriching the environment or removing a stress; by definition, endogenous changes are more difficult to understand and address. Some hints that most manifestations of this condition are motivated by endogenous rather than exogenous processes come from feline sensory physiology.

The feline cutaneous response generated by Types 1 and 2 slow-adapting (SA) epidermal units is characterized by a rate of discharge that is proportional to the amount of displacement of the hair or the indentation of the skin (76). These SA units interact with rapid-adapting (RA) units in the vibrissae around the face, lips, mouth, and guard hairs to generate the classic biting response that follows vibrissae stimulation in predatory situations (77). This sensory response may be one reason why cats chew more frequently than dogs (who lick) when manifesting self-mutilation.

Feline postures and head attitude have profound effects on mediation of oral responses through descending spinal tracts. Cutaneous and proprioceptive feedback interact to program the relative timing of flexor and extensor activity (78). Many of the behaviors that cats exhibit during bouts of hyperesthesia resemble the classic chewing/aggression mediated by the ventromedial hypothalamus and the medial amygdala. Cholecystokinin-B (CCK-B; central brain) receptors are also involved in the firing of feline jaw musculature, suggesting a central role in SIB in cats involving neurochemical control of satiety and association of brain regions shown to be involved in predatory, consummatory behavior (79).

Taken together, the data on feline cutaneous responses, vibrissae stimulation, head posture, ventromedial hypothalamus and medial amygdala responses in predatory/consummatory situations, and CCK-B activity in jaw-firing suggest a testable hypothesis regarding the mechanism of SIB in cats. This is not to imply that one should disregard more obvious, and perhaps parsimonious, exogenous explanations for the behavior; however, to assume that these are instructional is an oversimplification. Self-licking, biting, and hair loss are nonspecific symptoms. Any conditions, behavioral or dermatologic, that enhance these symptoms will render the condition and its treatment more complex.

Canine Acral Lick Dermatitis/Granulomas

Many dogs that are anxious lick themselves. General physical and physiological signs of anxiety are the same as those previously discussed for cats. The association between anxiety and grooming behaviors is illustrated by dogs that are anxious when separated from certain people. Closer examination of dogs that have separation anxiety reveals a high incidence of saliva-stained carpi and recurrent lick granuloma. Lick granulomas are a good example of multifactorial disorders that may involve, in some cases, either anxiety or SIB associated with OCD. All lick granulomas are not due to the same underlying modality, as licking is a relatively nonspecific symptom. The pattern in which the licking occurs hints at the variation in putative underlying mechanisms requiring different treatments.

Medical causes of lick granulomas have been investigated and compose the first level of diagnostic rule-outs (61). Nerve conduction dysfunction has been implicated in cases of lick granuloma in dogs (80). Impediment is not common, but when conduction is impeded, the impediment is bilateral, while the mutilation is invariably unilateral. For animals with acral lick dermatitis and granulomas, the amplitude of sensory evoked potentials is no different in affected versus nonaffected limbs (80). This strongly suggests that the conduction velocity abnormality does not cause the behavior.

Sensory neuropathies may be more complex. Heritable sensory neuropathy has been noted for a family of pointers (79–83). Affected dogs mutilate and chew off their toes, have loss of nociceptive function, and have reduced substance-P activity. Fine alterations of sensory and substance-P function are seldom examined for patients with acral lick dermatitis and granuloma, but such deficits may play a role in the development of the pathology and may facilitate any anxiety associated with it.

Pruritus has been implicated in medical causes of lick granuloma (61) and also may have a role in obsessive skin-picking (84). Pruritus and anxiety are not unrelated at the biochemical level (85), but pruritus is best understood as a primary sensory modality. Various types of itching may play a significant role in self-mutilation.

SIB with lick granuloma appears to fit the OCD profile for increased frequency in families of animals for which another OCD has been diagnosed. Given this, it is not surprising that some breeds appear more commonly afflicted than others. Examination of 98 biopsies submitted to the Surgical Pathology Laboratory at the Veterinary School of the University of Pennsylvania during a 17-month period indicated that, when compared with the total in-hospital pool of 44,960 cases seen in this period, Doberman Pinschers and Labrador Retrievers were significantly overrepresented in the acral lick dermatitis pool ($P < 0.0001$ and $P < 0.007$, respectively; Cochran Mantel Haenszel chi square (CMH test)) (61). This, coupled with data from the patient population of the Behavior Clinic for specific breeds (i.e., Doberman Pinschers, Great Danes, German Shepherds, Golden Retrievers), strongly supports the possibility of an underlying genetic component to the condition. OCDs are postulated to run in human families and to be heritable (73,74). Some proportion of acral lick dermatitis cases are likely to be due to OCD or an OCD-like disorder. The potential for developing an animal model of OCD is enormous, and development of such a model would greatly facilitate canine research in this area. Similar conditions occur in other species maintained and developed as pets.

Dogs and cats have been, to varying degrees and for thousands of years, selected to live with humans as part of their household. The social systems of dogs and cats have facilitated the extent to which this symbiotic relationship has developed. Accordingly, one could argue that, under good husbandry conditions, the general conditions of these pets' maintenance are not stressors, per se. The situation is certainly different for zoo and laboratory animals—their conditions of maintenance have been noted as stressors—and SIB is frequently reported in many species kept under these conditions (67,68,86,87). Horses and caged birds fall into an intermediate category.

Horses
Horses live in large social groups where harem and/or hierarchical systems are maintained by social challenges attendant with maturity. Horses kept as pets or working animals seldom have the opportunity to experience the range of social and physical stimuli that they would under free-ranging conditions. Accordingly, many stereotypic behaviors reported in horses respond well to adjustments made in response to physical and social needs (88,89).

Stallions and geldings appear to be at risk for SIB that involves flank-biting and other stereotypical behaviors of vocalization and movement (90–92). The behaviors manifest in SIB can be associated with grooming but may also be associated with species-specific herding, social, and sexual behaviors, and appear to be particularly obvious when the animal is confined (45,92).

These behaviors have been characterized as SIB, and their nonspecific signs have been postulated to be similar to those of SIB when it is exhibited in Tourette syndrome (92). It is unclear if these nonspecific signs are due to a condition in which mutilation may play a role (i.e., Tourette syndrome), or whether the problem is OCD manifesting partly as SIB. Given the pattern of the behaviors, the role played by perturbation of the social system, and the response to medications, including those used to treat OCD (88), it is likely that SIB in horses is related to OCD. The extent to which the social and physical environments play a role here should not be underestimated and may suggest that SIB in horses is not a good model for endogenous SIB or OCD.

Birds
Feather-picking in birds ranges from excessive grooming, to plucking, to picking and gouging (93,94). Avian species that have been adopted by humans for life in cages are generally social. Psittacines, in particular, are highly social and gregarious and can live in flocks of thousands. Their social relationships are complex and are modulated by extensive and intricate intraspecific posturing and vocalization. While psittacines exhibit many of the same social and court-

ship behaviors to their human handlers, this is actually evidence for lack of domestication through artificial selection and evolution, and for human anthropocentrism. Contrast this to the situation in truly domesticated animals like dogs, where specific behavioral patterns (e.g., guarding, herding) have been rigorously maintained through artificial selection.

Like horses, many of the stereotypic behaviors that these birds exhibit are associated with restricted social interactions and level of stimulation and physical confinement. In fact, the first attempts to redress the appearance of symptoms associated with SIB in birds involve social and physical environmental enrichment. At some point, this management strategy fails for some birds. There are insufficient data to conclude whether this failure is associated with the complexity of the social system from which the species was derived, or whether there are other factors that may predispose the condition to progress neurochemically. That some of these birds respond to the anti–obsessive-compulsive medication clomipramine (93,94) suggests that the SIB may be associated with OCD; however, because of the profound role played by the social and physical environment, it is arguable whether feather-picking in birds or self-mutilation in horses represents a model for the development of endogenous OCD that would be analogous or homologous to that exhibited by humans.

Treatment of SIB

Specific drugs should be chosen on the basis of specific inclusion and exclusion criteria rooted in a hypothesis of underlying mechanism (95,96). Drugs commonly used to treat SIBs are members of one or a few classes of psychotropic medications: tricyclic antidepressants (TCAs), narcotic agonists/antagonists, 5-HT agonists, and SSRIs. Effects of these medications are related to which neurochemical or receptor they affect and the functional location in the brain where such receptors are concentrated.

TCAs decrease the rate of firing of the locus coeruleus (LC), thereby decreasing norepinephrine (NE) release (97), although the therapeutic effects of these compounds can be regulated through enhancement of glutamine and 5-HT. All TCAs act by inhibiting 5-HT reuptake. It is postulated that the specific effect of clomipramine is to facilitate a localized increase in 5-HT in the region of the basal ganglia, particularly the caudate nucleus (98). The beneficial effects of 5-HT reuptake blockers in the treatment of stereotypies have been noted for individuals with autism, mental retardation, schizophrenia, stuttering, nail-biting, trichotillomania, self-mutilation syndrome, and anorexia nervosa (99). Clomipramine is relatively specific for treatment of OCDs, as it lacks the antidepressant properties of other TCAs (98). This drug is relatively specific for alleviation of obsessive-compulsive effects and has been successful in treating obsessive-compulsive spectrum conditions in humans, such as trichotillomania (100). Clomipramine has also been used successfully in the treatment of lick granuloma in dogs (101), and excessive motoric behavior associated with OCD in dogs (102) and cats (Overall KL, unpublished data, 1996). It is important to realize that conditions such as acral lick dermatitis and granuloma may represent diffuse syndromes with multiple causality, as discussed previously.

Fluoxetine and other SSRIs may not be better than imipramine and other TCAs for some patients with milder signs of OCD (103). Common SSRI side effects include nervousness, tremor, anxiety, insomnia, diarrhea, sexual dysfunction, nausea, anorexia, and weight loss. All SSRIs can interact with monoamine oxidase inhibitors, causing serotonin syndrome. The metabolism of TCAs is inhibited by fluoxetine via inhibition of liver enzyme CYP2D6 (97). Each intermediate metabolite may change the metabolism of another so that excretion of both is prolonged; hence, treatment using a combination of drugs is becoming popular in refractory cases.

Up to 40% to 60% of human patients with OCD do not get full relief of symptoms solely from the administration of SRIs (104). Addition of partial 5-HT1A agonists, like buspirone, does not seem to help, suggesting that multiple modalities of function contribute to the condition. Buspirone, a partial, but nonselective, 5-HT1A agonist, increases the rate of firing of the LC (105). Its effects are mediated through both dopamine and serotonin receptors (106). But no additional improvement is seen in most patients with OCD, and depressive or anxiety symptoms are common with the addition of buspirone to a stable dose of fluoxetine (107). Anxiety and depression associated with OCD are considered secondary to it; therefore, treating them without treating the OCD will not produce complete resolution. These sequelae often resolve if the OCD is successfully treated (108).

Clearly, it is not appropriate to treat the presumed underlying cause of any symptom of SIB without also treating local lesions. Lesions should be cultured and treated with antibiotics as indicated. Should there be localized scratching, the addition of an antipruritic medication may be hepful. All TCAs have joint antipruritic and anti-anxiety components, the extent of which varies according to the drug formulation. Amitriptyline has been occasionally successful in treating trichotillomania (109) and some stereotypies in companion animals (58), possibly—in part—as a result of this dual action. As an H1 receptor antagonist, doxepin is 880 times more potent than diphenhydramine, and 67 times more potent than hydroxyzine (110).

Other drugs that may be helpful in the treatment of SIB include clozapine (a tricyclic antipsychotic) and carbamazepine (a tricyclic anticonvulsant) (111,112). In addition, thioridazine (a phenothiazine derivative) has been used successfully to control aberrant motor behavior and SIB in the dog, and lithium and opioid antagonists have been used successfully in humans (18,113,114). Tryptophan deficiencies may potentiate depression, while dietary supplementation with tryptophan (a 5-HT precursor) may potentiate the action of antidepressants, suggesting serotonergic dysfunction in depression (115). Recent work has indicated that CCK is present in large concentrations in the limbic system of the brain and may mediate perception of anxiety. The CCK-B receptor, which is restricted to the brain, appears to have anxiolytic effects when stimulated (79). This paves the way for novel treatment of SIB associated with anxiety and may be particularly relevant with regard to the cat model discussed previously.

Treatment of SIB Associated with OCD

NONTREATMENTS: SHOCK AND RESTRAINT

Caution is urged in using punishment, including shock, to suppress normal or abnormal fearful responses to stimuli. Shock increases the anxiety level of animals and so may worsen the anxiety-related behavior. However, competitive inhibition of one anxiety with another could result in a behavioral or phenotypic change in the type of behavior exhibited (see Table 9.1, Level 1), but may not ameliorate the neurochemical pathology (see Table 9.1, Level 3). This effect has been noted across a wide variety of species (chicks (116), dogs (117), monkeys (118)). Alternatively, if shock is precisely controlled and used to cue the individual to inhibit SIB (i.e., operant conditioning), both learning and altered brain chemistry (involving changes in endogenous opioids) can be associated with a reduction in SIB (119).

Restraint may prohibit further injury from occurring, but it does nothing to address the mechanism facilitating SIB. Tail-chasing in Scottish Terriers is worsened by restraint (120). If these behaviors are truly anxiety-related, the worsening effect of restraint makes sense, as it only hinders access and raises the animal's anxiety level. Restraint does nothing to treat the condition at any level, it merely prevents the behavior. This should make us question the use of restraint devices like Elizabethan collars. As aids to prevent further mutilation and infection, they may have some role, but they are clearly inappropriate as the sole form of treatment for any anxiety-related condition or OCD.

RATIONAL TREATMENT

The general paradiagm for treatment of SIB is similar to that for the treatment of any anxiety-related disorder. A combination of behavior modification (primarily counterconditioning and desensitization) and pharmacologic intervention will usually be successful if the stereotypic behavior is due to an underlying anxiety. Counterconditioning is usually unsuccessful without antianxiety medication to break the psychological trigger for the cycle (121).

When using drugs to treat SIB, which either occurs alone or in association with OCD, it is important to remember the following:

1. Not all agents commonly used affect the same neurochemicals; some alter brain concentrations of NE and 5-HT, while others are more specific for 5-HT.
2. Even agents that affect the same neurotransmitter system may not affect all receptor subtypes identically. This characteristic accounts for much of the variation in the effects of, for example, the SSRIs (95,97,99,105).
3. Little is known about how specific agents change actual neuronal metabolism. Most antianxiety agents act either as presynaptic agonists, neurotransmitter reuptake inhibitors, or as agonists at postsynaptic receptors. Given neurochemical and receptor heterogeneity between individuals with apparently similar conditions, it is hardly surprising that there is considerable variation in response to treatment even when an identical pharmacologic agent is employed. Making an effort to identify and group the behavioral subtypes of the activity in question may lead to a more specific mechanistic understanding of the condition (see Table 9.1).

A specific example of this approach is provided by acral lick dermatitis and granuloma. The pattern of the *behavioral* development of the lick lesion may provide an important clue about the level of underlying dysfunction and which medication might work best. For example, lick granulomas, in general, respond to treatment with anti–obsessive-compulsive medication only about 60% of the time (122,123); this is the same percentage that responds to all other treatments (61,124–126). Regardless, at the Veterinary Hospital of the University of Pennsylvania (VHUP), dogs responding *best* to such medications are those whose lesions develop after sudden, furious, continuous and non-interruptible mutilation, and whose lesions worsen concomitant with continuous and noninterruptible licking (i.e., a behavior that has become obsessive and compulsive).

On the basis of behavioral signs alone, it may be possible to make a phenotypic classification of acral lick dermatitis and granuloma. At the Behavior Clinic at VHUP this classification includes:

1. Licking associated with injury or irritation
2. Licking associated with seasonal exposure to allergens
3. Licking associated with gradual onset that may or may not be chronic
4. Licking associated with environmental change
5. Licking that is continuous and noninterruptible
6. Licking and/or chewing that is violent and sudden in its appearance.

Preliminary results suggest that narcotic antagonists have worked best for dogs in category 6 (the sudden violent population), who may also be helped by SSRIs, specific TCAs, and antiepileptic agents (e.g., carbamazepine). TCAs that are also potent H1 antagonists (e.g., doxepin) are most efficacious for patients in the categories 1, 2, and 3, while antianxiety medications (e.g., amitriptyline, imipramine, clomipramine) appear to be most beneficial for animals in categories 3, 4, and 5. Note that combination treatment with agents affecting pruritus and anxiety may be required to control the symptoms of the condition. That this condition can have discrete sets of behaviorally recognizable phenotypic presentations that cluster with treatment suggests a variable underlying neurochemical mechanism.

The general SIB treatment paradigm mandates the following:

1. Identification of any actual stressors, and manipulative tests of the hypothesis that they are involved.
2. Use of behavior modification to encourage cessation of the inappropriate behavior, to encourage general relaxation that will be competitive with the undesirable behavior and will encourage alterations in neurotransmitters, and to teach the animal new behaviors that will help to abort the inappropriate behavior and will encourage general relaxation spontaneously.
3. Use of pharmacologic intervention as an aid to implementing behavior modification (see Table 9.1, Level 1) and to address the putative pathophysiologic basis of the behavior (see Table 9.1, Level 3). The more specific the drug mechanism, the more accurately a hypothesis can be tested. Even without the aid of specific agents, however, medications can be selected that are best suited to the particular constellation of symptoms.
4. Premedication physical and laboratory examination of any animal that is to be treated with any agent. The minimum data include a complete blood count and a serum biochemistry profile. This is important, particularly in the United States, where use of most of the medications discussed here is considered "extra-label." Under this label the law (1996 AMDUCA) specifies compliance with all data bases routinely used in human medicine.

DOSING CAVEATS

Most of the drugs discussed in this text are contraindicated in humans and animals with renal or hepatic disease, as they may experience altered clearance and potentiation if there is any impairment in renal and hepatic function. Hence, premedication laboratory evaluation is mandatory (and subject by law in the United States). Electrocardiography is warranted for any animal that may be predisposed to a conduction disturbance. Tests for necessary medical (somatic or organic) rule-outs should also be encouraged.

Most psychotropic medication may affect thyroid hormone concentrations, potentiate arrhythmias, engender epileptiform seizures, and increase most hepatic-associated enzyme activities, particularly that of alkaline phosphatase. Treatment with TCAs at high dosages has been associated with sick euthyroid syndrome. Transient effects that may potentiate other behavior problems include altered thirst and appetite (127).

Rational pharmacologic treatment mandates frequent patient monitoring. This is especially true if the medication is to be continued long-term. Clients should be aware that these conditions are not cured, they are only controlled. Recidivism rates may be high, and the best treatment may require continued use of medication. If clients wish to withdraw their pet from medication, withdrawal should be sufficiently gradual so that clients can learn if there is some minimum dose required by the animal. Withdrawal of medication should only be attempted if the animal has maintained peak improvement for a time period at least equal to and preferably greater than the withdrawal time. For some medications like clomipramine or fluoxetine, which require 3 to 5 weeks to display efficacy, withdrawal times are as long, or longer, if dosages are titrated as part of a program of gradual withdrawal (127).

A list of drugs useful in the treatment of fears and anxiety-related conditions is provided in Table 9.5. Again, it is important to remember that an accurate diagnosis is essential in choosing an appropriate medication, and that the most specific but least restrictive drug is generally the medication of choice.

Table 9.5. Psychopharmacologic agents that may be useful in the treatment of anxiety disorders

Animal/Disorder	Drug (form)	Dosage
Cat/OCD and hyperesthesia	Alprazolam (tablets: 0.25, 0.5, 1, 2 mg [1 and 2 mg tablets are scored])	0.125–0.25 mg/kg PO q12h
	Amitriptyline (tablets: 10, 25, 50, 75, 100, 150 mg)	0.5–2.0 mg/kg PO q12–24h
	Buspirone (tablets: 5, 10 mg)	0.5–1.0 mg/kg PO q8–12h
	Clomipramine (capsules: 25, 50, 75 mg)	0.5 mg/kg PO q24h
	Clorazepate (tablets: 3.75, 7.5, 11.25, 15, 22.5 mg; capsules: 3.75, 7.5, 15 mg)	0.5–2.0 mg/kg PO prn for profound distress; 0.2–0.4 mg/kg PO q12–24h
	Diazepam (tablets: 1, 2 mg; solution: 5 mg/mL)	0.2–0.4 mg/kg PO q12–24h
	Fluoxetine (capsules: 10, 20 mg; solution: 5 mg/mL)	0.5–1.0 mg/kg PO q24h
	Hydrocodone (tablets: 5 mg)	0.25–1.0 mg/kg PO q8–12h
	Naltrexone (tablets: 50 mg [scored])	2.2 mg/kg PO q24h (up to 25–50 mg *per cat*)
	Nortriptyline (capsules: 10, 25, 50, 75 mg)	0.5–2.0 mg/kg PO q12–24h
	Oxazepam (tablets: 15 mg; capsules: 10, 15, 30 mg)	0.2–0.5 mg/kg PO q12–24h (1.0–2.5 mg *per cat* PO q12–24h)

Table 9.5. *Continued*

Animal/Disorder	Drug (form)	Dosage
Dog/OCD and acral lick dermatitis	Alprazolam (tablets: 0.25, 0.5, 1, 2 mg [1 and 2 mg tablets are scored])	0.01–0.1 mg/kg PO prn for phobic or panic attacks; *not* to exceed 4 mg per dog per day (0.75–4.0 mg per dog per day) Start with 1–2 mg for a 25-kg dog
	Amitriptyline (tablets: 10, 25, 50, 75, 100, 150 mg)	1–2 mg/kg PO q12h
	Buspirone (tablets: 5, 10 mg)	1 mg/kg PO q8–24h
	Carbamazepine (tablets: 200 mg [scored]; chewable tablets: 100 mg [scored])	4–8 mg/kg PO q12h; 0.5–1.25 mg/kg PO q8h
	Clomipramine (capsules: 25, 50, 75 mg)	1 mg/kg PO q12h × 2 wk; then 2 mg/kg PO q12h × 2 wk; then 3 mg/kg PO q12h × 4 wk
	Clorazepate (tablets: 3.75, 7.5, 11.25, 15, 22.5 mg; capsules: 3.75, 7.5, 15 mg)	0.55–2.2 mg/kg PO q24h (*or* prn for storms and noises)
	Doxepin (capsules: 10, 25, 50, 75, 100, 150 mg; solution: 10 mg/mL)	3–5 mg/kg PO q8–12h
	Fluoxetine (capsules: 10, 20 mg; solution: 5 mg/mL)	1 mg/kg PO q12–24h
	Haloperidol (tablets: 0.5, 1, 2, 5, 10, 20 mg; solution: 2 mg/mL)	1–4 mg PO q12h
	Hydrocodone (tablets: 5 mg)	1 mg per 4 kg PO q8h
	Hydroxyzine (tablets: 10, 25, 50, 100 mg; capsules: 25, 50, 100 mg; solution: 10 mg/mL; suspension: 25 mg/5 mL)	2.2 mg/kg PO q8h
	Imipramine (tablets: 10, 25, 50 mg; capsules: 75, 100, 125, 150 mg)	2.2–4.4 mg/kg PO q12–24h
	Naloxone (injectable only: 0.4 mg/mL in 1-mL ampules, 1-mL disposable syringes, or 10-mL vials; 0.02 mg/ml in 2-mL ampules)	11–22 μg/kg IV (SC, IM) prn
	Naltrexone (tablets: 50 mg [scored])	2.2 mg/kg PO q12–24h
	Nortriptyline (capsules: 10, 25, 50, 75 mg; solution: 10 mg/5 mL)	1–2 mg/kg PO q12h
	Thioridazine (tablets: 10, 15, 25, 50, 100, 150, 200 mg; solution; 25 mg/5 mL, 30 mg/mL, 100 mg/mL)	1.1–2.2 mg/kg PO q12–24h

Solution = a drug incorporated into an aqueous or alcoholic solution; suspension = undissolved drug dispersed in a liquid for oral or parenteral use.

Summary

SIB in humans is restricted to a diagnosis that is associated with cognitive impairment. This represents a problem for assessment for self-injury in animals. Regardless, the diagnosis of self-mutilation and/or SIB, either alone or associated with a diagnosis of OCD, appears to be multifactorial and heterogeneous. Environmental and behavioral stressors can contribute to the underlying neuropharmacology of these conditions. Two specific conditions, feline hyperesthesia and canine acral lick granuloma—which can involve broad-sense SIB in animals and that may be analogous or homologous to the condition when it appears in humans—demonstrate the extent to which the symptoms can be variable. When SIB is demonstrated in these conditions, it often—but not always—fits a profile compatible with OCD. Seizure activity has also been implicated in these and similar conditions, particularly in the cat, for which stimulation of the amygdala and ventromedial hypothalamus produces stereotypic aggressive behavior that may be self-directed (128–130). Various neurochemical mechanisms, including those associated with endorphin metabolism (131), have been implicated in this feline behavior pattern. This heterogeneity suggests that the conditions should be evaluated based on the overall pattern of behavior (i.e., compulsive behavior that involves mutilation), rather than on the basis of a solitary clinical sign (i.e., the presence of a granuloma). Such an approach will allow for treatment of more benign conditions like situation-associated anxiety early in the course of the development of clinical signs.

Manifestation of these conditions can also be influenced by phylogeny. Cats, as part of their adaptation as small, largely solitary predators, have a cutaneous response that is proportional to the amount of displacement of hair or the indentation of the skin. Their head postures also affect timing of extensor and flexor activity. These adaptations to their predatory style may influence the form taken by the abnormal SIB/OCD behaviors that they display. Most SIBs exhibited by dogs are concentrated on their distal extremities and tail. This is also where atopic disease is commonly manifest, and the relationship at the neurochemical level between pruritus and anxiety should not be ignored. Also, humans have selected, through breeding, dogs that are configured differently than their canine ancestors. Such historical effects doubtless play a role in the form taken by abnormal behavior when it develops.   ·

The longer the situation has been ongoing, the more likely it is that the underlying neurophysiology has progressed. These are not static conditions: they change with experience, treatment, and the interaction of the two. Accordingly, dogs that are anxious in general may be at greater risk for the development of OCD under certain circumstances. Pharmacologic agents that seek to address changes in central opioid, dopamine, and serotonin metabolism have all been employed with varying degrees of success. Drugs that are more specific (some of the SSRIs and agonists) can also help in the test of mechanistic hypotheses. SSRIs and newer anti-anxiety agents under development hold the most hope for future understanding and treatment of these conditions.

References

1. Luescher UA, McKeown DB, Halip J. Stereotypic or obsessive-compulsive disorders in dogs and cats. Vet Clin North Am Sm Anim Pract 1991;21:401–413.
2. Overall KL. Recognition, diagnosis, and management of obsessive-compulsive disorders, Part I. Canine Prac 1992;17:40–44.
3. Kiley-Worthington M. Behavioural problems of farm animals. Stockfield, England: Oriel Press, 1977.
4. Swedo SE, Leonard HL, Rapoport JL, et al. A double-blind comparison of clomipramine and desimpramine in the treatment of trichotillomania (hair pulling). N Engl J Med 1989;321:491–501.
5. Lipinski JF. Clomipramine in the treatment of self-mutilating behaviors. N Engl J Med 1991;324:1441.
6. Perse T. Obsessive-compulsive disorder: a treatment review. J Clin Psychiatry 1988;49:48–55.
7. American Psychiatric Association. Diagnostic and Statistical Manual of Mental Disorders, 4th ed. Washington, DC: American Psychiatric Association, 1994.
8. Clutton-Brock J. A natural history of domesticated animals. Cambridge: British Museum (Natural History), Cambridge University Press, 1987.
9. Coppinger R, Glendenning J, Torop E, et al. Degree of behavioral neoteny differentiates canid polymorphs. Ethology 1987;75:797–108.
10. Overall KL. Terminology in behavioral medicine: necessary and sufficient conditions for behavioral diagnoses. Am Vet Soc Anim Behav Newsletter 1995;17:3–7.
11. Overall KL. Clinical behavioral medicine for small animals. St. Louis: Mosby, 1997.
12. Casner JA, Weinheimer B, Gualtieri CT. Naltrexone and self-injurious behavior: a retrospective population study. J Clin Psychopharmacol 1996;16:389–394.
13. Gualtiere CT. The differential diagnosis of self-injurious behavior in mentally retarded people. Psychopharmacol Bull 1989;25:358–363.
14. Thrush DC. Congenital insensitivity to pain: a clinical, genetic, and neurophysiological study of four children from the same family. Brain 1973;96:369–386.
15. Aman MG. Efficacy of psychotropic drugs for reducing self-injurious behavior in the developmental disabilities. Ann Clin Psychiatry 1993;5:171–188.
16. Farber JM. Psychopharmacology of self-injurious behavior in the mentally retarded. J Am Acad Child Adolesc Psychiatry 1987;26:296–302.
17. Overall KL. Stereotypic and ritualistic behaviors. Proc N North Amer Vet C 1994;8:55–57.
18. Gualtieri CT. The measurement of self-injurious behavior. J Neuropsychiatry 1991;3:S30–S34.
19. Buitelaar JK. Self-injurious behaviour in retarded children: clinical phenomena and biological mechanisms. Acta Paedopsychiatr 1993;56:105–111.
20. Hellings JA, Warnock JK. Self-injurious behavior and serotonin in Prader-Willi syndrome. Psychopharmacol Bull 1994;30:245–250.
21. Winchel RM, Stanley M. Self-injurious behavior: a review of the behavior and the biology of self-mutilation. Am J Psychiatry 1991;148:306–317.
22. Breese GR, Baumeister AA, McCown TJ, et al. Behavioral differences between neonatal and adult-6-hydroxydopamine treated rats to dopamine agonists: relevance to neurological

symptoms in clinical syndromes with reduced brain dopamine. J Pharmacol Exp Ther 1984a;231:343–354.

23. Breese GR, Naumeister AA, Napier TC, et al. Neonatal-6-hydroxydopamine treatment: model of susceptibility for self-mutilation in the Lesch Nyhan syndrome. Pharmacol Biochem Behav 1984b;235:287–295.

24. Breese GR, Criswell HE, Mueller RA. Evidence that lack of brain dopamine during development can increase the susceptibility for aggression and self-injurious behavior by influencing D_1-dopamine receptor function. Prog Neuropsychopharmacol Biol Psychiatry 1990;14:S65–S80.

25. Goldstein M, Kuga S, Kusano N, et al. Dopamine agonist self-mutilative biting behaviors in monkeys with ventromedial tegmental lesions of brainstem, possible pharmacological model for Lesch-Nyhan syndrome. Brain Res 1986;367:104–150.

26. Lloyd KG, Hornykiewicz O, Davidsons L, et al. Biochemical evidence of dysfunction of brain neurotransmitters in the Lesch-Nyhan syndrome. N Engl J Med 1981;305:1106–1111.

27. Eichelmann B. Catecholamines and aggressive behavior. In: Usdin E, ed. Neuroregulators and psychiatric disorders. New York: Oxford University Press, 1977.

28. Richardson JS, Zaliski WA. Naloxone and self-mutilation. Biol Psychiatry 1983;18:99–101.

29. Coid J, Allilo B, Rees LH. Raised plasma metencephalin in patients who habitually mutilate themselves. Lancet 1983;2:545–546.

30. Perse TL, Greist JH, Jefferson, et al. Fluvoxamine treatment of obsessive-compulsive disorder. Am J Psychiatry 1987;144:1543–1548.

31. Dantzer R. Behavioural, physiological and functional aspects of stereotyped behaviour: a review and a reinterpretation. J Anim Sci 1986;62:1776–1786.

32. Swedo SE, Pietrini P, Leonard HL, et al. Cerebral glucose metabolism in childhood-onset obsessive-compulsive disorder: revisualization during pharmacotherapy. Arch Gen Psychiatry 1992;49:690–694.

33. Insel TR. Toward a neuroanatomy of obsessive-compulsive disorder. Arch Gen Psychiatry 1992;49:739–744.

34. Baxter LR, Schwartz JM, Bergman KS, et al. Caudate glucose metabolic rate changes with both drug and behavior therapy for obsessive-compulsive disorder. Arch Gen Psychiatry 1992;49:681–689.

35. Coon H, Plaetke R, Holik J, et al. Use of a neurophysiological trait in linkage analysis of schizophrenia. Biol Psychiatry 1993;34:277–289.

36. Luxenberg JS, Swedo SE, Flament MF, et al. Neuroanatomical abnormalities in obsessive-compulsive disorder detected with quantitative X-ray computed tomography. Am J Psychiatry 1988;145:1089–1093.

37. Cronin GM, Wiepkema PR, van Ree JM. Endorphins implicated in stereotypies of tethered sows. Experientia 1986;42:198–199.

38. Gilham SB, Dodman NH, Shuster L, et al. The effect of diet on cribbing behavior and plasma β-endorphin in horses. Appl Anim Behav Sci 1994;41:147–153.

39. Goodman I, Zacny J, Osma A, et al. Dopaminergic nature of feeling induced behavioral stereotypies in stressed pigeons. Pharmacol Biochem Behav 1983;18:153–158.

40. Davis GC, Buchsbaum MS, Naber D, et al. Altered pain perception and cerebrospinal endorphins in psychiatric illness. Ann NY Acad Sci 1982;398:366–373.

41. Pitman RK. Animal models of compulsive behavior. Biol Psychiatry 1989;26:189–198.

42. Soubrie P. Reconciling the role of central serotonin neurons in human and animal behavior. Behav Brain Sci 1986;9:319–335.

43. Rolf LH, Haarmann FY, Grotenmeyer K-H, Kehrer H. Serotonin and amino acid context in platelets of autistic children. Acta Psychiatr Scand 1993;87:315–316.

44. Gillberg C, Terenius L, Lönnerholm G. Endorphin activity in childhood psychosis. Arch Gen Psychiatry 1985;42:780–783.

45. Dodman NH, Shuster L, Court M, Patel J. Use of narcotic antagonist (nalmefene) to suppress self-mutilative behavior in a stallion. J Am Vet Med Assoc 1988;192:1585–1586.
46. Terenius L, Wahlstrom A, Lindstom L, et al. Increase CSF level of endorphins in chronic psychosis. Neurosci Lett 1976;3:157–162.
47. Brown SA, Crowell-Davis S, Malcolm T, Edwards P. Naloxone responsive compulsive tail chasing in a dog. J Am Vet Med Assoc 1987;190:884–886.
48. Dodman NH, Shuster L, White SD, et al. Use of narcotic antagonists to modify stereotypic self-licking, self-chewing, and scratching behavior in dogs. J Am Vet Med Assoc 1988; 193:815–819.
49. Pickar D, Vartanian F, Bunney WE, et al. Short-term naloxone administration in schizophrenic and manic patients. Arch Gen Psychiatry 1982;39:313–319.
50. Greenberg D, Marks I. Behavioural psychotherapy of uncommon referrals. Br J Psychiatry 1982;141:148–153.
51. Lienemann J, Walker FD. Naltrexone for treatment of self-injury. Am J Psychiatry 1989;146:1639–1640.
52. Schwartz S. Naltrexone-induced pruritus in a dog with tail-chasing behavior. J Am Vet Med Assoc 1993;202:278–280.
53. Rossier J, French ED, Rivier C, et al. Foot-shock induced stress increases β-endorphin levels in blood but not brain. Nature 1977;270:618–620.
54. Sampson D, Willner P, Muscat R. Reversal of antidepressant action by dopamine antagonists in an animal model of depression. Psychopharmacology 1991;104:491–495.
55. Zuckerman S. Serotonin, impulsivity, and emotionality. Behav Brain Sci 1986;9:348–349.
56. Ricketts RW, Goza AB, Ellis CR, et al. Fluoxetine treatment of severe self-injury in young adults with mental retardation. 1993;32:865–869.
57. Fontaine R, Chouinard G. Fluoxetine in the long-term maintenance treatment of obsessive-compulsive disorders. Psychiatric Ann 1989;15:88–91.
58. Voith VL. Behavioral disorders. In: Ettinger SJ, ed. Textbook of veterinary internal medicine. Philadelphia: Saunders, 1989:227–228.
59. Overall KL. Recognition, diagnosis, and management of obsessive-compulsive disorders, Part II. Canine Pract 1991;17:25–27.
60. Overall KL. Recognition, diagnosis and management of obsessive-compulsive disorders, Part III. Canine Pract 1992;17:39–43.
61. Shanley KS, Overall KL. Psychogenic dermatoses. In: Kirk RW, Bonagura JD, eds. Kirk's current veterinary therapy. XI: Small animal practice. Philadelphia: Saunders, 1992:552–558.
62. Beaver BV. Animal behavior case of the month. J Am Vet Med Assoc 1993;203:651–652.
63. Hansen CPB. Stereotypies in ranch mink: the effect of genes, litter size and neighbours. Behav Proc 1993;29:165–178.
64. Blackshaw JK, Sutton RH, Boyan MA. Tail chasing or circling behavior in dogs. Canine Pract 1994;19:7–11.
65. Dantzer R, Mormède P. Behavioural consequences of frustration and conflict in pigs. In: Bessei W, ed. Disturbed behavior in farm animals. Stuttgart, Germany: Verlag Eugen Ulmer, 1982:87–100.
66. Fraser AF, Broom DM. Farm animal behavior and welfare, 3rd ed. London: Balliere Tindall, 1990.
67. Goosen C. Some causal factors in autogrooming behavior of adult stump-tailed macaques (*Macaca arctoides*). Behavior 1974;49:111–159.
68. Raab A, Dantzer R, Michaud B, et al. Behavioral physiological and immunological consequences of social status and aggression in chronically coexisting resident and intruder dyads of male rats. Physiol Behav 1986;36:223–228.
69. Sharman DF, Mann SP, Fry JP, et al. Cerebral dopamine metabolism and stereotyped behavior in early-weaned piglets. Neuroscience 1982;7:1937–1941.

70. Fraser D. Observations of the behavioural development of suckling and early-weaned piglets during the first six weeks after birth. Anim Behav 1978;26:22–30.

71. Delius JD. Preening and associated comfort in birds. Ann NY Acad Sci 1988;525:40–55.

72. Van Putten G, Elsof WJ. Inharmonious behavior of veal-calves. In: Bessei W, ed. Disturbed behavior in farm animals. Stuttgart, Germany: Verlag Eugen Ulmer, 1982:61–71.

73. Robins LN, Helzer JE, Weisman MM. Lifetime prevalence of specific psychiatric disorders in three sites. Arch Gen Psychiatry 1984;41:949–958.

74. Thyer BA, Parrish RT, Curtis GC, et al. Ages of onset of DSM-III anxiety disorders. Comp Psychiatry 1985;26:113–152.

75. Shell LG. Feline hyperesthesia syndrome. Feline Pract 1994;22:10.

76. Iggo A. Cutaneous receptors with a high sensitivity to mechanical displacement. In: de Reuch ABS, Knight J, eds. Touch, heat, and pain. London: CIBA Foundation, 1966:237–256.

77. Siegal A, Pott CB. Neural substrates of aggression in flight in the cat. Prog Neurobiol 1988;31:261–283.

78. Carlson Kuhta P, Smith JL. Scratch response in normal cats: hindlimb kinematics in muscle synergies. J Neurophysiol 1990;64:1654–1667.

79. Singh L, Lewis AS, Field MJ, et al. Evidence for involvement of the brain cholecystokinin B receptor in anxiety. Proc Natl Acad Sci USA 1991;88:1130–1133.

80. van Nes JJ. Electrophysiological evidence of sensory nerve dysfunction in 10 dogs with acral lick dermatitis. J Am Anim Hosp Assoc 1986;22:157–160.

81. Cummings JF, de Lahunta A, Winn SS. Acral mutilation and nociceptive loss in English Pointer dogs: a canine sensory neuropathy. Acta Neuropathol 1981;53:119–157.

82. Cummings JF, de Lahunta A, Braund KG, et al. Animal model of human disease: hereditary sensory neuropathy, nociceptive loss and acral mutilation of pointer dogs—canine hereditary sensory neuropathy. Am J Pathol 1983;115:136–138.

83. Cummings JF, de Lahunta A, Simpson ST, et al. Reduced substance P-like immunoreactivity in hereditary canine sensory neuropathy of pointer dogs. Acta Neuropathol 1984;63:33–40.

84. Garney MJ, Tollefson GD. Association of affective disorder with migraine headaches and neurodermatitis. Gen Hosp Psychiatry 1988;10:148–149.

85. Shanley K. Pathophysiology of pruritus. Vet Clin North Am Sm Anim Pract 1988;18:971–981.

86. Lawler CP, Cohen PS. Paw grooming induced by intermittent positive reinforcement in rats. Ann NY Acad Sci 1988;525:417–419.

87. Kraemer GW, Clarke AS. The behavioral neurobiology of self-injurious behavior in rhesus monkeys. Prog Neuropsychopharmacol Biol Psychiatry 1990;14:S141–S168.

88. Houpt KA, McDonnell SM. Equine stereotypies. Comp Cont Ed Pract Vet 1993;15:1565–1571.

89. McClure S, Chaffin MK, Beaver BV. Nonpharmacologic management of stereotypic self-mutilative behavior in a stallion. J Am Vet Med Assoc 1992;200:1975–1977.

90. Houpt KA. Domestic animal behavior for veterinarians and animal scientists, 2nd ed. Ames, IA: Iowa State University Press, 1991.

91. Houpt KA. Self-directed aggression: a stallion behavior problem. Equine Pract 1983;5:6–8.

92. Dodman NH, Normile JA, Shuster L, Rand W. Equine self-mutilation syndrome (57 cases). J Am Vet Med Assoc 1994;204:1519–1523.

93. Grindlinger H, Ramsay E. Compulsive feather picking in birds (letter). Arch Gen Psychiatry 1991;48:857.

94. Ramsay EC, Grindlinger H. Treatment of feather picking with clomipramine. Proc Assoc Avian Vet 1992:379–382.

95. Elkin I, Pilkonis OA, Docherty JP, Sotsky M. Conceptual and methodological issues in comparative studies of psychotherapy and pharmacotherapy. I. Active ingredients and mechanisms of change. Am J Psychiatry 1988;145:909–917.

96. Elkin I, Pilkonis OA, Docherty JP, Sotsky M. Conceptual and methodological issues in comparative studies of psychotherapy and pharmacotherapy. II. Nature and timing of treatment effects. Am J Psychiatry 1988;145:1070–1076.

97. Rang HP, Dale MM, Rittner JM, Gardner P. Pharmacology. New York: Churchill Livingstone, 1995.

98. Ananth J. Clomipramine: an antiobsessive drug. Can J Psychiatry 1986;31:253–258.

99. Messiha FS. Fluoxetine: a spectrum of clinical applications and postulates of underlying mechanisms. Neurosci Biobehav Rev 1993;17:385–396.

100. Flament MF, Rapoport JL, Berg CF, et al. Clomipramine treatment of childhood obsessive-compulsive disorder. Arch Gen Psychiatry 1985;42:977–983.

101. Nesbitt GH, Kedan GS. Differential diagnosis of feline pruritus. Comp Cont Ed Pract Vet 1985;7:163–168.

102. Overall KL. Use of clomipramine to treat ritualistic stereotypic motor behavior in three dogs. J Am Vet Med Assoc 1994;205:1733–1741.

103. Gram LF. Fluoxetine. N Engl J Med 1994;331:1354–1361.

104. McDougle CJ, Goodman WK, Leckman JF, et al. Limited therapeutic effect of addition of buspirone in fluvoxamine-refractory obsessive-compulsive disorder. Am J Psychiatry 1993;150:647–649.

105. Rickels K, Schweizer E. Clinical overview of serotonin reuptake inhibitors. J Clin Psychiatry 1990;51(suppl):9–15.

106. Teicher M. Biology of anxiety. Med Clin North Am 1988;72:791–814.

107. Grady TA, Piggott TA, L'Heureux F, et al. Double-blind study of adjuvant buspirone for fluoxetine-treated patients with obsessive-compulsive disorder. Am J Psychiatry 1993;150:819–821.

108. Montgomery SA, Bullock T, Fineberg N. Serotonin selectivity for obsessive-compulsive and panic disorders. J Psychiatry Neurosci 1991;16:30–35.

109. Snyder AH. Neurotransmitters and CNS disease: schizophrenia. Lancet 1982;319:970–973.

110. Gupta M, Gupta AK, Ellis CN. Antidepressant drugs in dermatology. Arch Dermatol 1987;153:647–652.

111. Suria A, Killam EK. Carbamazepine. Adv Neurol 1980;27:563–575.

112. Uhde TW, Boulenger J-P, Roy-Byrne PP, et al. Longitudinal course of panic disorder. Prog Neuropsychopharmcol Biol Psychiatry 1988;9:39–51.

113. Jones RD. Use of thioridazine in the treatment of aberrant motor behavior in a dog. J Am Vet Med Assoc 1987;191:89–90.

114. Crews WD Jr, Bonaventura S, Rowe FB, Bonsie D. Cessation of long-term naltrexone therapy and self-injury: a case study. Res Dev Disabil 1993;14:331–340.

115. Delgado PL, Charney DS, Price LH, et al. Serotonin function and the mechanism of anti-depressant action: reversal of anti-depressant induced remission by rapid depletion of plasma tryptophan. Arch Gen Psychiatry 1990;47:411–418.

116. Hess EH. Imprinting. New York: Van Nostrum, 1973.

117. Stanley WC, Elliot O. Differential human handling as reinforcing events and as treatments influencing later social behavior in Basenji puppies. Psychol Rep 1962;10:335–343.

118. Harlow HF, Harlow MK. Experimental psychopathology. New York: Academic Press, 1971.

119. Linscheid TR, Pejeay C, Cohen S, Footo-Lenz M. Positive side effects in the treatment of SIB using the self-injurious behavior inhibiting system (SIBIS): implications for operant and biochemical explanations of SIB. Res Dev Disabil 1994;15:81–90.

120. Thompson WR, Melzack R, Scott TH. "Whirling behavior" in dogs as related to early experience. Science 1956;153:939.

121. Rachman S, Levitt K. Panic, fear reduction, and habituation. Behav Res Ther 1990;26: 199–206.

122. Goldberger E, Rapoport JL. Canine acral lick dermatitis: response to the anti-obsessional drug clomipramine. J Am Anim Hosp Assoc 1991;27:179–188.

123. Rapoport JL, Ryland D, Kriete M. Drug treatment of canine acral lick: an animal model of obsessive-compulsive disorder. Arch Gen Psychiatry 1992;49:517–521.

124. Bullock JE. Acupuncture treatment of canine lick granuloma. Cal Vet 1978; April:14–15.

125. Rivers B, Walter PA, McKeever PJ. Treatment of canine acral lick dermatitis with radiation therapy: 17 cases (1979–1991). J Am Anim Hosp Assoc 1993;29:541–544.

126. White SD. Naltrexone for treatment of acral lick dermatitis in dogs. J Am Vet Med Assoc 1990;196:1073–1076.

127. Kaplan HI, Sadock BJ. Pocket handbook of psychiatric drug treatment. Baltimore: Williams & Wilkins, 1993;190–193.

128. Adamec RE. Behavioral and epileptic determinants of predatory behavior in the cat. Can J Neurol Sci 1975;2:457–466.

129. Adamec RE. Does kindling model anything clinically relevant? Biol Psychiatry 1990a; 27:249–279.

130. Adamec RE. Role of the amygdala and medial hypothalamus in spontaneous feline aggression and defense. Aggressive Behav 1990b;16:207–222.

131. Shaikh MB, Dalsass M, Siefel A. Opioidergic mechanisms mediating aggressive behavior in the cat. Aggressive Behav 1990;16:191–206.

132. Fraser D. Abnormal behaviour. Appl Anim Ethol 1980;6:311–313.

133. Hinde RA. Animal behaviour, 2nd ed. New York: McGraw-Hill, 1970.

134. Wiepkema PR. Developmental aspects of motivated behavior in domestic animals. J Anim Sci 1987; 65:1220–1227.

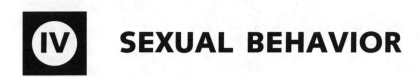

IV SEXUAL BEHAVIOR

Progestins: Indications for Male-Typical Problem Behaviors

10

Benjamin L. Hart

Robert A. Eckstein

Progestins, such as medroxyprogesterone acetate (MPA; Depro-Provera) and megestrol acetate (MA; Ovaban), are synthetic compounds that mimic the effects of the naturally secreted female hormone, progesterone. As such, progestins have powerful influences on various organ systems, most notably associated with the reproductive system (1), and are a mainstay of human oral or depository birth-control drugs (2,3). Progestins are used in treatment of breast cancer in women and in management of benign prostatic hyperplasia in men. The progestin MPA was explored as early as 1970 for its effectiveness in suppressing pathologic sexual behavior in human males (4). The drug, now employed in injectable form, clearly has effectiveness in a variety of abnormal manifestations of sexual drive in human males (5–9).

Following a report by Gerber and Sulman (10) that a progestin was effective in suppressing urine-marking, roaming, and mounting in companion dogs and cats, a number of veterinary clinicians studied the effectiveness of progestins in countering problem behavior in cats and dogs (11,12). In more structured clinical testing, the promise of these drugs for reducing urine-spraying in cats (13) and intermale aggression in male dogs (14) was documented by clinical surveys. The original concept set forth for animal use was that one should expect progestins to be of value in treating problem behaviors typically associated with males (15,16).

Two widely acclaimed review articles by Pemberton (17,18) touted the value of progestins for treatment of a variety of canine behavior problems including raucous behavior, biting, hyperkinesis, obsessive barking, timidity, destructiveness, phobias, night howling, and killing poultry, but neither case details nor data from clinical surveys were mentioned in these reports. The one behavior problem for which Pemberton did refer to data was urine-spraying in cats. For this condition, he claimed a success rate of up to 80%, an estimate which, in retrospect, was probably overly optimistic (19). It has been known for a long time that progesterone, its metabolites, and progestins, in large doses, are nonspecific sedatives and anesthetics (1,20) and that some behavioral effects are undoubtedly brought about by this action. Pemberton (18) mentions excessive timidity and temporal lobe epilepsy in cats as being responsive to the tranquilizing or sedative effects of high doses of progestins. Experimental evidence points to a barbiturate-like action of progesterone and its metabolites that may partially control epileptic seizures (21).

Currently, the main indications for progestin therapy in animals are for problem behaviors typically associated with males, such as urine-marking, aggression, and objectionable sexual mounting. However, currently available anxiolytic drugs may also alter these behaviors. Because progestins induce undesirable physiologic changes in other hormonal systems (e.g., adrenal cortex; see under Adverse Side Effects), they should probably be reserved for cases where anxiolytics have proven ineffective.

Progestins and testosterone both modulate male-typical behavior, though in different ways. The medial preoptic area and anterior hypothalamus are the principal sites of action of both of these steroids (22), and these brain regions are critical areas controlling male sexual and urine-marking behavior (23). However, progestins generally suppress male-typical sexual behaviors, whereas testosterone activates or maintains them. Male-typical behaviors are usually reduced or eliminated by removal of testosterone.

Some background information regarding the concept of sexually dimorphic behavior and the effects of testosterone on behavior is helpful in understanding the clinical use of progestins. As a historical perspective, it is interesting to note that the hormonal alteration of undesirable, sex-typical behavior of male animals is almost as old as the domestication process itself. For thousands of years, castration of cattle, sheep, goats, and swine has been a routine husbandry practice. It is testimony to the effectiveness of testosterone elimination in reducing aggression and undesirable sexual responses of males that the operation was so widely adopted and remains a current practice. The castration of male companion animals is a more recent development, but it is now routine to castrate immature male cats to prevent urine-spraying, roaming, and aggression, and to castrate male horses to prevent stallion-like sexual behavior and aggressiveness toward humans. However, in contrast to the reliable morphologic effects of castration in causing atrophy of accessory sex glands, such as the prostate gland or seminal vesicles, even casual observation of farm animals and pets reveals that castration does not uniformly alter male-typical behavior in all animals. The implications of such observations with regard to progestin therapy are discussed in this chapter.

Sexually Dimorphic Behaviors

Late in the prenatal life of male dogs and cats there is a surge of gonadal testosterone that acts on the brain to bring about gender-specific cytoarchitectural changes in the hypothalamus and other areas of the brain related to the display of male-like behavior. These neuroanatomic changes predispose males to urine-marking, mounting, roaming, and some aspects of aggressive behavior, especially after activation by testosterone at the time of puberty (24). Hypothalamic areas of the female brain are organized in a female direction due to the lack of prenatal testosterone, and females are less predisposed to engage in male-typical behavior even if given testosterone. Both males and females have the neural circuitry for behavioral patterns typical of both sexes, however, and the behavioral differences between males and females are not absolute but are of probability or frequency. Females can, and do, show male-typical patterns of urine-marking, mounting, and aggressive behavior, and males can show the female-typical responses (23).

Effects of Castration

There are experimental studies of castration in laboratory dogs and cats, as well as owner surveys, that yield information regarding species differences in the effects of castration. This information is also pertinent to the use of progestin therapy. Laboratory studies have shown that only 50% of male cats still showed copulatory behavior 5 weeks after castration, whereas 80% of male dogs showed copulatory behavior even 15 weeks after castration. Fifty percent of male dogs still showed the ejaculatory pattern of the genital lock 1 year after castration (25). Differences between cats and dogs appear to be a function of the sensitivity of the neural tissue to androgen withdrawal.

In addition to species differences, there are pronounced individual differences within a species illustrated by the fact that following castration some individuals retain the complete pattern of copulation for over 1 year, while others with the same sexual experience no longer show any sexual behavior after a few weeks. Experience in performing copulatory behavior has no predictive value as to whether or not the animal will continue to show the behavior following castration (25).

Laboratory studies revealing the efficacy of castration in altering sexual behavior in cats are consistent with a clinical survey of the use of castration in tom cats to reduce fighting with other males, urine-spraying, and roaming (26). In the latter survey, castration was effective in reducing these behaviors in 80 to 90% of cats. Among the cats in which the behaviors were changed, about half were reported to have changed rapidly (within 1 or 2 weeks) and the other half more gradually.

In accordance with the laboratory studies showing that castration does not change sexual behavior as readily in male dogs as male cats, two clinical surveys indicated a smaller percentage of male dogs showing changes in male-typical behavior following castration than male cats. In one of these reports (a retrospective case survey), urine-marking, mounting, and intermale fighting were reduced in only 50 to 60% of adult male dogs, although roaming was reduced in 90% (27). In a more recent retrospective survey of 57 owners of male dogs (age range 2–10 yr), owners were questioned about nine different behavior patterns and were asked to estimate the percentage improvement in these behaviors following castration (28). There were statistically significant decreases in urine-marking in the house, mounting, aggression toward human family members, aggression toward other dogs in the household, aggression toward unfamiliar dogs, and aggression toward human territorial intruders. There were no significant changes in fears of inanimate stimuli and aggression toward unfamiliar people (away from the home). The three behavior patterns showing the greatest probability of improvement were urine-marking, mounting, and roaming, in which about two-thirds of the dogs improved by at least 50% and one-third of dogs improved by at least 90%. Less than one-third of males showed a reduction of at least 50% in aggressive behaviors. Thus, while castration may affect a number of male-typical behavior patterns in dogs, the chances of altering the behavior vary depending on the behavior in question. A noteworthy finding of this survey was the complete absence of any statistical correlation between age of the dog, or duration of problem behavior at time of castration, and percent improvement following castration.

There is no way of knowing how many of the reported behavioral changes associated with castration reflect a placebo effect. Owners may have believed the operation had more effect than it really did, or they may have instituted environmental changes or behavior modification that altered behavior (29). Of course, such placebo effects are also possible with progestin therapy, as with any psychotropic drug treatment. With this caveat in mind, concepts from research on the effects of castration that would be anticipated to apply to progestin treatment are:

1. The behavior patterns that one expects to be altered are those that are sexually dimorphic and characteristic of males.
2. Progestins are more likely to change objectionable male-typical behavior in cats than in dogs.
3. Some behavior patterns are more likely to be altered by progestins than others. For example, in dogs, one would expect a lower efficacy in the treatment of aggression toward a human family member than in urine-marking in the house.
4. There are likely to be pronounced individual differences in the response to progestin treatment.
5. The age of the animal and the experience it has had in performing the behavior prior to treatment will not predict the response to progestin treatment.

Bearing in mind that both sexes have the neural circuitry for male-typical behavior, progestins may be given to both males and females that are displaying objectionable male-like behavior. Because progestins can induce cystic endometrial hyperplasia, mucometria, and pyometria, they are not recommended for intact females.

Mechanisms of Action

A well-known effect of progestins is to suppress the production of testosterone in gonadally intact males through the gonadotropic negative feedback mechanism. Suppression of testosterone is thought to be one of the mechanisms by which MPA lowers the deviant sex drive of treated male sex offenders (5–7). One would expect that this anti-sex drive effect would be less pronounced than castration because androgen levels are merely suppressed and not reduced to castration levels. However, as documented in clinical trials in cats, progestins suppress male-like behavior (e.g., urine-spraying) in already castrated male animals, so testosterone reduction obviously does not entirely account for the suppressant action of progestins on male behavior.

The neural mechanism of action of progesterone and progestins was initially thought to occur primarily by binding to cytosolic receptors, with effects on male behavior mediated by inhibition of 5-alpha steroid reductase (30,31). More recent research reveals that behavioral and physiologic effects can be brought about by diverse modes of action, sometimes with multiple mechanisms responsible for the same behavioral or physiologic endpoints. Evidence exists now for at least three types of effects of progestins: 1) altering the binding of a transcription factor to DNA, 2) affecting membrane fluidity, and 3) acting on $GABA_A$ receptors to produce effects similar to those observed after administration of benzodiazepines (1). A report suggesting increased beta-endorphin and met-enkaphalin levels in the hippocampus following progesterone administration is also intriguing (32).

Clinical Use

Two types of long-acting progestins are conventionally used on animals, and these are the same as those frequently used in human medicine, namely MPA, an injectable form, and MA, an oral medication form. The half-life of MA in the blood of human patients has been estimated at 8 days (33). In contrast, the blood concentration of MPA in humans is estimated to plateau at 3 months and decline gradually thereafter (34). This information profiles the differences in pharmacokinetics between MA and MPA but is not directly applicable to domestic species. No pharmacokinetic data are currently available for progestins in domestic animals.

Virtually all behaviors for which progestins are indicated are influenced by environmental factors, management, behavior modification, and/or pet-owner interactions. Thus, unless one is planning to maintain an animal on the drug therapy indefinitely, simultaneous environmental adjustments and behavior modification are required.

Of the clinical trials on progestin therapy to date, the most extensive data are provided by Cooper and Hart (19) who report on 60 cats treated for urine-marking (35 males, 25 females). Treatment was judged to be successful if

Table 10.1. Recommended dosage regimen for progestin therapy

Drug	Dosage
Medroxyprogesterone Acetate	
Cat	100 mg per male cat, SQ or IM, one injection
	50 mg per female cat, SQ or IM, one injection
Dog	5–10 mg/kg, SQ or IM, one injection
Megestrol Acetate	
Cat	5 mg per cat sid × 2 mo
Dog	0.5–1.0 mg/kg sid × 2 mo

problem urine-marking ceased or was markedly reduced. In this study, there was no indication of a difference in effectiveness between MPA and MA. Overall, 42% of the cats treated with progestin responded favorably. A significantly higher percentage of males than females responded to this treatment. The effectiveness of progestins in females was less than that reported for diazepam and buspirone, but in male cats progestins were about as effective as the two anxiolytics.

A small-scale clinical survey showing the effectiveness of MPA on intermale aggression in 8 dogs found that 75% of problem males responded (14). With regard to the effectiveness of progestins on dominance aggression in dogs and aggression in cats, the only information available is in the form of individual case reports (35,36). Until additional clinical trials are conducted, one can tentatively assume progestins may be clinically effective in some animals that exhibit problem urine-marking, mounting, or aggressive behavior (Table 10.1).

Returning to the castration model for predicting the effects of progestins on objectionable male-typical behavior, it is clear that the most sexually dimorphic behaviors, for example, urine-marking and mounting, are more easily treatable than aggressive behavior, though not all treated animals will respond. The castration model also suggests that comparable problem behaviors of cats will be more readily altered than in dogs. Extrapolating from clinical findings on urine-spraying in cats, a higher probability of success is expected with males (castrated) than females. Finally, there is no reason to believe that the age or experience of the animal in performing the behavior will influence the likelihood of success when progestins are employed for the treatment of sexually dimorphic behaviors.

Adverse Side Effects

The potential adverse side effects of progestins have received a good deal of attention. The most serious potential effect is probably adrenal cortical suppression, with a decrease in resting cortisol and a decrease in cortisol elevation after adrenocorticotropic hormone (ACTH) stimulation. This impairment is reversible even after 6 to 12 months of MA administration in cats (37). The effect of MA on cortisol was somewhat more severe than that in cats given prednisolone (38). The effects of MA on cortisol are mirrored by a reduction of adrenal cortex thickness (39).

Another side effect, noted in both cats and humans, is precipitation of diabetes mellitus, especially in prediabetic cats (40) and chronically ill human patients (41). Glucose tolerance is compromised in MA-treated cats (37,42). In some cats, mammary gland hyperplasia and tumors have been reported (43), and benign tumors have occurred in dogs treated with MPA (39).

An interesting side effect of progestins is appetite stimulation, noted frequently in cats (13) and in human patients (44). In human patients with diseases that produce anorexia and/or cachexia, MA has been shown to stimulate appetite (45,46).

Conclusion

Behavior problems for which progestins are indicated are often so serious as to threaten the animal's existence in a household as a companion pet. Therefore, as long as the clinician takes precautions, as one would with the administration of other synthetic steroids that affect the adrenal cortex, the long-acting progestins would appear to have their place in behavioral pharmacology. No adverse effects have been seen in humans after years of treatment (2,3); however, the doses used in animal behavior therapy are relatively larger than those used in humans for contraception or in treating sexual deviancy. The potential value of using progestins for treatment of objectionable male-like behavior, especially when anxiolytics have been ineffective, takes advantage of the concept that the progestins act in brain areas specific to the mediation of male-typical behavior and through cellular mechanisms different than those of commonly used anxiolytics.

References

1. Mahesh VB, Brann DW, Hendry LB. Diverse modes of action of progesterone and its metabolites. J Steroid Biochem Mol Biol 1996;56:209–219.
2. Westhoff C. Depot medroxyprogesterone acetate contraception: metabolic parameters and mood changes. J Reprod Med 1996;41:401–406.
3. Hickey M, Fraser I. The contraceptive use of depot medroxyprogesterone acetate. Clin Obstet Gynecol 1995;38:849–858.
4. Money J. Use of an androgen-depleting hormone in the treatment of male sex offenders. J Sex Res 1970;6:165–172.
5. Kravitz HM, Haywood TW, Kelly J, et al. Medroxyprogesterone treatment for paraphiliacs. Bull Am Acad Psychiatry Law 1995;23:19–33.
6. Gottesman HG, Schubert DS. Low-dose oral medroxyprogesterone acetate in the management of the paraphilias. J Clin Psychiatry 1993;54:182–188.

7. Cooper AJ, Sandhu S, Losztyn S, Cernovsky Z. A double-blind placebo controlled trial of medroxyprogesterone acetate and cyproterone acetate with seven pedophiles. Can J Psychiatry 1992;37:687–693.

8. Cordoba OA, Chapel JL. Medroxyprogesterone acetate antiandrogen treatment of hypersexuality in a pedophiliac sex offender. Am J Psychiatry 1983;140:1036–1039.

9. Gagne P. Treatment of sex offenders with medroxyprogesterone acetate. Am J Psychiatry 1981;183:644–646.

10. Gerber HA, Sulman FG. The effect of methyloestrenolone on oestrus, pseudopregnancy, vagrancy, satyriasis and squirting in dogs and cats. Vet Rec 1964;76:1089–1092.

11. Hart BL. Evaluation of progestin therapy for behavioral problems. Feline Pract 1979;9:3:11–14.

12. Hart BL. Indications of progestin therapy for problem behavior in dogs. Canine Pract 1979;6:5:10–14.

13. Hart BL. Objectionable urine spraying and urine marking in cats: evaluation of progestin treatment in gonadectomized males and females. J Am Vet Med Assoc 1980;177:529–533.

14. Hart BL. Progestin therapy for aggressive behavior in male dogs. J Am Vet Med Assoc 1981;178:1070–1071.

15. Hart BL. Problems with objectionable sociosexual behavior of dogs and cats: therapeutic use of castration and progestins. Comp Cont Ed 1979;1:461–465.

16. Hart BL, Hart LA. Canine and feline behavioral therapy. Philadelphia: Lea & Febiger, 1985:134–145.

17. Pemberton PL. Feline and canine behavior control: progestin therapy. In: Kirk R, ed. Current veterinary therapy VII: small animal practice. Philadelphia: Saunders, 1980:845–853.

18. Pemberton PL. Canine and feline behavior control: progestin therapy. In: Kirk R, ed. Current veterinary therapy VIII: small animal practice. Philadelphia: Saunders, 1983:62–71.

19. Cooper LL, Hart BL. Comparison of diazepam with progestins for effectiveness in suppression of urine spraying behavior in cats. J Am Vet Med Assoc 1992;200:797–801.

20. Gyermek L. Pregnenolone: A highly potent naturally occurring hypnotic-anesthetic agent. Proc Soc Exp Biol Med 1967;125:1058–1062.

21. Tauboll E, Lindstrom S. The effect of progesterone and its metabolite 5 alpha-pregnan-3 alpha-ol-20-one on focal epileptic seizures in the cat's visual cortex in vivo. Epilepsy Res 1993;14:17–30.

22. Rees HD, Bonsall RW, Michael RP. Pre-optic and hypothalamic neurons accumulate (-sup-3H) medroxyprogesterone acetate in male cynomolgus monkeys. Life Sci 1986;39:1353–1359.

23. Hart BL, Leedy MG. Neurological bases of males sexual behavior: a comparative analysis. In: Adler N, Pfaff D, Goy R, eds. Handbook of behavioral neurobiology, vol. 7. Reproduction. New York: Plenum Press, 1985:373–422.

24. Hart BL, Eckstein RA. The role of gonadal hormones in the occurrence of objectionable behaviours in dogs and cats. Appl Anim Behav Sci 1997;52:331–344.

25. Hart BL. Gonadal androgen and sociosexual behavior of male mammals: a comparative analysis. Psychol Bull 1974;81:383–400.

26. Hart BL, Barrett RE. Effects of castration on fighting, roaming, and urine spraying in adult male cats. J Am Vet Med Assoc 1973;163:290–292.

27. Hopkins SG, Schubert TA, Hart BL. Castration of adult male dogs: effects on roaming, aggression, urine marking, and mounting. J Am Vet Med Assoc 1976;168:1108–1110.

28. Neilson JC, Eckstein RA, Hart BL. Effects of castration on behavior of male dogs with reference to the role of age and experience. J Am Vet Med Assoc 1996 (in press).

29. Hart BL, Cliff KD. Interpreting published reports of extra-label drug use with special reference to reports of drug use to correct problem behavior in animals. J Am Vet Med Assoc 1996;209:1382–1385.

30. Gupta C, Bullock LP, Bardin CW. Further studies on the androgenic, anti-androgenic, and synandrogenic actions of progestins. Endocrinology 1978;102:736–744.
31. Siegel HI, Senatore A, Rogers S, Ahdieh HB. Cytosolic progestin receptors after single and multiple steroid treatments and during the estrous cycle. Horm Behav 1989;23:173–184.
32. Gordon FT, Soliman MR. Diurnal variation in the acute effects of estradiol and progesterone on beta-endorphin and met-enkephalin levels in specific brain regions of ovariectomized rats. Pharmacology 1994;49:192–198.
33. Chainey D, McCoubrey A, Evans JM. The excretion of megestrol acetate by beagle bitches. Vet Rec 1970;86:278–288.
34. Mishell DR Jr. Pharmacokinetics of depot medroxyprogesterone acetate contraception. J Reprod Med 1996;41:381–390.
35. Borchelt PL, Voith VL. Dominance aggression in dogs. In: Voith VL, Borchelt PL, eds. Readings in companion animal behavior. Trenton, NJ: Veterinary Learning Systems, 1996:230–239.
36. Borchelt PL, Voith VL. Aggressive behavior in cats. In: Voith VL, Borchelt PL, eds. Readings in companion animal behavior. Trenton, NJ: Veterinary Learning Systems, 1996:208–216.
37. Petersen ME. Effects of megestrol acetate on glucose tolerance and growth hormone secretion in the cat. Res Vet Sci 1987;42:354–357.
38. Middleton DJ, Watson AD, Howe CJ, Caterson ID. Suppression of cortisol responses to exogenous adreno hormone. Can J Vet Res 1987;51:60–65.
39. Selman PJ, van Garderen E, Mol FA, van den Ingh TS. Comparison of the histological changes in the dog after treatment with the progestins medroxyprogesterone acetate and proligestone. Vet Q 1995;17:128 133.
40. Romatowski J. Use of megestrol acetate in cats. J Am Vet Med Assoc 1989;194:700–702.
41. Henry K, Rathgaber S, Sullivan C, McCabe K. Diabetes mellitus induced by megestrol acetate in a patient with AIDS and cachexia. Ann Intern Med 1992;116:53–54.
42. Middleton DJ, Watson AD. Glucose intolerance in cats given short-term therapies of prednisolone and megestrol acetate. Am J Vet Res 1985;46:2623–2625.
43. Frank DW, Kirton KT, Murchison TE, et al. Mammary tumors and serum hormones in the bitch treated with medroxyprogesterone acetate or progesterone for four years. J Fert Steril 1979;31:340–346.
44. Aisner J, Parnes H, Tait N, et al. Appetite stimulation and weight gain with megestrol acetate. Semin Oncol 1990;17:2–7.
45. Donnelly S, Walsh TD. Low-dose megestrol acetate for appetite stimulation. J Pain Sympt Manag 1995;10:182–183.
46. Von Roenn JH. Randomized trials of megestrol acetate for AIDS-associated anorexia. Oncology 1994;1:19–24.

Pharmacologic Approaches to Urine-Marking in Cats

Robert A. Eckstein

Benjamin L. Hart

The most common category of feline behavior problems for which veterinary consultation is sought is problem elimination (1). When a cat is presented for problem urination, three main diagnostic categories must be considered and differentiated by the clinician. These categories are organic disease, inappropriate elimination, and urine-marking.

A wide variety of organic diseases may be manifested as an elimination problem. Cats with lower urinary tract disease may eliminate in unusual locations associated with pain, urgency, and/or increased urination frequency. Additionally, any cause of polyuria in the cat, such as diabetes mellitus or renal insufficiency, may lead to problem urination. Cats should be medically examined to rule out underlying organic disease before treating problem urination as a behavior problem.

The term *inappropriate elimination* denotes urination or defecation away from acceptable locations when there is no identifiable organic disease, and a communication function (marking) is not being served. For most cats, this means eliminating outside the litter-box. The most common cause of inappropriate elimination is litter-box aversion due to inadequate hygiene. Unpleasant experiences associated with the litter-box (such as being harassed by a puppy while in the box) also may lead to litter-box aversions. Additionally, cats may form elimination preferences for alternate locations or surfaces. Most cases of inappropriate elimination can be treated by behavioral means alone, without the use of psychoactive drugs. *Urine-marking* (spraying) is the deposition of urine in the environment which, in nature, would be a form of chemical communication with other cats. This chapter focuses on the diagnosis and treatment of this form of problem urination.

Diagnosis

It is of primary importance to distinguish between inappropriate urination and urine-marking, as the treatments differ. Table 11.1 may be useful in differentiating these two problems. Inappropriate elimination may involve urination,

Table 11.1. Differentiating inappropriate urination from urine marking

Behavioral Signs	Inappropriate Urination	Urine Marking
Posture	Squatting posture, fully emptying bladder	Standing, not fully emptying bladder; can be squatting
Litter box usage	Usually stops using box	Continues to use litter box for normal urination
Target areas	Suitable substrate such as carpet	Target areas, usually vertical, may have behavioral significance
Preliminary signs	Signs of aversion to box such as straddling box, shaking paws	Preceded by provoking stimuli such as new cats
Defecation behavior	Often accompanied by inappropriate defecation	Defecation behavior remains in box

defecation, or both. The litter-box or appropriate toilet area may no longer be used or may be used sporadically. When urination occurs, the normal squatting posture is used, and relatively large volumes of urine are typically deposited.

Urine-marking is usually performed from the standing position, tail up and quivering, while the cat alternately steps with the back legs and sprays urine on a vertical surface. Frequent targets are kitchen appliances, stereo speakers and walls. Using the same posture, urine may also be directed toward horizontal surfaces. Less frequently, objects, such as the owner's bed or clothing, may be marked from the squatting posture without spraying, but in the same context as spraying. According to available data, marking involves a vertical surface about 70% of the time and a horizontal surface about 30% of the time (2). Because urine-marking usually involves spraying, the terms urine spraying and urine-marking are often used interchangeably (as they will be here). With urine-marking behavior, the litter-box is usually still used for defecation and some urination. Often anxiety-provoking stimuli, such as the introduction of a new cat to the household, conflict between cats, or moving to a new household, can be identified as precipitating factors. There may be seasonal influences on the occurrence of urine-marking, stemming from stimuli associated with the breeding season.

Role of Hormones

Urine-marking reflects the interaction of several factors, including behavioral context, anxiety, and hormonal influences. Understanding the role of each of these factors is necessary when interpreting the cause of problem urine-marking. Urine spraying is a normal behavior of tom cats and presumably reflects an aspect of territoriality related to maintaining access to resources and repelling competing males. The behavior is under androgenic control, and there is some indication of seasonal fluctuations in the behavior. When blood testosterone levels are high (springtime) urine spraying is more prevalent in tom cats (3). Tom cats urine-mark prominent vertical objects within their territory, apparently with a view toward attracting the attention of neighboring cats venturing into the territory. It has been suggested that the reason why objects near territorial boundaries are often marked is not because perimeter marking delineates the territory, but because it is at territorial boundaries that animals frequently encounter competing conspecifics. In turn, these encounters provoke anxiety that may be manifested by urine spraying (4).

Although urine-marking is more typical of male cats, the behavior is also seen in females. The occurrence of urine-marking in females reflects the fact that the basic neural circuitry for this behavior exists in both sexes, although the behavior is more easily and intensively activated in males (5). A survey of over 154 owners of female cats spayed between 6 and 12 months of age revealed that 4% of the animals became frequent urine markers later as adults (6).

Therapeutic Approaches

CASTRATION

Customarily immature males are castrated between 6 and 12 months of age to control reproduction and to prevent undesirable male-typical behaviors, such as urine-marking, fighting, and roaming. However, the hormone-sensitive neural system responsible for the prevalence of these behaviors in males is organized late in fetal development under the influence of gonadal androgen secretion. Removal of testosterone by castration at 6 months of age does not eliminate the neural circuitry for urine-marking and does not completely eliminate the predisposition of male cats to urine-mark; castration simply removes the source of postpubertal activation of the underlying neural system (7). Nonetheless, castration of male cats before 10 months of age is quite effective in preventing urine-marking. A survey of 134 owners of male cats castrated between 6 and 10 months of age revealed that urine-marking occurred frequently in 12% of the cats as adults and on an occasional basis in 30% (6). The persistence of urine-marking in tom cats following castration is not due to residual amounts of testosterone, because testosterone is metabolized within hours of orchiectomy (8). Although not specifically studied in cats, work on laboratory rodents reveals that the maintenance of male-like behavior is not due to compensatory secretion of adrenal androgen (7).

In formulating a prognosis with regard to the effectiveness of treatments for urine-marking, the question arises as to whether male cats castrated before adulthood should respond to pharmacologic treatment more readily than cats not castrated until they are experienced urine-markers. Some perspective on this issue comes from survey data on the effects of castration performed in adulthood after urine-marking had become a problem and where the surgery eliminated or markedly reduced the problem in all but 13% of the animals (9). As mentioned previously, 12% of prepubertal castrates became frequent urine-markers as adults. Thus it would appear that castration at an earlier age is no more effective in preventing the behavior than in resolving the behavior in older males. By the same token, drug treatment of experienced males should be as effective as treatment of younger, less experienced males (assuming the drugs are working on the hormone-sensitive mechanisms).

PHARMACOLOGIC TREATMENT

Because antianxiety drugs are often used to successfully treat urine-marking, there is reason to believe that anxiety-evoking situations predispose cats to the initiation of urine-marking and that antianxiety drugs facilitate the cat's habituation to the anxiety-evoking circumstances, thus resolving the problem. Although the emphasis of this chapter is on pharmacologic treatment, behavior modification and environmental management approaches should be used in conjunction with pharmacologic treatment to increase the probability of pharmacologic therapy having the desired effect. Behavior modification possibilities are addressed after the discussion of pharmacologic treatment.

Pharmacologic treatment for urine-marking has evolved over the last two decades, starting with long-acting progestins (10,11), moving to benzodiazepine antianxiety drugs, particularly diazepam, and more recently involving serotonergic agents such as buspirone, amitriptyline and clomipramine. The progestins still have a role in treating urine-marking when anxiolytics prove ineffective. Progestins appear to be less effective for urine-marking in females than the commonly used anxiolytics, buspirone and diazepam, but are as effective in male cats (Figure 11.1).

COMPARISON OF DIAZEPAM AND BUSPIRONE

The problem of feline urine-marking which is often difficult to resolve with behavioral approaches alone, has prompted more clinical trials with pharmacologic treatment than any other clinical behavior problem. However, given the variety of possible psychoactive drugs currently available, there is still relatively little information from published clinical trials or case reports to guide the clinician as to the most useful or appropriate drug.

Open-label trials conducted with diazepam and buspirone provide some conceptual information that may apply to benzodiazepines and serotonergic drugs in general. In published trials, both drugs resulted in a reduction or cessation of urine-marking in 55 to 75% of cats (2,12,13). A higher percentage of cats from multiple-cat households respond to buspirone than those from single-cat households (2), perhaps as a reflection that living with other cats can be an anxiety evoking situation; this effect was not examined in the studies using treatment with diazepam.

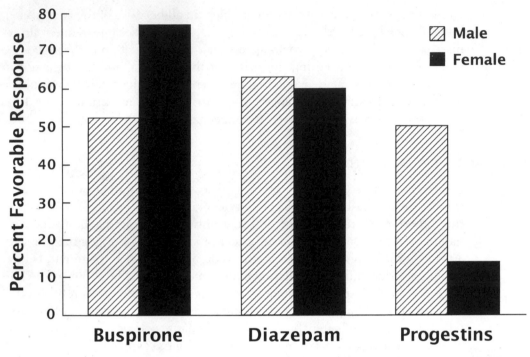

Figure 11.1.
Percentage of male and female cats from multiple-cat households responding favorably to buspirone, diazepam, or progestin. The difference in the responsiveness of the sexes was significantly ($P < .05$) different between buspirone and progestin, and between diazepam and progestin. (Modified from Hart BL, Eckstein RA, Powell KL, et al. Effectiveness of buspirone on urine spraying and inappropriate urination in cats. J Am Vet Assoc 1993;254–258.)

In comparing diazepam and buspirone, there is more than just efficacy to consider. Treatment with diazepam often causes a transient sleepiness and ataxia that does not occur with buspirone. Like other benzodiazepines, diazepam is dependency-producing with long-term use and can be associated with withdrawal reactions, an effect not seen in serotonergic drugs.

A recent report of acute hepatic necrosis in some cats treated with diazepam indicates that caution should be used in prescribing this drug (14). Diazepam should be discontinued and the cat examined medically if anorexia or vomiting occurs during treatment. Anorexia is a particularly useful marker of hepatic dysfunction, as diazepam typically acts as an appetite stimulant in cats. Lethargy and ataxia are less useful markers of this serious idiopathic reaction, because they are common side effects of diazepam therapy. A more intensive monitoring approach for this problem has been suggested, including biochemical screening for serum alanine transaminase and aspartase transaminase activity before and 3 to 5 days after diazepam therapy is initiated. However, some clinicians feel that this intensive and costly approach may not be currently justifiable given the apparent very low incidence of this idiopathic reaction.

A side effect noted with buspirone is an increase in aggression toward other cats, which was observed in 13% of treated cats. These cats were primarily from multi-cat households where the treated cat was previously reserved and avoided confrontations with the other cats. Apparently the drug resulted in a reduction of anxiety or fearfulness, and the treated cat then fought back when approached by the other cats.

The tendency for cats to resume marking once medication is discontinued is an important consideration in pharmacologic treatment of urine-marking. There is a major difference between the recidivism rates of buspirone and diazepam. In one survey 90% of animals successfully treated with diazepam for 8 weeks began urine-marking when the drug was discontinued (12). By comparison, only 50% of cats successfully treated with buspirone resumed urine-marking when this drug was discontinued (2). This difference probably reflects the fact that diazepam produces behavioral and physiological dependency, and discontinuing drug treatment results in emotional distress that predisposes cats to resume spraying. Conversely, buspirone is *not* a dependency-producing drug. Both buspirone and diazepam may suppress urine-marking in cats that were previously treated with progestins but failed to respond.

Like buspirone, amitriptyline and clomipramine, which are two other serotoneric drugs frequently used for urine-marking, do not produce dependency. Until further information is available, one could assume a treatment profile similar to that of buspirone with these other serotonergic drugs.

THERAPEUTIC PROTOCOLS

The treatment regimen suggested for any antianxiety drug is to conduct an initial 2- to 3-week trial to determine if the drug suppresses or reduces urine-marking (Figure 11.2). The dosage suggested for buspirone is 5 to 7.5 mg per cat, twice daily. The dosage range for diazapam is 1 to 2 mg per cat, twice daily. Treatment with amitriptyline is 5–10 mg per cat once daily, and clomipramine 0.5–1.5 mg per kg once daily. The initial trial is to determine if the drug will be effective. If the urine-marking behavior is significantly reduced, the cat should be treated for at least an additional 8 weeks before the drug is gradually reduced. Discontinuing the antianxiety drug will result in some cats resuming marking, while in others the behavior will remain suppressed (see Figure 11.2). Cats that resume urine-marking should receive long-term treatment for 6 to 12 months. After the drug is tapered off again, some animals can be expected to remain suppressed while others again will resume marking; these latter cats should be placed on the drug for even longer treatment.

If the clinician chooses to try progestin therapy, a recommended dose of the injectable progestin, medroxyprogesterone acetate (Deproprovera) is 25 mg for females and 50 to 100 mg for males; a single injection is given subcutaneously or intramuscularly. This should produce an effective pharmacologic blood level lasting for 1 to 2 months (15). An alternative form of progestin treatment

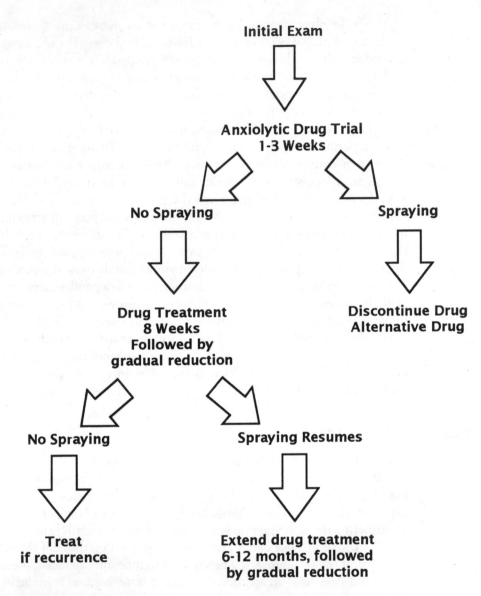

Figure 11.2.
Flow chart for suggested treatment regimen of urine-spraying by an anxiolytic drug.

is the orally administered megestrol acetate (Ovaban), given 5 mg per cat per day for 1 week. If effective, this drug should be continued for 1 to 2 months, before the dosage is decreased over 2 week intervals. Potential side effects of progestin treatment include: increased appetite, depression, adreno-cortical suppression, increased incidence of diabetes mellitus, and mammary gland tumors (16–21).

MECHANISMS OF ACTION

The three drugs that have been examined in clinical surveys for effectiveness on urine-marking (i.e., progestins, diazepam, and buspirone), have effects on different mechanisms in the brain. Progestins affect CNS activity through several possible mechanisms, one of which is to bind to cytosolic androgen receptors with a direct inhibiting effect on 5 alpha-steroid reductase in nerve cell bodies that are located within the hypothalamus and limbic system (22,23). Diazepam is bound by specific benzodiazepine receptors throughout the neuraxis and induces depression of neural activity through enhancement of gamma-amino butyric acid (GABA), an inhibitory neurotransmitter (24). Buspirone acts on serotonergic neurons by stimulating pre- and postsynaptic 5-HT_{1A} receptors. Because buspirone, diazepam, and progestins all use different neurotransmitter systems in regulating neural activity, one could justify attempting to use all of these drugs sequentially or in combination in different trials if necessary. For example, if buspirone seems to be ineffective after a 2 week trial, one could wait for a brief washout period and then administer diazepam.

Although not yet surveyed for effectiveness in clinical surveys, two drugs classified as antidepressants, amitriptyline (Elavil) and clomipramine, (Anafranil) have reportedly been useful for the treatment of feline urine-marking. They block the presynaptic re-uptake of bioactive amines, including serotonin, norepinephrine, and dopamine; clomipramine has a relatively greater effect on serotonin. Although buspirone also effects serotonergic neurons, it does so by acting on specific receptor types. Due to this difference in mechanism, it is reasonable to consider utilizing amitriptyline and clomipramine as therapeutic alternatives to buspirone and diazepam, as previously discussed.

ENVIRONMENTAL MANAGEMENT AND BEHAVIOR MODIFICATION

Although in many instances pharmacologic treatment may bring about resolution of a urine-marking problem without concomitant behavior modification approaches and environmental management, the simultaneous application of behavioral approaches to the problem can be expected to increase the probability and duration of the resolution effected by drug treatment (25). The behavioral approaches discussed here may be employed in an attempt to alter objectionable urine-marking prior to administration of pharmacologic treatments or concomitantly with the initiation of pharmacologic therapy (26). These alternative approaches are illustrated in Figure 11.3.

Environmental management is based on the fact that, with urine-marking, cats are attracted to the old target areas to maintain olfactory prominence by repeatedly marking the same area. By cleaning such areas with an enzymatic cleaner, it appears that the motivation is reduced for cats to remark

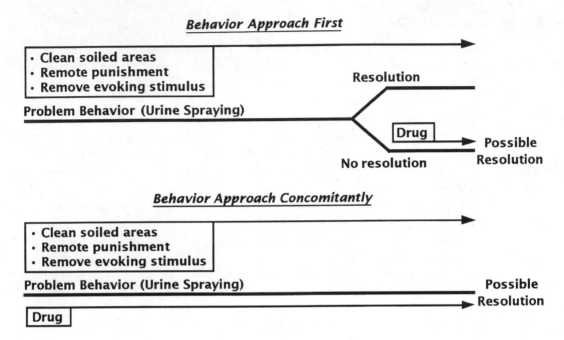

Figure 11.3.
Model of two approaches to treatment of urine-marking involving the integration of an anxiolytic drug with behavioral approaches. One may institute behavior approaches first, followed by drug treatment if necessary (top), or one may institute drug treatment and behavior approaches concomitantly under more urgent circumstances. (Modified from Hart BL. Behavioral and pharmacological approaches to problem urination in cats. Vet Clin North Am Small Anim Pract 1996;26:651–658.)

previously soiled areas. For some reason, kitchen appliances and stereo speakers seem to be common targets for urine-marking behaviors. Perhaps the chemical volatiles given off by electric insulating materials in the speakers and appliances attract cats to urine mark these areas as though another cat had previously visited and marked these objects. Such targeted appliances should be removed or covered for the duration of treatment.

Placing food or water near previously marked areas (after enzymatic cleaning) may help to control the problem. Remote punishment in the way of sticky tape (sticky side up) or electronically triggered alarms may be used to produce an aversion to marked sites if only one or two sites are targeted (27). The main problem with using remote punishment, or feeding and watering the cat at one or two marked sites, is that the cat is likely to switch its marking behavior to a new target. Thus, there is some rationale for using the pharmacologic approach to lower the motivation or reduce the anxiety involved in urine-marking together with selected use of behavioral approaches that reduce the strength of the anxiety provoking stimuli.

Interactive punishment, such as physically handling the cat, should be avoided, as this increases the level of perceived conflict and may actually increase the cat's motivation to mark. Most cat caretakers will want to use all means possible to resolve the marking problem, including both behavioral and pharmacological approaches.

One general concept in environmental management of urine-marking in multi-cat households is to reduce conflict between cats. This can be accomplished by increasing access to resources (food, water, litter), providing alternative routes to and from resources, and providing multiple perches for the cats. Sometimes visual stimuli from cats outside the house are involved in precipitating urine-marking behavior. In such cases, blocking the cat's visual access to the outdoors may be useful. This may mean covering up a window or restricting the cat's access to a room where it would otherwise see outdoor cats. For cats that mark only during the cat breeding season, one might plan to pharmacologically treat these animals each year as the breeding season begins.

A Model for Neural Mediation of Urine-marking

The fact that a variety of antianxiety drugs and progestins will eliminate urine-marking in some but not all cats, and that sometimes a cat that does not respond to one type of medication will respond to another, points to the possibility that there is more than one underlying neural substrate mediating urine-marking and that antianxiety drugs and progestins act differently (Figure 11.4).

Evidence of at least two different neural substrates comes from neurophysiologic studies showing that brain lesions in cats appear to have gender-specific effects on marking. Bilateral medial preoptic-anterior hypothalamic lesions, which typically inhibit male sexual behavior patterns (5), eliminated problem urine-marking in client-owned male cats but not in female cats (28). Olfactory tractotomy, on the other hand, eliminated urine-marking in female cats much more frequently than in male cats (29). While olfactory tractotomy eliminates an animal's sense of smell, the operation also induces neurologic changes in the limbic system in ways unrelated to the loss of olfaction (30,31). This could bring about changes in urine-marking through effects other than loss of olfaction.

In male cats the neural substrate involving the medial preoptic-anterior hypothalamic axis would be the predominant system driving urine-marking behavior. The system would be primarily suppressed by progestin administration as well as by the induction of lesions in the medial preoptic-anterior hypothalamic area. If this system is more active in males than females, one might expect this system to respond to progestin treatment more frequently in males than females, and this is what has been reported (10,12).

The neural substrate activated by anxiety would be affected primarily by antianxiety drugs. Anxiety mediated urine-marking should be observed about equally in male and female cats, and both genders would respond about the same to treatment with anxiolytics. This, too, is what has been reported

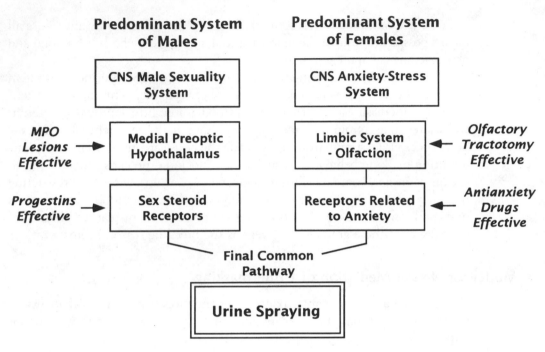

Figure 11.4.
Hypothetical model of a dual neuronal system of activating urine-spraying behavior. The differential effects of clinical neurosurgical procedures, namely medial preoptic hypothalamic lesions (MPO lesions) and olfactory tractotomy, as well as envisioned loci of actions of progestins in antianxiety drugs, are portrayed.

(10,12). It is possible that urine-marking in any particular cat may reflect the activation of just one system or the interaction of both mediating substrates.

Conclusion

The clinician's first task when presented with a cat who urinates out of the litter-box is to rule-out the possibility of underlying organic disease, and to distinguish between inappropriate elimination and urine-marking. Once the diagnosis of urine-marking is made, the clinician may combine the therapeutic approaches of neutering, behavior modification, and behavioral pharmacology. If the patient is not neutered, this is the best first step. Further treatment should include a combination of behavior modification and appropriate drug therapy for the best chance of problem resolution.

The psychoactive drugs currently in use for feline urine-marking include the serotonergic drugs buspirone, amitriptyline, and clomipramine, and the antianxiety drug diazepam. Progestins have been used historically and may still have their place when treating this problem when the serotonergic and antianxiety drugs have proven unsuccessful. All of the drugs mentioned come from diverse classes, with distinct mechanisms of action. Even the three serotonergic drugs differ in their specific mechanisms. Therefore, it is reasonable to try the recommended drugs in sequence, until one is found that helps to control the problem.

References

1. Borchelt PL. Cat elimination behavior problems. Vet Clin North Am Small Anim Pract 1991;21:257–264.
2. Hart BL, Eckstein RA, Powell KL, et al. Effectiveness of buspirone on urine spraying and inappropriate urination in cats. J Am Vet Med Assoc 1993;203:254–258.
3. Verberne G, Leyhausen P. Marking behavior of some viverridae and felidae. Time-interval analysis of marking pattern. Behavior 1976;58:192–253.
4. Ewer RF. The Carnivores. Ithaca, NY: Cornell University Press, 1973.
5. Hart BL, Leedy MG. Neurological bases of male sexual behavior. A comparative analysis. In: Adler N, Pfaff D, Goy R, eds. Handbook of behavioral neurobiology, vol. 7. Reproduction. New York: Plenum, 1985:373–422.
6. Hart BL, Cooper LL. Factors relating to urine spraying and fighting in prepubertally gonadectomized cats. J Am Vet Med Assoc 1984;184:1255–1258.
7. Hart BL, Eckstein RA. The role of gonadal hormones in the occurrence of objectionable behaviours in dogs and cats. Appl Anim Behav Sci 1997;52:331–344.
8. Hart BL. Problems with objectionable sociosexual behavior of dogs and cats: Therapeutic use of castration and progestins. Compend Cont Educ Small Anim Pract 1979;1:461–465.
9. Hart BL, Barrett RE. Effects of castration on fighting, roaming, and urine spraying in adult male cats. J Am Vet Med Assoc 1973;163:290–292.
10. Hart BL. Objectionable urine spraying and urine-marking in cats: Evaluation of progestin treatment in gonadectomized males and females. J Am Vet Med Assoc 1980;177:529–533.
11. Pemberton PL. Canine and feline behavior control: Progestin therapy. In: Kirk R, ed. Current Veterinary Therapy, vol. 8. Small Animal Practice. Philadelphia: Saunders, 1983.
12. Cooper LL, Hart BL. Comparison of diazepam with progestins for effectiveness in suppression of urine spraying behavior in cats. J Am Vet Med Assoc 1992;200:797–801.
13. Marder AR. Psychotropic drugs and behavioral therapy. Vet Clin North Am Small Anim Pract 1991;21:329–342.
14. Center SA, Elston TH, Rowland PH, et al. Fulminant hepatic failure associated with oral administration of diazepam in 11 cats. J Am Vet Med Assoc 1996;209:618–625.
15. Nash HA. Depo-Provera: A review. Contraception 1975;12:377–393.
16. Middleton DJ, Watson AD, Howe CJ, Caterson ID. Suppression of cortisol responses to exogenous adrenal hormone. Can J Vet Res 1987;51:60–65.
17. Romatowski J. Use of megestrol acetate in cats. J Am Vet Med Assoc 1989;194:700–702.
18. Middleton DJ, Watson AD. Glucose intolerance in cats given short-term therapies of prednisolone and megestrol acetate. Am J Vet Res 1985;46:2623–2625.
19. Petersen ME. Effects of megestrol acetate on glucose tolerance and growth hormone secretion in the cat. Res Vet Sci 1987;42:354–357.
20. Frank DW, Kirton KT, Murchison TE, et al. Mammary tumors and serum hormones in the bitch treated with medoxyprogesterone acetate or progesterone for four years. J Fert Steril 1979;31:340–346.
21. Selman PJ, can Garderen E, Mol FA, can den Ingh TS. Comparison of the histological changes in the dog after treatment with the progestins medroxyprogesterone acetate and proligestone. Vet Q 1995;17:128–133.
22. Gupta C, Bullock LP, Bardin CW. Further studies on the androgenic, anti-androgenic, and synandrogenic actions of progestins. Endocrinology 1978;102:736–744.

23. Henrik RA, Olson PN, Rosychuk RAW. Progestogen therapy in cats. Compend Contin Educ Pract Vet 1985;7:132–142.

24. Haefely W, Pieri L, Polc P, et al. General pharmaco-dynamics and neuropharmacology of benzodiazepine derivatives. In: Hoffmeister F, Stille G, eds. Psychotropic agents, Part 2. Anxiolytics, gerontopsychopharmacological agents, and psychomotor stimulants. Berlin: Springer-Verlag 1981:13–262.

25. Hart BL. Behavioral and pharmacological approaches to problem urination in cats. Vet Clin North Am Small Anim Pract 1996;26:651–658.

26. Hart BL, Cooper LL. Integrating use of psychotropic drugs with environmental management and behavioral modification for treatment of problem behavior in animals. J Am Vet Med Assoc 1996;163:1549–1551.

27. Hart BL, Hart LA. Canine and Feline Behavioral Therapy. Philadelphia: Lea & Febiger, 1985.

28. Hart BL, Voith VL. Changes in urine spraying, feeding and sleep behavior of cats following medial peptic-anterior hypothalamic lesions. Brain Res 1978;145:406–409.

29. Hart BL. Olfactory tractotomy for control of objectionable urine spraying and urine-marking in cats. J Am Vet Med Assoc 1981;179:231–234.

30. Edwards DA. Non-sensory involvement of the olfactory bulbs in the mediation of social behavior. Behav Biol 1974;11:287–302.

31. Wenzel BM. The olfactory system and behavior. In: DiCara LV, ed. Limbic and autonomic nervous systems research. New York: Plenum, 1974:1–33.

GERIATRIC BEHAVIOR

Geriatric Behavior Problems

Nicholas H. Dodman

Almost 20% of all dogs that are brought to the shelters and pounds for surrender are delivered there because they are "too old" (1). Any one of a number of age-related behavior changes can be the catalyst for such a decision. Some of the changes may relate to progressively intensifying behavior problems with insidious dissolution of the human-companion animal bond (2), but many are due to progressive, organic aging changes that are physical in nature.

Etiology

CENTRAL DEGENERATIVE CHANGES

In Chapter 13, we will learn about the cognitive dysfunction syndrome, the canine equivalent of Alzheimer's disease, in which cerebral aging changes adversely affect thought processing and, consequently, the animal's interactions and functioning in its environment. Affected dogs are slow to learn, less active, less responsive, and gradually lose control of bodily functions, most relevantly, elimination of urine or feces. Of all the trials that the owners of problem dogs face, "inappropriate elimination" as it is euphemistically called, is the one that seems to try the patience of owners the most. Houpt (3) reported a case of lissencephaly in a Lhasa Apso that had many learning disabilities and visual deficits. These shortcomings were tolerable for the owners, who only gave up on the dog when it lost bladder and bowel control. Fortunately, a new and effective treatment, L-deprenyl (use detailed in Chapter 13) has become available for use in cognitive dysfunction syndrome.

Central degenerative changes, however, are responsible for only a proportion of the behavioral changes affecting elderly dogs. Other reasons for altered behavior in the "golden years" include systemic disease, pain, deafness, visual problems, and social problems related to deteriorating health or the addition of new animals to the household (2).

SYSTEMIC DISEASE

If an elderly dog or cat is brought to a veterinary clinic suffering from behavior problems of recent onset, systemic disease must be high on the list of suspected contributing factors and should be ruled out by proper testing before initiating attempts at behavior modification therapy or pharmacotherapy. Brain tumors, renal disease, and hepatic disease can cause altered mentation and neurological syndromes in all species and hormonal/metabolic problems, such as hyperthyroidism in cats, can also impact on behavior. A full physical examination, complete blood count, chemistry profile, thyroid screen, and urinalysis are indicated in many cases of geriatric onset behavior problems. Sometimes additional testing (e.g., bile acids, plasma insulin assay, radiography, electroencephalography [with or without brain-stem auditory response testing], CT scan) may be required.

Even so, not all physical diagnoses will be revealed by routine testing of this nature, and it may be necessary to treat an animal palliatively until the condition can be diagnosed. A case in point was a dog seen at Tufts that had a relatively sudden onset of nocturnal separation anxiety. No physical cause for the dog's problems was found during extensive clinical and laboratory evaluation. Treatment, with buspirone, was palliative. A few weeks later the dog spontaneously fractured a limb and following radiography and a bone scan was found to have a disseminated bone tumor. A similar scenario occurred in a herding dog that started to herd shoes, hide in closets, and, eventually, to destroy doors and furniture when left alone. This dog also sustained a spontaneous limb fracture and was subsequently diagnosed with osteosarcoma. When the leg was amputated, the dog's anxiety ceased.

Many other insidious yet pernicious diseases can cause late-onset separation anxiety in geriatric dogs including conditions such as retrobulbar tumor, spinal cord disease, vetebral disc disease, arthritis, and intra-abdominal tumors. Pain and dysphoria which seem to make dogs more needy are often the root of geriatric onset separation anxiety problems syndrome. Conventional behavior modification programs are not of much value for such cases.

Treatment

The best therapy is, if possible, to eliminate or treat the cause of the problem. If this is not possible and if pain/dysphoria is involved, then analgesics and anxiolytics should be used to make the animal more comfortable. Which analgesic is indicated and in what dosage depends on the response to treatment. We often begin treatment with aspirin, escalating through aspirin/low-dose cortisone combinations (Cortaba TM), finally graduating to opioids, if necessary. *Butorphanol*, at approximately 0.25 mg/kg bid or tid, is probably one of the best choices because it is effective yet free from the legal restrictions that apply to its dependence-producing congeners. *Buspirone* is an excellent anxiolytic that can be combined with the analgesics previously mentioned to control anxiety accompanying this geriatric syndrome. Buspirone has no organ toxicity and few troublesome side effects to complicate treatment in these older patients. *Amitryptyline* is another useful agent for treating geriatric separation anxiety because it alleviates anxiety and, in addition, produces excellent analgesia (4). Benzodiazepines may be helpful to control separation anxiety in older patients.

Pain not only increases anxiety in previously timid or anxious animals, it can also exacerbate aggression in more dominant animals that are trying to protect themselves or that are irritable. Arthritis caused by, for example, hip dysplasia provides a classic example of a disease that causes pain in an aging dog. Other degenerative conditions, however, such as spinal disc protrusions or chronic ear disease, may also result in protective aggression. Painful conditions that elicit or aggravate agonistic responses are not limited to older animals, but wear-and-tear lesions of this type are more likely in this group of patients and should be suspected when an elderly animal starts to display increased irritability or frank aggression.

Sensory Loss

Sensory loss also may contribute to increasing aggression in older dogs. Cataracts or deafness, for example, may cause an animal to be surprised by the approach of others and thus to react disproportionately to their apparently sudden presence. Dominant dogs may be challenged by such rude awakenings; fearful dogs may be threatened. Either way, the retaliative response is practically the same. Also, because old dogs tend to sleep more, there will be more opportunity for supposed challenges of these semiconscious, sensorily deprived canine senior citizens. Treatment includes avoidance of threatening circumstances by a metered and well-advertised approach.

Phobias/Compulsive Behaviors

Other conditions that are prevalent in older dogs but not confined to them include various phobias, especially thunderstorm phobia, and some compulsive behaviors. Many fear- and anxiety-related conditions build over time and, if untreated, may attain their zenith in old age. Thunderstorm phobia can be compounded by comorbid separation anxiety, which itself may intensify in the face of age-related disability and pain. Treatment of phobias and compulsive behaviors is detailed in Chapters 5 and 6.

Social Problems

Social problems sometimes emerge as older dominant animals become less able to maintain their position in the hierarchy, especially if new, younger, and potentially dominant animals are added to the household. This scenario applies most commonly to domestic dogs and occurs when youngsters reach the challenging stage of adolescence while an older dominant dog is trying to preserve its social position. Any incapacitation of the older dog may cause the balance of power to swing in favor of the younger dog and may exacerbate interspecific aggression. Behavior modification and medical solutions to this problem are the cornerstone of treatment, but sometimes pharmacologic supportive therapy is also indicated.

Conclusion

Behavior problems in older dogs often arise from combined medical and psychologic disturbances. A thorough physical examination of such patients is always indicated, along with ancilliary diagnostic testing, to elucidate possible medical contributions to the problem. Unfortunately, there are no definitive tests for the all-too-common cognitive dysfunction syndrome, discussed in the next chapter, though finally a clearer clinical picture is beginning to emerge. Formal (FDA) approval of L-deprenyl for the treatment of this syndrome is likely to happen soon.

References

1. Rowan A. Shelter Statistics. Proceedings of Center for Animals Symposium at Tufts University Veterinary School, Boston, 1990.
2. Houpt KA, Beaver B. Behavioral problems of geriatric dogs and cats. Vet Clin North Am Small Anim Pract 1981;11:643–652.
3. Houpt KA. Learning. In: Domestic Animal Behavior for Veterinarians and Animal Scientists, 2nd ed. Ames, IA: Iowa State University Press, 1991:256.
4. Potter WZ, Husseini K, Manji HK, Rudorfer MV. Tricyclics and tetracyclics. In: Schatzberg AF, Nemeroff CB, eds. Textbook of Psychoparmacology. Washington, DC: American Psychiatric Press, 1995:141–160.

13 Canine Cognitive Dysfunction

William W. Ruehl

Benjamin L. Hart

Thanks to improvements in medical care, dogs, like people, are living longer; in fact, there are now more than 7.3 million pet dogs aged 10 years or older in the United States (1). Thus, a substantial number of elderly pet dogs are at risk for developing age-related medical and behavior disorders. Veterinary practitioners have long been aware of the occurrence of geriatric behavior problems in pet dogs, such as disturbance of normal sleep-wake cycles and housetraining. Such problems are usually referred to by pet owners and veterinarians as part of the "old dog syndrome," or, when severe, as "senility," and are incorrectly attributed by pet owners to "simple aging" or "normal aging." As discussed below, these behavior problems can sometimes be associated with histologic lesions in the brains of affected dogs that are very similar to lesions observed at autopsy in humans with dementia of the Alzheimer's type (DAT) (2).

Regardless of the cause of these behavior problems, many pet owners are frustrated by a perceived deterioration in the quality of life of their pets (who are often highly valued members of the family) as well as by the impact of sequelae exhibited by the dog, such as house soiling or nocturnal anxiety, on the human members of the family. As background for discussing possible pharmacologic approaches that hold promise for ameliorating geriatric behavior changes in dogs, we review a number of recent studies pertaining to age-related behavior changes in both dogs and human patients. New findings pertinent to practicing veterinarians include clinical presentation and course of the age-related behavior changes, prevalence, etiopathogenesis, results from neuropsychologic laboratory studies, and pharmacotherapy clinical trials in pet dogs. Building on this scientific foundation, pragmatic guidelines are presented to help veterinary practitioners diagnose and pharmacologically manage patients with cognitive dysfunction.

In this chapter, we use the term *cognitive dysfunction* (CD) to refer to the age-related or geriatric onset behavior changes that are not attributable to a general medical condition such as neoplasia or organ failure. In aging human patients, severe cognitive dysfunction, also referred to as dementia, is a clinical syndrome that involves a general decline of cognitive ability sufficient to produce functional disability in the workplace, socially, and/or as a family member (3). The diagnosis of human dementia specifies that a patient who was previously fully functional exhibits various signs of cognitive deficits that, in aggregate, "cause significant impairment in social or occupational functioning" (4). The cognitive deficits typically include signs of memory impairment, language disturbance, impaired ability to carry out motor tasks, failure to recognize familiar objects, and decreased ability to plan.

These signs in humans cannot all be directly applied to aging dogs, but some analogies to decrements or abnormalities in behaviors that were previously normally displayed are appropriate. As currently used in animal behavior, *cognition* refers to mental processes that are occurring within animals and cannot be directly observed; these include memory, learning, awareness, and perception (5). Behavior that in dogs would involve spatial orientation, memory, learning, housetraining, and recognizing and reacting to human family members are external manifestations of cognition. Age-related onset of impairment in these behaviors in dogs, which cannot be wholly attributed to sensory or motor impairment or general medical conditions, will be referred to as CD. From our experience collecting data on hundreds of aging dogs, we have found that many behavior changes can be assigned to the following categories: 1) disorientation, 2) decreased or altered social interactions or responsiveness to family members, 3) loss of prior housetraining, 4) disturbances of the sleep/ wake cycle, 5) and decreased activity.

Clinical Presentation and Course

As noted previously, veterinarians have long been aware of problematic behavior changes in elderly pet dogs (6–10). Several studies have explored brain pathology related to such behavior changes. In one study, for example, some dogs showed decreased exploratory behavior, decreased affection toward people and interaction with kennelmates, confusion, inability to locate food trays, loss of bearing, inability to localize sounds, difficulty with simple learning tasks, and/or loss of fastidious eating habits. Necropsy revealed ceroid lipofuscinosis, a mark of age-related neurodegenerative change (11). Similarly, a study found that elderly pet dogs whose brains exhibited lipofuscinosis and other neurodegenerative lesions at necropsy had displayed a variety of behavioral abnormalities, including disorientation and loss of housetraining (12).

Recent work utilizing clinical studies in pet dogs, as well as surveys of pet owners and practicing veterinarians, has been conducted to better define the presenting clinical features of canine CD. One study examined in detail 69 elderly pet dogs that were nominated for inclusion in the study by their owners according to the presence of one or more of the problems listed in Table 13.1 (6). Based on signalment, history, physical and neurologic examinations, complete blood count, and serum chemistry profile, dogs were excluded if they

Table 13.1. Incidence, severity, and response to 0.5 mg/kg once daily L-deprenyl treatment of behavior and cognitive problems in 69 elderly dogs, as reported by their owners. Source: (6).

| Problem | Percent of dogs affected at enrollment | | | | Response to L-deprenyl |
	Mild	Moderate	Severe	Total	
Housetraining	18	22	27	67	Improved**
Interest in food	26	12	4	42	Improved**
Activity, or attention to environment, including people or other animals	26	26	25	77	Improved**
Awareness and/or orientation to surroundings	17	28	23	68	Improved**
Ability to recognize familiar places, people, or other animals	25	22	16	63	Improved**
Ability to recognize/respond to commands or when called by name	17	19	44	80	Improved**
Hearing	7	12	68	87	Improved**
Climbing up or down stairs	22	31	25	78	Improved**
Tolerance to being alone	19	16	9	44	Improved
Development of compulsive behavior	25	32	12	69	Decreased*
Circling	13	10	6	29	Decreased**
Tremor or shaking	16	28	13	57	Decreased**
Wakes owner more at night and/or sleeps more in daytime	16	19	32	67	Decreased*
Inappropriate, persistent vocalization	19	7	16	42	Decreased
Increased stiffness or weakness	16	29	30	75	Decreased**

* P < .05; ** P < .01.

exhibited evidence of a concurrent systemic or debilitating general medical condition. The dogs that qualified for the study were 7 to 19 (mean = 13.5) years of age, with 73% older than 13 years, pointing to an increased prevalence with increasing age. Virtually all the dogs exhibited more than one of the problems listed in Table 13.1, with 46% manifesting eleven or more problems. The most commonly occurring signs included apparent hearing impairment, decreased activity and attention, and reduced ability to navigate stairs in the absence of musculoskeletal or visual impairment.

Typical of the dogs in the study was a 12-year-old female spayed English bulldog that had been showing signs for 6 months prior to being presented to a veterinarian for evaluation. Complete physical, neurologic, hematologic, and serum biochemical examinations did not explain the behavior problems, nor were any external influences identified to explain the problem behaviors. The signs included apathy, progressively decreasing activity, and an overall attitude suggesting that nothing could interest the dog any longer. She frequently became lost in the house and yard, and would often stare into space. There was also a severe hearing loss. Several sources of great frustration for the owner were that this previously well-housetrained dog started urinating in the house on an almost daily basis, was seen whining without obvious cause, and compulsively licked the floor. Small animal practitioners will recognize this case as representative of the commonly seen behavioral senility of dogs and what we refer to here as *severe CD*. This is also the type of patient in which the behavioral signs in aggregate correspond (with allowances for species differences) to those commonly recognized in people diagnosed with moderate or severe DAT (2–4,6).

For most human patients with DAT the onset is insidious, though the family often presents the patient because of the occurrence of some particularly noteworthy event or complaint. The course is generally slow, with progressive, usually stepwise deterioration of cognitive function (13,14). A typical case might span 15 to 20 years, from first evidence of memory impairment to death. The clinical diagnosis of DAT might not be made until approximately midway through the course. In advanced stages, the disease is characterized by loss of toilet hygiene, wandering, and uncooperative social behavior. During the latter stage, institutionalization for several years is customary. Death may result directly from neurologic deterioration but more frequently from sequelae such as aspiration pneumonia, urinary tract infection, or septicemia. Alternatively, the DAT patient might succumb to a concurrent general medical condition such as cancer or organ failure. The prevalence of DAT markedly increases with age, ranging from 1 to 3% of people ages 65 to 70 years, to as high as 47% in people over 85 years (15).

The similarity in behavioral signs of dogs diagnosed as having CD and human patients with DAT raises several questions of importance with regard to possible treatment. One obvious question is demographic: What percent of dogs at various ages exhibit CD? The analogy with human DAT predicts a positive correlation between age and the percentage of animals in a population showing CD. The second question relates to longitudinal changes in dogs that eventually are diagnosed as having CD. Is there a progression from initial behavioral signs, such as memory lapses, to signs of severe memory deficits or disorientation, along with increasingly antisocial behavior and failure of normal fastidiousness in toilet habits? Finally, there is the question of a neurologic cause. Are there clinicopathologic correlates that exist in dogs analogous to those seen in human DAT? The questions dealing with prevalence and neurologic cause or correlates have been, and are being, investigated. Preliminary findings from a prevalence study are presented next, followed by correlation of neuropsychologic study results with changes in brain histology.

Prevalence

In an ongoing study, we have addressed the prevalence of signs associated with CD in companion dogs that had been receiving adequate veterinary care (Neilson, Hart, and Ruehl, cited in 16). To date, 139 dogs, ages 11 to 16 years, which had been patients of the Veterinary Medical Teaching Hospital at the University of California—Davis have been selected; only those dogs for which there were no major debilitating general medical conditions or drug therapy that might explain the occurrence of the behavioral signs (evident from either the recorded history or from a screening interview with the client) were included.

A client interview form was developed using findings from the previous study of 69 dogs. Behavior changes examined to date were allotted a priori to four categories:

1. Changes in the usual sleep-wake cycle, such as increased daytime sleeping and less nighttime sleeping.
2. Changes in social interactions with the owner, such as decreased greeting behavior.
3. Signs of disorientation, such as becoming trapped in corners or behind furniture or staring into space.
4. Impairment in normal housetraining, with loss of signaling to go outdoors and house soiling.

There were specific questions under each of these categories, and depending on the category, criteria were established for the number of signs in each required for a positive score in that category. Figure 13.1 presents the data currently available.

Sixty-two percent of all dogs in the study (11–16 years) were scored positively in at least one of the four behavioral categories, but there was an increase from 32% in 11-year-old dogs to 100% in 16-year-olds. We also examined subsets of dogs who fulfilled the criteria for the category of disorientation and at least one additional category. For example, the criterion for

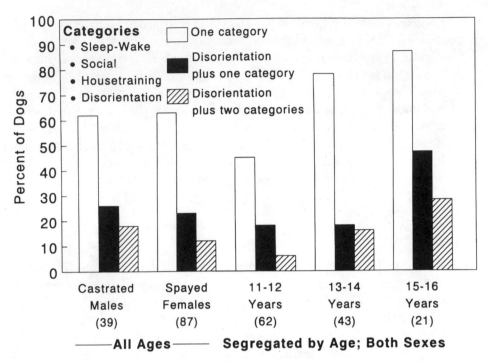

Figure 13.1.
Percent of dogs showing at least one behavioral category associated with cognitive dysfunction, and percent of dogs with each of two levels of cognitive dysfunction, expressed as having disorientation plus at least one other category, or disorientation plus at least two other categories. Source: Neilson, Hart, and Ruehl, (cited in 16).

scoring positive for disorientation plus one other category was met by 13% of 11-year-olds, but by 50% of 16-year-olds. The increase in the prevalence of CD categories with advancing years is clearly evident, reminiscent of the age-related increase in prevalence observed in elderly people. Within each age group the prevalence of CD signs in spayed females was similar to the prevalence in castrated males. At this time, there is an insufficient number of intact subjects for evaluation.

Systematic longitudinal studies of the course of CD in individual dogs have not yet been conducted. However, in surveys of more than 250 veterinarians throughout the United States and Canada, the practitioners reported that approximately 7% of pet owners who presented their otherwise healthy, elderly dogs for routine examination and immunization reported (without being prompted) that their pet exhibited one or more geriatric behavior problems typical of CD (Ruehl WW, unpublished data, 1996). The veterinarians also reported that from the time the signs of CD were brought to their attention by pet owners, or were sufficiently severe that they were evident at the time of physical examination, the dogs survived on average 18 to 24 months, typically with linear or stepwise deterioration of function. Dogs were ultimately euthanized due to clinical manifestations of CD, such as wandering or loss of housetraining, or due to physical signs of unrelated general medical conditions, such as cancer or organ failure. These observations, in addition to the data from Figure 13.1, indicate that elderly dogs, like elderly humans, often exhibit signs of CD and that the prevalence increases with advancing age.

The course of the condition in dogs is much shorter than in humans with DAT. Presumably this reflects the compressed lifespan of dogs. Furthermore, during routine examinations, unless the veterinarian specifically questions the owner regarding the occurrence of behavior changes in his or her elderly pet, the owner is likely to underreport the signs. This may be due in part to the owner's incorrect perception that the signs are due to "normal aging" and that "nothing can be done." In addition, the canine patients are often euthanized when housetraining is lost, which might be several months or years before death would otherwise occur.

In summary, the clinical course of CD in dogs is progressive and similar in nature to that seen in humans with DAT. Although the history and clinical presentation is unique for each dog with CD, as it is for each person suffering from DAT, a consistent set of behavioral patterns has emerged. This has allowed categorization of the behavioral signs, thus facilitating consistency in diagnosis, clarifying communication between veterinarians, and providing a framework for research in the clinically important areas of pathogenesis, prevalence, and efficacy of therapy. To address the question regarding clinicopathologic correlation, age-related cognitive changes in dogs were explored under controlled laboratory conditions and correlated with changes in brain histology.

Neuropsychologic Studies

Age-related declines in various aspects of cognition have been documented in humans and nonhuman primates as well as in laboratory rodents (17–20). Recent studies by Milgram et al have revealed a similar age-related decline of cognitive function in dogs in a variety of cognitive tasks known to be age-related in nonhuman primates, including object discrimination, reversal, object-recognition memory, and spatial memory (2,21,22).

The performance of young dogs was compared to that of elderly dogs for both pound-source animals and beagles born and housed exclusively in an institutional setting. The evaluation required the dog to solve progressively more difficult cognitive tasks. The findings confirmed that dogs, like other species, suffered age-dependent cognitive deterioration and, at advanced ages, were deficient in all tests except the simplest. In general, dogs that performed poorly on the object discrimination test also performed poorly on reversal and failed to solve the object-recognition task. With increasing age, there was a greater individual variability in cognitive performance. Interestingly, the performance variability of the elderly dogs largely reflected the existence of two subpopulations: those with cognitive impairment and those that were unaffected. The latter dogs may correspond to companion dogs—as well as to people—who remain cognitively intact into old age, sometimes referred to as "successful agers" (2).

Etiology and Pathogenesis

There are more than 60 recognized causes of dementia in humans, the most common of which is Alzheimer's disease, followed by vascular disease (23). The etiologies of these disorders and other age-related brain changes are unknown. Recent findings have emphasized the remarkable similarities between the brains of elderly dogs with CD and people with Alzheimer's disease (2,24,25). Additional work has established that the performance of dogs on some neuropsychologic tasks correlates strongly with the severity of Alzheimer's-like pathology present in the brains of affected dogs (26). A similar correlation between brain amyloid load and cognitive test scores exists in humans (27).

HISTOPATHOLOGY

The Alzheimer's-like neuropathology in dogs occurs primarily in the cerebral cortex and hippocampus, which are the same regions affected as in humans with Alzheimer's disease (2,24). The types of lesions in human Alzheimer's disease have been extensively documented, especially with respect to beta-amyloid accumulation, formation of plaques and neurofibrillary tangles, and other changes (28).

Neuropathology of aging dogs, but lacking behavioral history, was first reported in 1914 (29). A more recent study of brains obtained from elderly pet dogs with urinary incontinence, disorientation, and various other geriatric onset behavior problems showed meningeal fibrosis, lipofuscinosis, generalized gliosis, and ubiquitin-containing granules in white matter (12). Additional studies have described further histologic features including age-related cerebral vascular changes (30), thickening of the meninges, dilation of the ventricles, and age-related reactive gliosis (31). Other investigators have also documented Alzheimer's-like pathology in aged canine brains (32,33). At least some of the pathologic changes in aged canine brains may be genetically linked because, in a study of laboratory beagles, Russell et al (34) found congruence of pathology within 15 of 16 litters.

Perhaps the most significant histopathologic observations in old dog brains pertain to accumulations of beta-amyloid and its formation of plaques. Cummings et al (24) studied the pathology of elderly dog brains, focusing on plaque morphology and patterns of amyloid deposition, and confirmed that the lesions are very similar, although not identical, to those in the brains of humans with late-stage Alzheimer's disease. The subtle differences in plaque formation between humans and dogs, two species sharing the same environment and hence many of the same risk factors, may provide clues as to the cause(s) of CD and brain aging, perhaps ultimately leading to better management or prevention of CD in both species (2,6).

Because greater accumulation of beta-amyloid is associated with greater cognitive impairment in both dogs and humans, studies are under way to investigate mechanisms by which beta-amyloid might affect or correlate with cognitive impairment (26,27). The beta-amyloid present in the brain is different from the types of amyloid associated with diseases of other organs such as the kidney, liver, or pancreas. The amino acid sequences for the beta-amyloid proteins of dogs, cats, and humans have been ascertained to be identical (35). Beta-amyloid is neurotoxic and has numerous other properties, such as effects on ion channels, synaptic potentials, neurochemistry, and neuronal metabolism (2).

PATHOPHYSIOLOGY

A variety of neurotransmitter abnormalities have been described in Alzheimer's patients, including depletion or imbalances of acetylcholine, serotonin, norepinephrine, and dopamine. Depletion of catecholamines (norepinephrine and dopamine) from the prefrontal cortex has been correlated with CD in monkeys (36). The effects of norepinephrine are mediated via alpha-2 receptors, while the effects of dopamine appear to be mediated through D1, and possibly D2, receptors. Loss of norepinephrine and dopamine may substantially contribute to cortical cognitive deficits in aged monkeys and perhaps in other species as well. Intact cortical machinery appears to be necessary for full effect of catecholaminergic agonists, which may limit the clinical response to such drugs in patients severely affected with the degenerative changes of late-stage Alzheimer's-like pathology.

The enzyme monoamine oxidase B (MAOB) catalyzes dopamine breakdown, resulting in the production of free radicals. In a variety of species, brain MAOB activity is higher in the aged than in the young, and MAOB activities can be extremely high in patients with neurodegenerative disorders such as parkinsonism and Alzheimer's disease (37). These findings suggest a role in the treatment of CD for drugs that inhibit MAOB, facilitate dopaminergic tone, and/or decrease free radical burden.

ENDOCRINE ASPECTS

Endocrine and metabolic disorders can cause dementia in humans. For example, hypothyroidism is a recognized cause of dementia in people, but its role, if any, in canine CD is unclear. Interestingly, while recruiting dogs for a chemotherapeutic clinical trial in progress, we have encountered numerous dogs with signs of CD and documented dysregulation of the hypothalamic pituitary adrenal (HPA) axis, including elevated urinary cortisol/creatinine and lack of suppression of plasma cortisol concentration subsequent to intravenous administration of 0.01 mg/kg dexamethasone (38). These dogs did not exhibit clinical signs typical of Cushing's syndrome, such as polyuria, polydipsia, polyphagia, alopecia, or changes in body conformation. Studies of humans with DAT have revealed that 27 to 52% of these patients also exhibit HPA axis dysregulation, such as lack of suppression subsequent to dexamethasone administration (39,40). In a recent prospective study in humans with mild cognitive impairment, the existence of "subclinical" imbalance of the HPA axis was associated with subsequent further deterioration of cognitive ability (41).

Conversely, behavioral manifestations have been well described in humans with Cushing's syndrome (42). Dogs with pituitary-dependent hyperadrenocorticism (PDH) also exhibit behavioral or cognitive signs, such as lethargy, panting, and alterations of sleep/wake cycle, as well as changes in greeting behavior and decreased responsiveness to their owners (43,44).

Dysregulation of the HPA axis in dogs is associated with hypothalamic dopamine depletion (45). Further work is needed to determine the extent to which HPA axis dysregulation, dopamine depletion, or other endocrine imbalances might be related to CD in canine patients.

Pharmacotherapy—General Considerations

STRATEGIES

For dogs with behavioral signs due at least in part to a general medical condition (e.g., neoplasia, infection, organ failure) or display of problematic, yet normal behavior, treatment is directed toward the specific cause. In other dogs with geriatric behavior problems, the above-mentioned causes are not present or may not account completely for the behavior problems; presumably the CD signs in these patients are related to Alzheimer's-like pathology (2,24–27). Therapeutic strategies for these dogs should parallel those for humans with DAT and should be focused on two areas (46). The first approach is symptomatic and seeks to replace depleted neurotransmitters and facilitate their metabolism; the second approach seeks to slow or reverse the progression of the disease process.

Interest in repleting neurotransmitter levels or promoting their metabolism increased greatly following demonstration that brains of DAT patients are depleted of several neurotransmitters including dopamine, serotonin, norepinephrine, and especially acetylcholine (46). These neurotransmitters are involved in numerous critical brain functions of memory, behavior, and mood. Neurotransmitter function can be enhanced by increasing synthesis, inhibiting degradation, promoting release, decreasing reuptake after nerve firing, or providing replacement with agonists.

The first neurotransmitter targeted in DAT pharmacotherapy development was acetylcholine (ACh), due to its role in memory storage and its deficiency in the brains of Alzheimer's disease patients. A major effort has met with limited success (47). The cholinergic agent tacrine (Cognex) was the first drug approved by the U.S. Food and Drug Administration specifically for DAT treatment. Unfortunately, reported benefits were quite modest and consisted primarily of a slowing of the cognitive decline; common adverse events included elevation of serum liver enzyme activities, as well as nausea, vomiting, diarrhea, and headache (48). We are unaware of any reports of the use of tacrine in dogs with CD.

With respect to the second strategy, one way to slow the progress of CD may be by modulating the inflammatory or immune responses (46). Another approach is to alter amyloidogenesis by rendering the beta-amyloid molecule less toxic, decreasing its accumulation by inhibiting synthesis, altering its processing, or by promoting its removal (46). Alternatively, nerve conduction or neuron metabolic processes can be normalized. Finally, neuroprotection can be attempted by abrogating apoptosis or programmed cell death of damaged neurons, or by enhancing neuron regeneration (49).

DEVELOPMENT OF DRUGS

In the veterinary literature, there are few articles devoted to therapy of behavior problems in geriatric pet dogs (10). Nicergoline, a drug with alpha-adrenolytic effects and producing cerebral vasodilation along with increased metabolic activity of cerebral neurons, has been reported to significantly increase activity in aging dogs by 75% compared with placebo, which increased activity by 23% (50). The drug is available in several European countries but not in North America.

Considerable evidence indicates that L-deprenyl HCl (selegiline HCl; Anipryl) may help dogs with CD by both mitigating neurotransmitter depletion (especially dopamine) enhancing catecholaminergic activity and slowing neurodegenerative disease progression.

L-Deprenyl

The compound L-deprenyl is typically characterized as a selective, irreversible inhibitor of MAOB. Although L-deprenyl's success as an antidepressant, for which it was originally proposed, has been limited, it has clinical utility for a variety of neurodegenerative disorders, including Parkinson's disease and DAT in humans (37,51–53), and is also effective for treatment of canine PDH (Cushing's disease). It is approved and marketed for use in dogs in the United States, Canada, and France (43,44). During the past several years, we have studied L-deprenyl's performance for treatment of canine CD in formal prospective clinical trials and corroborative studies conducted under an

Investigational New Animal Drug (INAD) exemption by the FDA Center for Veterinary Medicine. Pertinent findings follow.

The precise mechanisms by which L-deprenyl produces clinical response in dogs with CD are not fully understood but may be due in part to the drug's enhancement of brain dopamine concentrations and metabolism. A variety of neurodegenerative disorders in humans, as well as canine PDH and perhaps canine CD, are characterized by depletion of dopamine within the brain (45). In the CNS, dopamine is rapidly metabolized by monoamine oxidases. MAOB activity levels are known to increase not only with age but particularly in certain neurodegenerative disorders such as Parkinson's disease and Alzheimer's disease (37). L-deprenyl is a selective and irreversible inhibitor of MAOB, as demonstrated in humans, nonhuman primates, mice, and rats (54). It also inhibits MAOB in the canine brain. When administered to healthy dogs orally once daily for 3 weeks at doses of 0.1 to 1.0 mg/kg, L-deprenyl inhibited brain (hippocampal and cortical) MAOB in a dose-dependent fashion, with peak inhibition approximating 92% (55).

L-deprenyl also increases dopamine concentrations in the synaptic cleft by several additional mechanisms. The first is by enhancing the impulse-mediated release of catecholamines (56). The drug also decreases presynaptic dopamine reuptake. An additional consequence of the inhibition of MAOB is an increase in the concentration of another of this enzyme's substrates, phenylethylamine, which potentiates the action of dopamine. L-deprenyl also increases the synthesis of the enzyme aromatic *l*-amino acid decarboxylase, which in turn increases dopamine synthesis (54,57). By these actions, L-deprenyl should help restore dopaminergic balance in the cortex, hippocampus, and other brain regions of an individual with CD and thus ameliorate clinical signs.

Effects of L-deprenyl on metabolism of free radicals may also play a therapeutic or prophylactic role in geriatric patients. Free radicals are highly reactive oxygen-containing molecules that can cause damage to vital cell structures, such as membrane constituents and DNA. Many investigators believe free radicals contribute to aging processes and to pathogenesis of neurodegenerative disorders (58). L-deprenyl decreases free radical production by inhibiting MAOB. Within the canine brain, the drug also increases the activity of the free radical–scavenging enzyme superoxide dismutase (SOD) (59).

Interestingly, L-deprenyl also exerts neuroprotective effects. Experiments in laboratory rodents demonstrated that L-deprenyl enhanced the survival of dopaminergic neurons after exposure to dopaminergic neurotoxins (49). The neuroprotective effect also occurs in peripheral cholinergic neurons after trauma (60). The precise mechanism(s) of neuroprotection is unknown but at least two possibilities have been proposed: 1) L-deprenyl may decrease or alter apoptosis (programmed cell death) of injured neurons. As noted earlier, apoptosis in the dog brain increases with age and correlates with signs of CD

(26); 2) alternatively, L-deprenyl may promote synthesis or release of nerve growth factors (61). Whatever the mechanism, it is important to note that the neuroprotective effects are clinically relevant, as L-deprenyl was proven to slow the progression of Parkinson's disease and Alzheimer's disease rather than merely provide symptomatic relief (53,62).

PHARMACOKINETICS

Until recently, pharmacokinetic analyses for L-deprenyl were complicated by lack of availability of an assay that could detect the intact molecule at concentrations less than 10 ng/mL. Mahmood et al (63) developed an in vitro fluorometric assay for use with human and canine plasma that can detect L-deprenyl concentrations as low as 0.25 ng/mL, and described L-deprenyl kinetics in a study of four female mongrel dogs. Tablets were crushed and dissolved in water. Dogs were fasted overnight, then administered 1 mg/kg L-deprenyl by gavage. The L-deprenyl was absorbed rapidly, with a maximum concentration of 5.2 ± 1.36 ng/mL attained 25 ± 5.8 minutes after administration. Absolute bioavailability in the dog was 8.51 ± 3.31%. The L-deprenyl compound is stable in heparinized canine whole blood for at least 1 hour when maintained at 37°C, and in canine plasma for at least 10 days when stored at −20°C.

SAFETY STUDIES

We examined the safety of chronic L-deprenyl administration in 82 beagle dogs aged 3 to 16 years at the time dosing began. During more than 2 years of administration, no clinically significant differences between the L-deprenyl and placebo groups were seen with respect to routine laboratory parameters (complete blood counts, serum biochemistry profiles), liver function tests (serum bile acid concentrations), neurologic and behavior examinations, ophthalmic examinations, and blood pressure measurements (6,64).

In clinical trials involving 132 dogs with PDH treated with L-deprenyl for as long as 18 months, only six dogs (5%) experienced adverse events that led either to discontinuation of therapy, dismissal from the study, or a reduction in dose: signs did not recur when L-deprenyl was reinstituted at a lower dose of 1.0 mg/kg/day. In the other dogs studied, no adverse events were reported that were thought likely to be due to L-deprenyl therapy, and no dogs required the dosage to be adjusted or the treatment to be discontinued (65).

EFFECTS ON HPA AXIS

The endocrine effect of chronic administration of L-deprenyl on the HPA axis was evaluated in a group of elderly (6–17 years) beagle dogs (66). Tests were performed on pairs matched by age, sex, and weight. One member of each pair had been treated orally with 1 mg/kg/day of L-deprenyl for 1 year; the other member received placebo. There were no statistical differences in the baseline or post-ACTH (adrenocorticotropic hormone) stimulation in cortisol concentrations between the L-deprenyl and placebo group, respectively. These results indicated that chronic administration of L-deprenyl does not result in glucocorticoid insufficiency.

To further evaluate the effects of chronic L-deprenyl administration on the canine HPA axis, corticotropin-releasing hormone (CRH) stimulation tests were performed on 58 beagle dogs (29 pairs). One member of each pair had been treated orally with 1 mg/kg/day of L-deprenyl for 1 year; the other received placebo. The results indicated that chronic L-deprenyl administration decreased the release of cortisol in response to CRH stimulation (67). These results complement those of earlier studies in which dopaminergic blockade resulted in enhanced CRH-mediated ACTH release in normal dogs (68).

Based on these findings as well as additional pathophysiologic concepts and evidence discussed previously, Bruyette et al (43,44,69) conducted a series of clinical trials to evaluate the efficacy and safety of L-deprenyl in pet dogs with PDH under investigational new animal drug exemptions by the Canadian Bureau of Veterinary Drugs (BVD) and the FDA Center for Veterinary Medicine. The trials were prospective and conducted according to protocols previewed by personnel at the BVD and FDA, and approved by the appropriate Institutional Animal Care and Use Committees (IACUCs). In each enrolled subject, the diagnosis was confirmed based on clinical signs, laboratory abnormalities, dexamethasone suppression, and other endocrine tests as needed. Dogs were treated with 1 to 2 mg/kg L-deprenyl orally once daily and monitored for 6 months. Therapy with L-deprenyl resulted in return toward normal of the dexamethasone suppression test results ($P < .0001$), as well as improvement ($P < .05$) at various time points in all common clinical parameters (44).

Cognitive Effects

Head et al (70) evaluated the effects of L-deprenyl on performance of laboratory housed dogs using the neuropsychologic tests discussed earlier under Neuropsychologic Studies. In one fully blinded, placebo-controlled trial, oral daily administration of L-deprenyl improved spatial short-term memory in aged dogs but not in young dogs (Figure 13.2). The effect of dose was also evaluated. The optimal dose varied by individual, with the best response at either 0.5 mg/kg or 1.0 mg/kg given orally once daily. Oral doses less than 0.5 mg/kg or greater than 1.0 mg/kg were less effective. This inverted parabolic dose-response curve is a well-known characteristic of numerous psychotropic and behavior drugs, and has been demonstrated for L-deprenyl cognitive effects in rat studies and in a trial of patients with DAT (71,72).

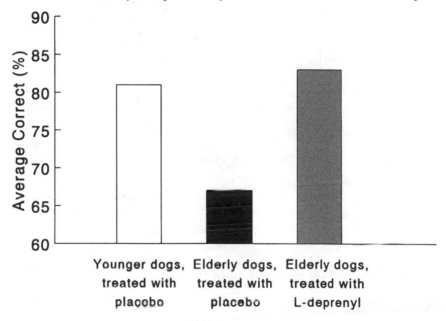

Spatial memory decline in elderly dogs, and its reversal with L-deprenyl in a placebo controlled study

Figure 13.2.
Spatial memory decline in elderly dogs and its reversal with L-deprenyl in a placebo-controlled study. Source: (70).

In another fully blinded study, the same investigators assessed effects of chronic daily administration of 1.0 mg/kg L-deprenyl versus placebo utilizing a battery of the neuropsychologic tests noted above. The dogs were assigned on the basis of pretreatment performance to one of two groups: cognitively intact or cognitively impaired. In the former group, L-deprenyl had no effect. The performance of dogs in the latter group was improved, although it did not attain statistical significance, perhaps due to the small subgroup sample size (73).

Taken together, these results suggest that L-deprenyl improves performance of cognitively impaired dogs. Based on these results and the pathophysiologic and pharmacologic points already mentioned, clinical trials in pet dogs with CD were indicated.

PROSPECTIVE CLINICAL TRIAL

Ruehl et al (6) conducted a prospective clinical trial in pet dogs to evaluate the safety and efficacy of L-deprenyl to treat CD, as well as to further characterize presenting complaints of owners of elderly dogs and to develop methodology for future trials. Client-owned dogs were nominated for preliminary evaluation based on the presence of one or more of the geriatric problems listed in Table

13.1. Nominated dogs were evaluated for suitability to be enrolled and treated with the study drug (L-deprenyl) by history, physical examination, neurologic examination, complete blood count, and serum biochemistry profile. Dogs were excluded if they exhibited evidence of a concurrent general medical condition. Sixty-nine dogs fulfilled the enrollment criteria and were administered 0.5 mg/kg L-deprenyl tablets once daily in open-label fashion; subjects were re-evaluated monthly during the 3-month study. At each re-evaluation the dog's owner completed a behavior questionnaire similar to that utilized at enrollment, and the subject was evaluated medically by the procedures used in determining suitability for the study. Dogs were 7 to 19 years of age (mean = 14 years), weighed 3.6 to 36 kg (mean = 14 kg), and at enrollment exhibited multiple signs of CD. Table 13.1 demonstrates that after 1 month of L-deprenyl therapy, the population was improved in all fifteen parameters evaluated ($P <$ .05 for thirteen parameters). Benefits were generally maintained at 2 and 3 months, with the percentages of individuals who improved with respect to global function at each month being 77%, 76%, and 78%, respectively.

Diagnosis and Management of Canine CD

DIAGNOSTIC CONSIDERATIONS

A veterinarian may observe geriatric behavior signs typical of CD at the time of physical examination of an elderly dog, or these problems may be reported spontaneously by the pet owner. As previously mentioned, the owners tend to underreport the occurrence of these signs unless specifically queried by the veterinarian or staff. To facilitate early recognition of geriatric behavior problems and diagnosis of CD, many veterinarians encourage owners to complete a senior dog checklist (Figure 13.3). If the owner notes the presence of one or more problems, then additional history is obtained to help characterize the geriatric behavior problems with respect to severity, duration, frequency of occurrence, and impact on the lifestyle and quality of life of both the pet and the owner.

It is important for two reasons to determine what medical problems, if any, may also be present. First, many patients with CD suffer from concurrent unrelated general medical conditions (e.g., arthritis, organ dysfunction, neoplasia), at the time of diagnosis of CD or shortly thereafter. In one study, more than half the pet dogs with CD, who otherwise appeared healthy when diagnosed with CD, developed clinical manifestations of unrelated medical problems within a period of 1 week to several months (Ruehl WW, unpublished data, 1997). Second, the medical condition may contribute to the behavior problems, in which case treatment of the former may mitigate or eliminate the latter.

In community veterinary practice, the medical workup of dogs with geriatric behavior problems often includes physical examination, neurologic examination focusing on cranial nerve function and evaluation of the perineal

Elderly Dog Checklist

	√ YES
Loss of house training	
Increased thirst	
Reduced activity	
Excessive panting	
Confusion or disorientation	
Less interaction with family	
Inability to recognize family	
Decreased hearing	
Sleeps more during day	
Altered appetite	
Weight change	
Difficulty climbing stairs	
Increased stiffness	

Figure 13.3.
Senior dog checklist.

reflex (especially in housesoiling dogs), and routine laboratory procedures such as complete blood count and biochemistry profile. Also often indicated are urinalysis and endocrine evaluation, such as resting T4 concentration and low-dose dexamethasone suppression (LDDS); urine culture may also be helpful. Some patients may require additional studies such as electrocardiography or imaging studies (e.g., radiology, ultrasound, MRI, or CT scan). Of note, brain imaging studies of human dementia patients help to rule out vascular and neoplastic causes of cognitive deterioration but cannot be used to confirm a diagnosis of Alzheimer's disease (3). The diagnosis of Alzheimer's disease can only be fully confirmed by histopathologic examination of brain tissue obtained by biopsy (rarely) or autopsy (3). Thus, human patients suspected of having Alzheimer's disease are classified as having DAT or "probable AD."

DOSAGE AND ADMINISTRATION

Following diagnosis of CD and appropriate medical evaluation, L-deprenyl therapy is initiated at a dose of 0.5–1.0 mg/kg (0.23–0.45 mg/lb) body weight orally once daily (6). Morning administration is preferable, especially in dogs with sleep/wake cycle disturbances. The veterinary formulation is well absorbed, and the tablet can be administered with or without food. Many owners typically report behavior improvements within the first 2 weeks of therapy, and some note that improvement begins within the first few days. By the end of the first month, approximately 77% have improved, but a few demonstrate improvement only in the second month of therapy. Further incremental improvement is often noted during the second or third month of therapy.

The rapidity of response as well as the ultimate magnitude and duration of benefit vary between individual dogs, possibly due to severity and duration of the brain pathology prior to treatment initiation, or to the presence of concurrent medical conditions. Husbandry, factors in the home environment, and the pet's behavior repertoire prior to the onset of CD may also modify the ultimate pharmacotherapeutic response.

Treated patients should be re-evaluated for behavior improvement periodically during the first month, which may be accomplished by interviewing the owner via telephone or, if warranted, by personal interview of the owner and physical examination of the patient. If no behavior improvement is evident after 1 month, the dose can be increased to 1 mg/kg once daily, and the dog should be re-evaluated in similar fashion 1 month later. If there is still no improvement or if at any time behavior signs progress, the patient should be re-evaluated for the presence of concurrent disorders, including performance of appropriate laboratory tests or other studies as warranted. Dogs whose CD signs are stable or improved and who are otherwise healthy should be re-examined every 3 to 6 months, as elderly dogs often manifest new medical problems in that time period. Dogs whose CD is stable or improved but who have concurrent medical disorders may need to be re-evaluated more frequently, as dictated by the particular medical problem.

During clinical trials, dogs treated with L-deprenyl for as long as 3 years were monitored for the occurrence of adverse drug interactions. No drug interactions were reported with a variety of antibiotics, anthelminthics, ectoparasiticides, heartworm medications, analgesics, and antihistamines (44). Concurrent use of L-deprenyl with ephedrine or other monoamine oxidase inhibitors, antidepressants, or medications where monoamine oxidase inhibition may play a role (amitraz; Mitaban) is not recommended (65).

In humans, L-deprenyl is contraindicated for use with meperidine, and this contraindication is often extended to other opioids (65). In humans, severe CNS toxicity, including death, has been reported with the combination of selegiline and tricyclic antidepressants and selegiline and selective serotonin reuptake inhibitors. Although no adverse drug interactions were reported in the field trials in dogs, it seems prudent to avoid the combination of L-deprenyl and tricyclic antidepressants and L-deprenyl and selective serotonin reuptake inhibitors. This warning is extended to include tetracyclic antidepressants and other antidepressants, including amoxapine, protriptyline HCl, trimipramine maleate, and venlafaxine HCl (65).

At least 14 days should elapse between discontinuation of L-deprenyl and initiation of treatment with a tricyclic antidepressant or selective serotonin reuptake inhibitor. Because of the long half-life of fluoxetine HCl and its active metabolites, at least 5 weeks should elapse between discontinuation of fluoxetine and initiation of treatment with L-deprenyl (65). The effect of L-deprenyl on breeding, pregnant, and lactating bitches and breeding dogs has not been determined, and L-deprenyl is contraindicated in patients with known hypersensitivity to this drug (65).

References

1. American Veterinary Medical Association. The veterinary service market for companion animals. Schaumburg, IL: American Veterinary Medical Association, 1992.
2. Cummings BJ, Head E, Ruehl WW, et al. The canine as an animal model of human aging and dementia. Neurobiol Aging 1996;17:259–268.
3. Morris JC. Diagnosis of Alzheimer's disease. In: Khachaturian ZS, Radebuagh TS, eds. Alzheimer's disease: cause(s), diagnosis, treatment and care. Boca Raton, FL: CRC Press, 1996:76–81.
4. Frances A, Pincus HA, First MB. Diagnostic and statistical manual of mental disorders, 4th ed. Washington, DC: American Psychiatric Association, 1994:133–143.
5. McFarland D. The Oxford companion to animal behaviour. Oxford. Oxford University Press, 1987.71–72.
6. Ruehl WW, Bruyette DS, DePaoli A, et al. Canine cognitive dysfunction as a model for human age-related cognitive decline, dementia and Alzheimer's disease: clinical presentation, cognitive testing, pathology and response to L-deprenyl therapy. Prog Brain Res 1995;106:217–225.
7. Houpt KA, Beaver B. Behavior problems of geriatric dogs and cats. Vet Clin North Am Small Anim Pract 1981;11:643–652.
8. Chapman B, Voith V. Behavior problems in old dogs. J Am Vet Med Assoc 1990;196:944–946.
9. Mosier JE. Effects of aging on body systems of the dog. In: Goldston RT, ed. Geriatrics and gerontology. Vet Clin North Am Small Anim Pract 1989;19:1–121.
10. Hunthausen W. Identifying and treating behavior problems in geriatric dogs. Vet Med 1994;89(suppl):688–700.
11. Koppang N. Canine ceroid lipofuscinsosis—a model for human neuronal ceroid lipofuscinsosis and aging. Mech Ageing Dev 1973;2:421–445.
12. Ferrer I, Pumarola M, Rivera R, et al. Primary central white matter degeneration in old dogs. Acta Neuropathol 1993;86:172–175.
13. Reisberg B, Ferris H. In: Crook T, Gershon S, eds. Diagnosis and treatment of adult onset cognitive disorders (AOCD). Old Saybrook, CT: Psymark Communications, 1991:37–48.
14. Brooks JO, Kraemer HC, Tanke ED, Yesavage JA. The methodology of studying decline in Alzheimer's disease. J Am Geriatr Soc 1993;41:623–628.
15. Evans DA, Funkenstein HH, Albert MS. Prevalence of Alzheimer's disease in a community population of older persons. JAMA 1989;262:2551–2556.

16. Hart BL, Hart LA. Selecting, raising, and caring for dogs to avoid problem aggression. J Am Vet Med Assoc 1997;210:1129–1134.

17. Arnsten AFT, Goldman-Rakic PS. Alpha-adrenergic mechanisms in prefrontal cortex associated with cognitive decline in aged nonhuman primates. Science 1985;230:1273–1276.

18. Bachevalier J, Landis LS, Walker LC, et al. Aged monkeys exhibit behavior deficits indicative of widespread cerebral dysfunction. Neurobiol Aging 1991;12:99–111.

19. Campbell BA, Krauter EE, Wallace JE. Animal models of aging: sensory-motor and cognitive function in the aged rat. In: Stein DO, ed. The psychobiology of aging: problems and perspectives. New York: Elsevier/North-Holland, 1980:201–226.

20. Willig F, Palacios A, Monmaur P, et al. Short-term memory, exploration and locomotor activity in aged rats. Neurobiol Aging 1987;8:393–402.

21. Milgram NW, Head E, Weiner E, Thomas E. Cognitive functions and aging in the dog: acquisition of nonspatial visual tasks. Behav Neurosci 1994;108:57–68.

22. Head E, Mehta R, Hartley J, et al. Spatial learning and memory as a function of age in the dog. Behav Neurosci 1995;109:851–858.

23. Katzman R. Alzheimer's disease. N Engl J Med 1986;314:964–973.

24. Cummings BJ, Su JH, Cotman CW, et al. β-amyloid accumulation in aged canine brain: a model of early plaque formation in Alzheimer's disease. Neurobiol Aging 1993;14:547–560.

25. Kiatipattanasakul W, Nakamura S, Nakayama H, et al. Apoptosis in the aged dog brain. Vet Pathol 1996;33:600.

26. Cummings BJ, Head E, Afagh AJ, et al. β-amyloid accumulation correlates with cognitive dysfunction in the aged canine. Neurobiol Learn Mem 1996;66:11–23.

27. Cummings BJ, Cotman DW. Image analysis of β-amyloid load in Alzheimer's disease and relation to dementia severity. Lancet 1995;346:1524–1528.

28. Cotman CW, Cummings BJ, Pike CJ. Molecular cascades in adaptive versus pathologic plasticity. In: Gloria A, ed. Neuroregeneration. New York: Raven, 1993:217–240.

29. Lafora G. Neoformaciones dendriticas en las neuronas y alteraciones de la neuroglia en el perro senil. Trab del Lab de Investig biol 1914;12(fasc):1.

30. Uchida K, Nakayama H, Tateyama S, Goto N. Immunohistochemical analysis of constituents of senile plaques and cerebrovascular amyloid in aged dogs. J Vet Med Sci 1992;54:1023–1029.

31. Shimada A, Kuwamura M, Awakura T, et al. Topographic relationship between senile plaques and cerebrovascular amyloidosis in the brain of aged dogs. J Vet Med Sci 1992;54:137–144.

32. Giaccone G, Verga L, Finazzi M, et al. Cerebral preamyloid deposits and congophilic angiopathy in aged dogs. Neurosci Lett 1990;114:178–183.

33. Uchida K, Okuda R, Yamaguchi R, et al. Double labeling immunohistochemical studies on canine senile plaques and cerebral amyloid angiopathy. J Vet Med Sci 1993;55:637–642.

34. Russell JR, White R, Patel E, et al. Familial influence on plaque formation in the beagle brain. Neuroreport 1992;3:1093–1096.

35. Cummings BJ, Satou T, Head E, et al. Diffuse plaques contain C-terminal $A\beta_{42}$ and not $A\beta_{43}$: evidence from cats and dogs. Neurobiol Aging 1996;17:653–659.

36. Arnsten AFT. Catecholamine mechanisms in age-related cognitive decline. Neurobiol Aging 1993;14:639–641.

37. Tariot PN, Schneider LS, Patel SV, Goldstein B. Alzheimer's disease and L-deprenyl: rationales and findings. In: Szelenyi I, ed. Inhibitors of monoamine oxidase B. Basel: Birkhauser Verlag, 1993:301–317.

38. Ruehl WW, Bruyette DS, Entriken TL, et al. Adrenal axis dysregulation in geriatric dogs with cognitive dysfunction (Abst.) J Vet Intern Med 1997;11:119.

39. Jenike MA, Albert MS. The dexamethasone suppression test in patients with presenile and senile dementia of the Alzheimer's type. J Am Geriatr Soc 1984;32:441–444.

40. Spar JE, Gerner R. Does the dexamethasone suppression test distinguish dementia from depression? Am J Psychiatry 1982;139:238.

41. Lupien S, LeCours A, Lussier I, et al. Basal cortisol levels and cognitive deficits in human aging. J Neurosci 1994;14:2893–2903.

42. Nieman LK, Cutler GB. Cushing's syndrome. In: DeGroot, ed. Endocrinology, 3rd ed. Philadelphia: Saunders, 1995:1741–1770.

43. Bruyette DS, Ruehl WW, Smidberg TL. Canine pituitary dependent hyperadrenocorticism: a spontaneous animal model for neurodegenerative disorders and their treatment with L-deprenyl. Prog Brain Res 1995;106:207–215.

44. Bruyette DS, Ruehl WW, Entriken T, et al. Management of canine pituitary-dependent hyperadrenocorticism with L-deprenyl (Anipryl®). Vet Clin North Am Small Anim Pract 1997;27:273–286.

45. Peterson ME, Palkovits M, Chiueh CC, et al. Biogenic amine and corticotropin-releasing factor concentrations in hypothalamic paraventricular nucleus and biogenic amine levels in the median eminence of normal dogs, chronic dexamethasone treated dogs, and dogs with naturally-occurring pituitary-dependent hyperadrenocorticism (canine Cushing's disease). J Neuroendocrinol 1989;1:169–171.

46. Shihabuddin L, Davis KL. Treatment of Alzheimer's disease. In: Khachaturian ZS, Radebuagh TS, eds. Alzheimer's disease: causes(s), diagnosis, treatment and care. Boca Raton, FL: CRC Press, 1996:258–269.

47. Growdon JH. Treatment for Alzheimer's disease? N Engl J Med 1992;327:1306–1308

48. Davis KL, Thal LJ, Gamzu ER, et al. A double-blind, placebo-controlled multicenter study of tacrine for Alzheimer's disease. N Engl J Med 1992;327:1253–1259.

49. Tatton WG, Greenwood CE. Rescue of dying neurons: a new action for deprenyl in MPTP Parkinsonism. J Neurosci Res 1991;30:666–672.

50. Postal JM, et al. RM302: a new treatment for aging dogs. Proceedings of the 24th World Veterinary Congress, Rio de Janiero, Brazil, August 18 20th, 1991.

51. Parkinson Study Group. Effect of deprenyl on the progression of disability in early Parkinson's disease. N Engl J Med 1989;321:1363–1371.

52. Parkinson Study Group. Effects of tocopherol and deprenyl on the progression of disability in early Parkinson's disease. N Engl J Med 1993;328:176–183.

53. Olanow CW, Hauser RA, Gauger L, et al. The effect of deprenyl and levodopa on the progression of Parkinson's disease. Ann Neurol 1995;38:771–777.

54. Heinonen EH, Lammintausta R. A review of the pharmacology of selegiline. Acta Neurol Scand 1991;84(Suppl 136):44–59.

55. Milgram NW, Ivy GO, Murphy MP, et al. Effect of chronic oral administration of L-deprenyl in the dog. Pharmacol Biochem Behav 1995;51;421–428.

56. Knoll J, Miklya I, Knoll B, et al. (−) Deprenyl and (−) 1-phenyl-2-propylaminopentane, [(−)PPAP], act primarily as potent stimulants of action potential-transmitter release coupling in the catecholaminergic neurons. Life Sci 1996;58:817–827.

57. Jurio AV, Li XM, Paterson A, Boulton AA. Effects of monoamine oxidase B inhibitors on dopaminergic function: role of 2-phenylethylamine and aromatic l-Amino acid decarboxylase. In: Lieberman A, Olanow CW, Youdim MBH, Tipton K, eds. Monoamine oxidase inhibitors in neurologic diseases. New York: Marcel Dekker, 1994:181–200.

58. Gerlach M, Riederer P, Youdim MH. The mode of action of MAO-B inhibitors. In: Szelenyi I, ed. Inhibitors of monoamine oxidase B: pharmacology and clinical use in neurodegenerative disorders. Basel: Birkhauser Verlag, 1993:183–201.

59. Carrillo MC, Milgram NW, Wu P, et al. L-deprenyl increases activities of superoxide dismutase (SOD) in striatum of dog brain. Life Sci 1994;54:1483–1489.

60. Salo PT, Tatton WG. Deprenyl reduces the death of motoneurons caused by axotomy. J Neurosci Res 1992;31:394–400.

61. Tatton WG, Ju WYH, Ansari KS, Seniuk NA. Reduction of nerve cell death by deprenyl without monoamine oxidase inhibition. In: Lieberman A, Olanow CW, Youdim MBH, Tipton K, eds. Monoamine oxidase inhibitors in neurologic diseases. New York: Marcel Dekker, 1994:217–248.

62. Sano M, Ernesto C, Thomas RG, et al. A controlled trial of selegiline, alpha-tocopherol, or both as treatment for Alzheimer's disease. N Eng J Med 1997;336:1216–1222.

63. Mahmood I, Peters DK, Mason WD. The pharmacokinetics and absolute bioavailability of selegiline in the dog. Biopharm Drug Dispos 1994;15:653–664.

64. Ruehl W, Bruyette D, Muggenburg B. Effects of age and administration of the monoamine oxidase inhibitor L-deprenyl on total fasting bile acid concentration in laboratory beagles. Vet Pathol 1993;30:432.

65. Deprenyl Animal Health, Inc. Anipryl® tablets insert. Overland Park, KS, 1997.

66. Bruyette D, Ruehl W, Muggenburg B. Effects of treatment with the monoamine oxidase inhibitor L-deprenyl on anterior pituitary function in geriatric beagle dogs. Vet Pathol 1993;30:436.

67. Bruyette D. Effects of chronic treatment with the monoamine oxidase inhibitor (L-deprenyl) on CRH stimulation testing in geriatric beagle dogs. J Vet Intern Med 1994;8:163.

68. Zerbe CA, Clark TP, Sartin JL, et al. Domperidone treatment enhances corticotropin releasing hormone stimulated ACTH release from the dog pituitary. Neuroendocrinology 1993;57:282–288.

69. Bruyette DS, Darling LA, Griffin D, Ruehl WW. L-deprenyl for canine pituitary dependent hyperadrenocorticism: pivotal efficacy trial. J Vet Intern Med 1996;10:182.

70. Head E, Hartley J, Kameka AM, et al. The effects of L-deprenyl on spatial short term memory in young and aged dogs. Prog Neuropsychopharmacol Biol Psychiatry 1996;20:515–530.

71. Brandies R, Sapir M, Kapon Y, et al. Improvement of cognitive function by MAO-B inhibitor L-deprenyl in aged rats. Pharmacol Biochem Behav 1990;39:297–304.

72. Tariot PN, Cohen RM, Sunderland T, et al. L-deprenyl in Alzheimer's disease. Arch Gen Psychiatry 1987;44:427–433.

73. Milgram NW, Ivy GO, Head E, et al. The effect of L-deprenyl on behavior, cognitive function, and biogenic amines in the dog. Neurochem Res 1993;18:1211–1219.

APPENDIX

Evaluation of Clinical Trials in Behavioral Pharmacology

Benjamin L. Hart
Kelly D. Cliff

The treatment of behavior problems in companion animals, like medical practice in general, involves the clinician's personal skills in interacting with clients as well as use of scientific knowledge gained through experimentation and clinical studies. As veterinarians increasingly prescribe drugs for problem behaviors, progress in the field of behavioral therapy depends on accurate evaluation of studies involving drugs. Drugs approved by the U.S. Food and Drug Administration's Center for Veterinary Medicine have been subjected to controlled trials that rigorously demonstrate efficacy. However, almost all of the drugs mentioned in this text are used in an extra-label fashion sanctioned by recent federal approval of extra-label use of drugs for non-food animals; these drugs generally have *not* been subjected to controlled clinical trials in animals. Some psychotropic drugs approved for human use have involved dogs and/or cats in product testing, but information is sparse regarding efficacy, adverse side effects, and long-term value in the treatment of problem behavior in companion animals (1,2). This chapter provides some guidelines for evaluating available published information concerning the effectiveness of various psychotropic drugs used in companion animals.

A major goal of clinical trials is to distinguish real drug effects from imagined or placebo effects and/or effects brought about by unplanned environmental management or behavior modification introduced by the client/owner. The importance of placebo effects in human medicine has been known and debated for decades and was profiled in 1955 in a classic paper by Beecher (3), who pointed out that placebo effects have been apparent since the 1800s. He reviewed literature showing that, on average, 35% of human patients treated for problems such as the common cold, wound pain, headache, cough, mood abnormalities, and anxieties showed a placebo effect. The surprising extent of the placebo effect was evident in recent studies, one of which revealed a decrease in size of the hyperplastic prostate gland in men receiving placebo (4). Another study showed significant improvement in menopausal symptoms and elevation of estradiol levels in women receiving placebo (5).

In veterinary behavioral pharmacology, treatment success is evaluated on the basis of reports made by the animal's owners rather than by physical examination or laboratory tests, which are the methods used to assess progress in other veterinary specialties such as dermatology or internal medicine. Because animals do not know they are being treated, per se, one could argue that a much smaller proportion of clinical trial data should reflect placebo effects. However, one could equally argue that it is easier to imagine positive results in animals because owners are anxious to see improvement in their pets. In addition to imagined results, owners may institute behavior modification or environmental management procedures that were not included in the treatment regimen, which then might appear as placebo effects (6). Such effects are especially likely to appear in data from retrospective surveys but could occur in prospective trials as well.

Typically, when a veterinarian treats an individual patient, a psychoactive drug is prescribed, presumably along with instructions that the client follow a program of behavior modification and/or environmental management (7). If there is a positive outcome, it does not really matter how much of the improvement is due to the drug and how much is due to the behavioral approaches, as long as the problem is resolved to the client's satisfaction. The tendency is to credit the drug, even for aspects of improvement brought about by behavioral approaches. However, progress in the field of behavioral pharmacology requires an attempt at distinguishing placebo effects from drug effects, and it is the task of clinical trials to separate these two aspects. The gold standard for distinguishing placebo from drug effects is the controlled randomized trial, which forms the basis for FDA approval of drugs. Because most drugs used for problem behaviors have not been subjected to such placebo-controlled trials, veterinarians must evaluate the literature available about these various drugs.

There are four general types of studies published in the literature that address drugs for behavioral and medical purposes: 1) double-blind clinical trials, 2) prospective open-label clinical trials, 3) retrospective case surveys, and 4) case reports. The strength of evidence that a particular drug will be effective for a particular problem varies from one type of study to another.

Double-Blind Clinical Trials

This type of trial provides the most accurate information on the effectiveness of drug treatment for problem behavior. The main feature of these trials is that they minimize the placebo effect through randomized assignment of animals to various groups, utilization of a control group, and standardization of behavior modification techniques. In these trials, at least two treatment groups are used in a *double-blind fashion* (i.e., neither the investigators nor the owners know which animals are in which groups). The experimental group receives the drug at the expected effective dose range (which has usually been worked out in preliminary trials and toxicity studies), and the control group may receive a placebo or the conventional standard treatment. There may be two experimental groups receiving different dosages of the drug under investigation. Selection bias in assigning animals to a group is avoided by a randomization procedure that may be balanced in terms of age or sex of the animals (stratified randomization design). Participating owners are given the same information and the same instructions regarding behavior modification. Evaluation of treatment may occur only at the end of the trial or periodically, for example, by interviewing clients on a weekly basis.

In human clinical trials, patients often are able to detect that they are assigned to the drug group rather than the placebo group, based on side effects of the treatment. Side effects may include physiologic signs, such as dry mouth, loss of appetite, or increased sleepiness. This, of course, could affect the results of the trial, because if the patient and investigator know which group the patient belongs to, the door is open for imagined effects. It is also possible for pet owners to know if their animal has been assigned to a drug group based on side effects, for example, if the drug increases appetite or sleepiness or produces transient ataxia as is common with diazepam treatment of cats. It may be quite difficult to avoid this type of influence in drug trials, as it is rarely feasible to give an "active" placebo that has the same physiologic effects as the drug being studied. In addition, an active placebo may actually enhance the placebo effect by reinforcing belief in the power of the drug (5).

Because some placebo effect is usually expected in clinical trials, the main object is to determine whether the drug has an effect beyond that of a placebo (8,9). As an example, one may find that 20% of animals receiving a placebo improve, whereas 75% of animals receiving the new drug improve. The difference between the percent responding to the placebo and the percent responding to the drug (i.e., 55% in this example) is an estimate of the number of animals for which the drug was effective. When a new drug is compared with conventional drug treatment, the study reveals whether the new treatment is at least as good or better than the conventional one. Such trials will not reveal whether the new treatment is actually better than placebo, however, because if the conventional drug has not been tested against placebo, neither drug may actually be better than placebo. Assuming that both the new drug and the conventional drug are more effective than placebo, but that the new drug is not significantly different than the conventional drug, the new drug may still be considered to have advantages if it produces fewer side effects or is less expensive.

The most common protocol for a controlled trial is the *parallel design* in which two groups receive treatment concomitantly, and the results are evaluated at the end of the trial. Some parallel trials may involve two or more experimental groups with different drug dosages being utilized in each group (Figure A.1). One variant of the parallel design uses a placebo-washout intro-

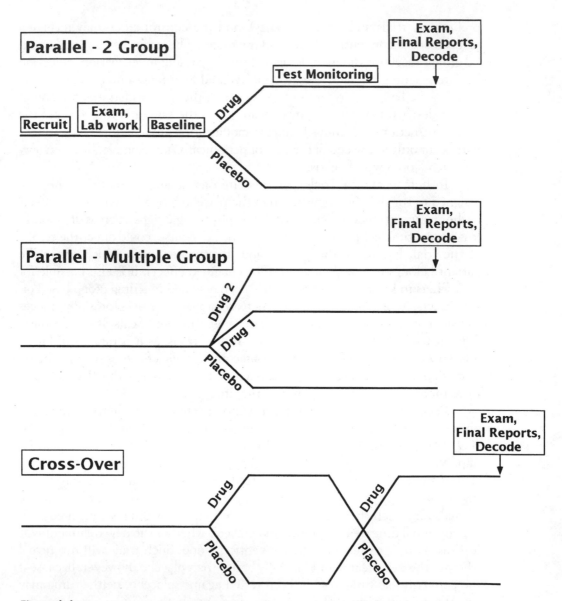

Figure A.1.
Schematic diagrams of various study designs for randomized, controlled clinical trials. In some trials, a group given an older standard treatment may replace the placebo group. All trials include recruiting participants, performing screening interviews and initial examinations, and collecting baseline laboratory data, as indicated for the parallel-2 group trials. The parallel-multiple group trials may include more than one drug or more than one dose of a single drug. (Modified from Hart BL, Cliff KD. Interpreting published reports of extra-label drug use with special reference to reports of drugs used to correct problem behavior in animals. J Am Vet Med Assoc 1996;209:1382–1385.)

ductory period during which owners are told that their animals may be receiving a drug when in fact all animals are being treated with placebo. Those subjects that readily respond to placebo are then removed from the trial, and the remaining subjects are assigned to the drug and placebo groups randomly (10,11). However, there has been little success in improving the results of controlled studies by attempting to identify and eliminate placebo responders (12). Moreover, by removing placebo responders, test subjects may no longer reflect the general population.

Parallel trials are usually planned to have a fixed duration. A variant of fixed duration is a sequential trial in which enrollment of subjects is staggered over a period of time, allowing for periodic comparison of drug and placebo groups. This method allows a decision to be made as to the number of cases required to achieve significant results when the new treatment is found to be superior (13). If the drug is clearly ineffective, the trial may be stopped sooner than initially anticipated (14).

In any clinical trial, there is considerable variability from subject to subject, reflecting differences in biologic sensitivity to pharmacologic treatment. For this reason, many subjects are often needed in each group. An experimental design that can minimize this variability is the *crossover trial*, which uses subjects as their own controls. In this type of trial, treatment for each group is switched partway through the trial, with those subjects that received placebo initially receiving the drug next, and those that received the drug receiving placebo next (see Figure A.1). Generally, crossover trials require fewer subjects because of reduced variability between groups (15). However, as animals are used as their own controls and given two types of treatment, crossover trials are generally longer in duration than parallel trials. Unfortunately, this increases the likelihood that some subjects will drop out of the trial or be excluded if owners become less compliant with the protocol.

Crossover designs cannot be used when the treatment may permanently change the subject. For example, in a trial testing a drug for separation anxiety, if an anxiolytic drug permanently changes an animal's anxiety about being separated, a crossover design could not give a fair comparison between placebo and drug treatment if the drug treatment was given first. The crossover design is appropriate if the behavior is an ongoing problem that is not permanently changed by drug treatment. For a stereotypy that is altered only while the subject is receiving the drug, the crossover design might work quite well. This was the design used in comparing serotonin reuptake blockers with other drugs for treatment of acral lick dermatitis in dogs (16). Crossover designs may also be used to help avoid the unblinding that can occur with a drug's side effects. A complex experimental design can be used that involves a crossover of patients from one group to the other without the investigator or the client knowing when they have been switched from one group to another (17).

Prospective Open-Label Clinical Trials

The distinguishing feature of this type of trial is that assignment to groups is *open-label*, meaning that the investigators, and often the animal owners, know which treatment is being given. This type of trial was used in examining the effects of a narcotic antagonist on self-licking, self-chewing, and scratching in dogs (18), and the effects of anxiolytics on urine-marking in cats (19,20). If the trial involves two different groups, one receiving placebo and one receiving drug, the trial may call for not telling the owners the type of treatment their animal is receiving (a *single-blind* trial), thereby presumably reducing the placebo effect. However, a placebo effect is still possible through the investigator. There are some examples of single-blind trials: a study comparing different drugs for the treatment of canine acral lick dermatitis (21); a study of the effect of dietary protein on behavior of dogs (22); and a variant of the single blind format for a study of the effectiveness of fluoxetine for treating aggressive dominance in dogs in which clients were told that the dog would be on placebo during one of five treatment weeks (23).

As with double-blind controlled trials, animals for open-label prospective trials are recruited and included in the study on the basis of specific criteria (24). The protocol is planned in advance, and all animals are treated similarly. Inclusion criteria may exclude animals that are not members of a certain subgroup. For example, enrollment may be restricted to only neutered male dogs in a test of drugs for aggressive behavior. Dogs with diseases that may account for the problem would also fall under exclusion criteria. Prospective trials differ from retrospective case surveys and case reports (see below), in that for retrospective studies, animals are not necessarily recruited with specific inclusion and exclusion criteria.

In prospective open-label trials in which all animals are treated only with the new drug, it is assumed that the treatment is comparative because the treatment will be compared theoretically with an older standard or historical treatment (if one has been used) or with no treatment at all. In the treatment of urine-marking in cats, for example, each animal was used as its own control by referring to the frequency of the behavior prior to treatment (19,20). When the animals were given a pharmacologic treatment, it was assumed that the reduction in the behavior, if any, reflected the effect of the drug.

One problem with this type of trial is that behavioral management between the two groups may vary substantially. This has caused some authorities to question the value of using historical controls (25). Another problem is that in an open-label trial with a placebo group, owners may not wish to participate if they feel there is only a 50% chance that their animal will receive the new drug. It is generally easier to find subjects for a trial if owners know their pets will receive the new treatment. As with double-blind, placebo-controlled trials, the investigator may offer to give the drug on a so-called compassionate-use basis at the end of the trial for those that did receive placebo.

Retrospective Case Surveys

Conducting a retrospective case survey involves reviewing hospital records on the use of a drug for a particular behavior and statistically evaluating this information (24). Specific criteria can be applied to determine which cases will be included or excluded and which will help the predictive value of the information. Case surveys may provide very useful information on the biologic variation in animal responsiveness and on the general efficacy of the drug (i.e., the portion of animals responding or degree of change in the animals that did respond) if the number of cases is large enough (e.g., ten or more subjects). From this data, one also gets a sense of the likelihood of adverse effects. Placebo effects may be possible since the drug was administered in an open-label fashion (8,26). Some examples of case surveys are studies of progestins to treat urine-spraying in cats (27) and aggression in dogs (28). Reports of effects of castration on problem behavior in cats and dogs represent retrospective case surveys, although the trials involve removal of an endogenous hormone rather than the administration of a drug (29,30,31).

One of the major problems with retrospective case surveys is that the treatment of animals could have varied as the attending clinicians became more accustomed to using the treatment, with animals treated later in the study faring better than those treated earlier (24). Of course, details of the treatment with regard to the parameters of drug administration and accompanying behavior modification could vary if more than one clinician is involved.

Case Reports

Case reports are published accounts of behavioral changes in one or just a few animals being treated, and involve usually just positive outcomes. They are presented in narrative form with no data. Naturally, they provide less information than retrospective surveys or prospective trials, because the biologic variation among animals cannot be represented with just one or very few animals. As in retrospective case surveys, case reports are open-label and therefore do not discriminate between improvement attributable to changes in management or behavior modification and improvement due to the drug. Usually, clinicians want to implement everything they can to improve a serious problem behavior, and they might erroneously ascribe the positive effects to the drug rather than to behavioral approaches. Case reports are the only type of information available for many of the psychotropic drugs (1), and while they do not provide reliable information on efficacy, side effects, or prospects for long-term resolution of the problem, they do stimulate further investigation and reveal the potential of using a drug for a particular problem behavior (8).

Conclusion

Behavioral pharmacology differs from other areas of pharmacology because the results rely on the owner's observations of the animal's behavior rather than on clinical data obtained from direct physical and laboratory examination of the animals (6). There has not yet been an established precedent for evaluating such data. Sometimes behavioral data may be reported in discrete events, such as number of urine-marks or frequency of growling per day, but more often it involves global measures of response to treatment, such as reduction in aggressive attitude or fearfulness.

As behaviorists gain experience in evaluating and conducting behavioral trials, we will learn more about the most reliable methodology for obtaining useful information. As veterinarians increasingly prescribe drugs for behavior problems, progress in this field depends on increasing accuracy in the evaluation of studies involving drugs, so that improvement resulting from pharmacologic influences can be distinguished from imagined improvement or improvement resulting from behavior modification or environmental management.

References

1. Dodman NH, Shuster L. Pharmacologic approaches to managing behavior problems in small animals. Vet Med 1994;89:960–969.
2. Marder AR. Psychotropic drugs and behavior therapy. Vet Clin North Am Small Anim Pract 1991;21:329–342.
3. Beecher HK. The powerful placebo. JAMA 1955;159:1602–1606.
4. Lepor H, Williford WO, Barry MJ, et al. The efficacy of terazosin, finasteride, or both in benign prostatic hyperplasia. N Engl J Med 1996;335:533–539.
5. Weiner M, Weiner GJ. The kinetics and dynamics of responses to placebo. Clin Pharmacol Ther 1996:60:247–254.
6. Hart BL, Cliff KD. Interpreting published reports of extra-label drug use with special reference to reports of drugs used to correct problem behavior in animals. J Am Vet Med Assoc 1996;209:1382–1385.
7. Hart BL, Cooper LL. Integrating use of psychotropic drugs with environmental management and behavioral modification for treatment of problem behavior in animals. J Am Vet Med Assoc 1996;209:1549–1551.
8. Rudorfer MV. Challenges in medication clinical trials. Psychopharmacol Bull 1993;29:35–44.
9. Benkert O, Maier W. The necessity of placebo application in psychotropic drug trials. Pharmacopsychiatry 1990;23:203–205.
10. Prien RF. Methods and models for placebo use in pharmacotherapeutic trials. Psychopharmacol Bull 1988;24:4–8.
11. Reimherr FW, Ward WF, Byerly WG. The introductory placebo washout: a retrospective evaluation. Psychiatry Res 1989;30:191–199.

12. Shapiro AK, Shapiro E. Patient-provider relationships and the placebo effect. In: Matazzaro JD, Weiss SM, Herd JA, Miller NE, eds. Behavioral health: a handbook for health enhancement and disease prevention. New York: Wiley-Interscience, 1984;371–383.

13. Whitehead J. The design and analysis of sequential clinical trials. New York: Halstead Press/ John Wiley & Sons, 1983.

14. Pocock SJ. When to stop a clinical trial. B Med J 1992;305:235–240.

15. Spilker B. Guide to clinical trials. New York: Raven, 1991.

16. Rapoport JL, Ryland DH, Kriete M. Drug treatment of canine acral lick: an animal model of obsessive-compulsive disorder. Arch Gen Psychiatry 1992;49:517–521.

17. Senn S. Crossover trials in clinical research. New York: John Wiley & Sons, 1993.

18. Dodman NH, Shuster L, White SD, et al. Use of narcotic antagonists to modify stereotypic self-licking, self-chewing, and scratching behavior in dogs. J Am Vet Med Assoc 1988;193:815–819.

19. Cooper L, Hart BL. Comparison of diazepam with progestin for effectiveness in suppression of urine spraying behavior in cats. J Am Vet Med Assoc 1992;200:797–801.

20. Hart BL, Eckstein RA, Powell KL, Dodman NH. Effectiveness of buspirone on urine spraying and inappropriate urination in cats. J Am Vet Med Assoc 1993;203:254–258.

21. Goldberger E, Rapoport JL. Canine acral lick dermatitis: response to the antiobsessional drug clomipramine. J Am Anim Hosp Assoc 1991;27:179–182.

22. Dodman NH, Reisner I, Shuster L, et al. Effect of dietary protein content on behavior in dogs. J Am Vet Med Assoc 1996;208:376–379.

23. Dodman NH, Donnelly R, Shuster L, et al. Use of fluoxetine to treat dominance aggression in dogs. J Am Vet Med Assoc 1996;209:1585–1587.

24. Pocock SJ. Clinical trials: a practical approach. Chichester, England: John Wiley & Sons, 1983.

25. Clark VA. Historical studies: should you believe the results? Plast Reconstr Surg 1990;4:793–795.

26. Rothman KJ. Modern epidemiology. Boston: Little, Brown, 1986.

27. Hart BL. Objectionable urine spraying and urine marking in cats: evaluation of progestin treatment in gonadectomized males and females. J Am Vet Med Assoc 1980;177:529–533.

28. Hart BL. Progestin therapy for aggressive behavior in male dogs. J Am Vet Assoc 1981;178:1070–1071.

29. Hart BL, Barrett RE. Effects of castration on fighting, roaming, and urine spraying in adult male cats. J Am Vet Med Assoc 1973;163:290–292.

30. Hopkins SF, Schubert TA, Hart BL. Castration of adult male dogs: effects on roaming, aggression, urine marking, and mounting. J Am Vet Med Assoc 1976;168:1108–1110.

Index

Encephalomyelitis of cattle, 73–74t
Encephalopathy, 85–86
Endocrine system
  aggression with disorders of, 88–95
  in cognitive dysfunction, 291–292
Endorphins. *See also* Beta-endorphins
  in aggressive behavior, 33–34
  in infantile autism, 229
  in self-injurious behavior, 230–231
Enkephalins
  in aggressive behavior, 33–34
  in compulsive behavior, 197
Environment
  management of for urine-marking in cats, 271–273
  modification for compulsive and self-injurious
      behaviors, 193
Epilepsy
  aggressive attacks with, 68
  temporal lobe, 68–71
Episodic behavior, 19
Episodic dyscontrol, 69–71
Equine alphavirus encephalitis, 73–74t
Equine fears, 128
Ergot alkaloids, 83t
Erythromycin, 160
Estrogen
  aggression and, 54–55, 94
  levels of, 9
Estrus-linked aggression, 42, 94
  ovariohysterectomy for, 55
Ethanol. *See* Alcohol
Ethology
  aggression model of, 18–21
  anxiety model of, 107
  theory in in behavior disorder classification
      systems, 3
Ethosuximide, 53
Evolutionary theory, 2–3
Excitatory amino acids, 29

Fear. *See also* Anxiety
  acquired. *See also* Phobia
    functional classification of, 143–144
    neurobiology of, 141–143
  clinical manifestations of, 125–128
  definition of, 122
  development of, 148–150
  drugs to alleviate, 130–131t
  etiology of, 122–123
  maladaptive, 149–150
  mechanisms of, 105

peripheral mechanisms of, 124–125
physiologic response to, 123–125
spontaneous, 148–149
treatment of conditions related to, 128–138
Fear response, 142–143
  affective and instrumental phases of, 143
Fear-based conditions, 128–138
Fear-potentiated startle response, 111–112
Fear-related aggression, 4, 41, 42
  opioid antagonists for, 54
  propranolol for, 50
Feather-picking, 2, 3, 238
  stereotypies of, 235
Feline fears, 127
Feline hyperesthesia syndrome, 71–72, 235–236
  psychopharmacologic agents for, 244t
  treatment of, 73
Feline immunodeficiency virus, 73–74t
Feline ischemic encephalopathy, 86
Fence running, 195
Fiddling, 142
Fight response, 142
Flight-flight response
  catecholamines in, 50
  noradrenergic system and, 124
Fighting stance, 65–66
Flesinoxan, 112
Flight response, 142
Flooding, 128
Fluid therapy, 84
Flumazenil, 31
Fluoxetine (Prozac)
  for aggressive behavior, 26, 57t
  bioavailability of, 214
  for canine acral lick dermatitis and OCD, 245t
  for cat hyperesthesia and OCD, 244t
  for compulsive disorder, 213–214
  for compulsive pacing, 187
  for fear and anxiety, 131t
  for feline hyperesthesia syndrome, 73
  future developments of, 117
  for Prader-Willi syndrome, 228
  for self-injurious behavior, 231, 240
  side effects of, 46, 214
Fluphenazine
  for aggression, 48–49
  for compulsive disorder, 209
Fluvoxamine
  for aggressive behavior, 26
  in fear-potentiated startle response, 112
  future developments of, 117
  for Prader-Willi syndrome, 228